Mental Health, United States, 2010

U.S. DEPARTMENT OF HEALTH AND HUMAN SERVICES
Substance Abuse and Mental Health Services Administration
www.samhsa.gov

This page intentionally left blank

ACKNOWLEDGMENTS

This report was prepared for the Substance Abuse and Mental Health Services Administration (SAMHSA) by RTI International under contract number HHSS283200700021I/ HHSS28342003T with SAMHSA, U.S. Department of Health and Human Services (HHS). Judith Teich of the Center for Behavioral Health Statistics and Quality (CBHSQ) served as the Government Project Officer.

Disclaimer

The views, opinions, and content of this publication are those of the authors and do not necessarily reflect the views, opinions, or policies of SAMHSA or U.S. Department of Health and Human Services (HHS).

Recommended Citation

Substance Abuse and Mental Health Services Administration. (2012). *Mental Health, United States, 2010*. HHS Publication No. (SMA) 12-4681. Rockville, MD: Substance Abuse and Mental Health Services Administration.

Originating Office

Center for Behavioral Health Statistics and Quality, Substance Abuse and Mental Health Services Administration, 1 Choke Cherry Road, Rockville, MD 20857. HHS Publication No. (SMA) 12-4681. Printed 2012.

This page intentionally left blank

CONTENTS

This page intentionally left blank

DETAILED CONTENTS

EXECUTIVE SUMMARY

Mental Health, United States, 2010 is the most recent edition of a publication issued by the Substance Abuse and Mental Health Services Administration (SAMHSA) of the U.S. Department of Health and Human Services biannually since 1980. The current volume serves as a comprehensive resource for mental health statistics at the national and State levels; it draws information from 35 different data sources and includes more than 25 exhibits and 130 tables. The volume presents national-level estimates on (1) the mental health of the population, (2) providers and settings for mental health services, and (3) payers and payment mechanisms. In addition, the 2010 volume presents State-level estimates of the mental health of each State's population, as well as provider and payment mechanisms for mental health services at this level.

The 2010 edition of *Mental Health, United States* provides mental health statistics using the most recent data available. This edition also includes several new tables that provide expanded information on some special populations of interest, such as children and members of the military; mental health service provision in nontraditional settings, such as the use of clubhouses to help integrate people with mental illness into the community; and estimates particularly relevant to States, such as the impact of the recent budget crisis on service provision.

This volume is organized into seven sections. Section 1 provides an introduction to the report and an overview of the current policy context relevant to the U.S. mental health service delivery system. Sections 2 through 5 present background information and exhibits pertinent to the mental health of the population, providers and settings, payers and payment mechanisms, and States, respectively. Section 6, Data Gaps, identifies key areas in which only limited information is available and for which further study may be indicated. Examples of gaps include the need for data that track the incidence and prevalence of mental illness, as well as the recovery process, and detailed estimates on the mental health of certain vulnerable populations, particularly children. Section 7 presents tables with detailed population, provider, payment mechanism, and State estimates.

The following are highlights of the data presented in *Mental Health, United States, 2010*:

1. Mental Health of the Population

- Approximately 11 million U.S. adults (4.8 percent) had serious mental illness (SMI) in 2009.
- More than one quarter of adults with SMI also had co-occurring substance dependence or abuse in 2009.
- During the 2001–2004 period, one out of eight U.S. children aged 8 to 15 (or 13.1

percent) had a mental health disorder in the past year.

- In 2007, more than 34,000 deaths in the United States were due to suicide.

2. Providers and Settings for Mental Health Services

- In 2009, more than one in eight U.S. adults received some type of mental health treatment in the past year.
- During the 2001–2004 period, more than half of all children with a mental health disorder received treatment in a hospital, clinic, or office within the past year.
- In 2009, 40 percent of adults with SMI reported not receiving any treatment.
- From 1996 to 2008, medication fills have increased considerably for mental health and/or substance abuse conditions. The categories of medication with the greatest growth have been antidepressant medications for adults and stimulant medications for children.

3. Payers and Payment Mechanisms

- Although mental health expenditures have increased (from $32 billion in 1986 to $132 billion in 2005), they have fallen as a share of all health expenditures (from 7.2 percent in 1986 to 6.1 percent in 2005).
- In 2005, public sources of coverage—such as Medicaid—accounted for more than 50 percent of all mental health expenditures.
- From 1986 to 2005, spending on prescription medications increased faster than any other type of mental health care.

4. States: People, Providers, and Payers

- During the 2005–2009 period, State-specific prevalence of past year major depressive episodes ranged from 5.2 to 9.5 percent in adults and 6.8 to 10.3 percent in youth aged 12 to 17.
- During the 2005–2009 period, State-specific utilization rates of outpatient specialty mental health treatment ranged from 3.0 to 9.5 percent for adults and from 8.0 to 16.9 percent for youth aged 12 to 17.
- States with a large proportion of the population living in rural areas have greater shortages of mental health professionals than States with a large proportion of the population living in urban areas.

The scope of the next volume in the series, *Behavioral Health, United States, 2012*, will be broadened to include information on substance use disorders, which co-occur frequently with mental health disorders. This larger perspective on behavioral health will help strengthen the series' utility as a key resource for decision making in a changing and challenging health care landscape.

1. INTRODUCTION

1.1 The *Mental Health, United States* Series

For more than 25 years, the *Mental Health, United States* series has presented nationwide measures of mental health. Published biannually by the Substance Abuse and Mental Health Services Administration (SAMHSA), the volume serves as the Nation's most comprehensive resource for mental health statistics. The data provide timely insights into the population's mental health status, the provision of mental health treatment, and funding for that treatment in the United States.

1.2 Organization

This volume is organized into seven sections. Section 1 provides an introduction to the report and an overview of the current policy context relevant to the U.S. mental health service delivery system. Sections 2 through 5 present background information and exhibits pertinent to the mental health of the population, providers and settings, payers and payment mechanisms, and States, respectively. Section 6, Data Gaps, identifies key areas in which only limited information is available and for which further study may be indicated. Examples of gaps include the need for data that track the incidence and prevalence of mental illness, as well as the recovery process, and detailed estimates on the mental health of certain vulnerable populations, particularly children. Section 7 presents tables with detailed population, provider, payment mechanism, and State estimates.

1.3 New Features

In addition to updating the data from *Mental Health, United States, 2008*, the 2010 volume contains a number of new features:

- ***State-level data.*** Perhaps the most significant addition is the State-level estimates section, which addresses the need for State-level data to inform day-to-day decisions on budgeting, planning, and care provision. Many of these tables and exhibits draw from SAMHSA's National Survey on Drug Use and Health (NSDUH).
- ***Needs of children.*** A number of tables focus specifically on the needs of and services for children.
- ***Impact of State budget crises.*** Results from a recent survey by NRI Inc. (2011) provide insight into the impact of the budget crises in States on mental health service provision.
- ***Services in nontraditional settings.*** The volume now provides key estimates for clubhouses—a nontraditional setting for nonclinical services—and inmates in Federal, State, and local facilities.
- ***Treatment gap.*** A number of tables consolidate the existing evidence on

treatment availability for people who need mental health services.

- *Data gaps.* The volume delineates key gaps in the available mental health data sources used as a basis for estimates to note potential areas for further study.

1.4 Policy Environment

The data from *Mental Health, United States* should be put into context before use. The policy environment will have influenced the data presented here, and the data in this volume also may influence the outcome of current policy and the formation of future policy. The mental health policy environment is currently dominated by the interconnected topics of health care reform, mental health parity, changes to Federal mental health block grants to States, and the economic recession.

Although several piecemeal reforms to the mental health and general health care system have occurred in recent years, health care reform legislation passed in 2010 is likely to have a profound effect on the treatment and financing of mental health. Based on two legislative acts in 2010—the Patient Protection and Affordable Care Act (Public Law 111-148) and the Health Care and Education Reconciliation Act of 2010 (Public Law 111-152), together referred to as the Affordable Care Act (ACA)—reform likely will change the provision of mental health care in numerous ways. Perhaps the most relevant changes are as follows:

- In 2010, adults with preexisting conditions were given access to insurance through a temporary, high-risk insurance pool called the Pre-Existing Condition Insurance Plan.
- In 2010, the age limit at which children could be covered by their parents' insurance was raised from age 22 to age 26.
- In 2011, out-of-pocket spending on prescription medication will be limited.
- In 2014, Medicaid will be expanded to cover an estimated 16 million individuals who were not covered previously and with incomes at or below 133 percent of the Federal poverty level (FPL) (Ku, 2010). Medicaid currently covers select groups of people with lower incomes and with disabilities and pays for about 28 percent of all mental health spending (SAMHSA, 2010a).
- In 2014, people ineligible for Medicaid and with incomes up to 400 percent of FPL will be allowed to receive premium subsidies through tax credits for health plans offered through State health insurance exchanges. These exchanges will be new entities that will reorganize the insurance market for health insurance—for example, by coordinating private insurance and Medicaid plans—and offer a choice of plans (HealthCare.gov, 2011).
- In 2014, Medicaid will cover medication such as barbiturates, benzodiazepines, and smoking cessation medications.

Historically, third-party coverage for treatment for behavioral health needs placed a greater burden on consumers than treatment for general medical needs. In recent years, this lack of parity has been addressed incrementally by different States and by the Federal government using various pieces of legislation, such as the Mental Health Parity Act of 1996 and the Mental Health Parity and Addiction Equity Act of

2008 (MHPAEA). This legislation should help improve access to care for people with mental illness (SAMHSA, 2010b). Moreover, as private and public coverage is expanded by health care reform, the impact of parity legislation will deepen because this legislation applies to people with existing coverage and those who are newly covered.

Since the move toward deinstitutionalization that began in the late 1960s, most mental health care has been provided in community settings (Frank & Glied, 2006). The main way by which the Federal government helps provide community-based mental health services for adults and children is through the Community Mental Health Services Performance Partnership Block Grant (CMHSPPBG) administered by SAMHSA. SAMHSA is working with States to change the block grant application, reporting, and planning requirements, starting with 2012 funding. The changes are intended to reduce the application burden on States and will likely direct funding to support people with gaps in coverage, cover treatment and support services not covered by third-party insurance, fund prevention activities, and collect data to assist in treatment planning (SAMHSA, 2011a, 2011b). With this flexibility, States may be able to target block grant funds toward needed wraparound services—such as employment or housing—that are not covered by third-party health insurance.

The economic recession in the United States and ongoing budget crises in many States have far-reaching policy implications for mental health because States play a particularly important role in underwriting mental health care provision. In 2005, State and local sources accounted for almost 20 percent of all mental health spending, whereas they accounted for 6 percent of spending on all health conditions (SAMHSA, 2010a). The impact on care is likely quite widespread. For example, a recent survey indicates that nearly 3,000 State psychiatric beds were closed in 2009 and 2010 and that 16 States and the District of Columbia planned to close State psychiatric hospital beds in the future (NRI Inc., 2011). Any requirements that health reform places on States in the future may further challenge State budgets. People who rely on State mental health resources may be in particular jeopardy, because they also often rely on other services through State-funded sources, such as those providing education, criminal justice, or housing.

1.5 Summary

This volume of *Mental Health, United States* provides a broad perspective on many complex components of the Nation's mental health system. The volume includes updated data with an increased focus on State-level estimates, children, mental health treatment in nontraditional settings, and levels of unmet mental health needs.

The face of the U.S. mental health service delivery system is changing. This is a period of tremendous financial pressure on State and federally sponsored programs, accompanied by the potential for unprecedented reform to the health care delivery system. Ongoing monitoring and research efforts must keep up with shifts in the U.S. population size and diversity; these efforts also must monitor the impact of policy changes and budget crises on the Nation's mental health service array and financing structures.

1.6 References

Frank, R. G., & Glied, S.A. (2006). *Better but not well: Mental health policy in the United States.* Baltimore, MD: Johns Hopkins University Press.

Ku, L. (2010). Ready, set, plan, implement: Executing the expansion of Medicaid. *Health Affairs, 29*(6), 1173–1177.

HealthCare.gov (2011). Coming in 2014: Affordable insurance exchanges. Retrieved from http://www.healthcare.gov/law/provisions/exchanges/index.html

NRI Inc. (2011). *State Mental Health Agency Budget Reductions Survey.* Falls Church, VA: NRI Inc.

Substance Abuse and Mental Health Services Administration (SAMHSA). (2010a). *National expenditures for mental health services and substance abuse treatment, 1986–2005* (DHHS Publication No. SMA 10-4612). Rockville, MD: Center for Mental Health Services and Center for Substance Abuse Treatment, SAMHSA.

Substance Abuse and Mental Health Services Administration (SAMHSA). (2010b). Parity: Landmark legislation takes effect. What are the implications for millions of Americans? *SAMHSA News, 18*(1), 1–2.

Substance Abuse and Mental Health Services Administration (SAMHSA). (2011a). SAMHSA FY 2012–2013 block grant application, frequently asked questions. Retrieved from http://www.samhsa.gov/grants/blockgrant/BG_FAQS_05-24-11.pdf

Substance Abuse and Mental Health Services Administration (SAMHSA). (2011b). SAMHSA news release: SAMHSA introduces guidance changing its block grant programs to reflect new opportunities provided by parity, health reform and emerging science. Retrieved from http://www.samhsa.gov/newsroom/advisories/1104110222.aspx

2. MENTAL HEALTH OF THE POPULATION

2.1 Narrative

2.1.1 Overview

Mental disorders are common, often serious, and treatable disorders that have a major impact on the U.S. population. An essential building block in the effort to prevent, treat, and assist in recovery from mental disorders is an understanding of the prevalence of mental disorders. Prevalence estimates contribute to developing an accurate picture of the level and type of mental health care needs for the overall U.S. population, as well as the risk of mental disorders within specific subpopulations of interest. National prevalence estimates can indicate the prevalence of any mental disorder or specific types of mental disorders, their severity or impairment level, and changes in the prevalence of the disorder over time.

This section presents mental disorder prevalence information for adults and children, rates of co-occurring health and substance abuse problems with mental health problems, suicide prevalence rates, and indicators of mental health status within selected special populations, including military personnel and children in the child welfare system. The tables present estimates from a variety of data sources, including the two national surveys that collect annual indicators of mental health status in the U.S. population: the National Survey on Drug Use and Health (NSDUH) and the National Health Interview Survey (NHIS). This section addresses several of the strategic initiatives of the Substance Abuse and Mental Health Services Administration (SAMHSA), which support its mission to reduce the impact of substance abuse and mental illness on America's communities (SAMHSA, 2011). For example, a number of tables specifically pertain to SAMHSA's strategic initiatives on Trauma and Justice and on Military Families.

2.1.2 U.S. Population: Adults

(Exhibits 1 through 3 and Tables 1 through 7)

Estimates relevant to the U.S. adult population include the prevalence of mental disorders, serious mental illness (SMI), and serious psychological distress (SPD). The first estimates presented are of any mental illness (AMI) and SMI, which refers to diagnosable mental disorders that result in serious functional impairment (Tables 1 and 2). Other estimates describe the prevalence of major depressive episode (MDE) (Tables 3 and 4) and past 30-day SPD (Tables 5 through 7). SPD does not represent a diagnosis; rather, it reflects the presence of mental health symptoms that may negatively affect a person's ability to participate in family, community, and work life. This construct is measured by a symptom scale designed to assess recent psychological distress (within the past 30 days). Whereas the concept of and term SMI is widely used by providers and policy makers, SPD is not as well known.

In 2009, 19.9 percent of the U.S. adult population experienced AMI (excluding substance use disorders) in the past year (Table 1). Prevalence of AMI was higher for females (23.8 percent) than males (15.6 percent). AMI also was higher for persons with Medicaid or Children's Health Insurance Program (CHIP) coverage (33.4 percent) or who are uninsured (24.9 percent) than for persons with private insurance (17.3 percent) or other coverage (16.1 percent). Exhibit 1 and Table 1 also indicate that 4.8 percent of adults had SMI, which equates to approximately 11 million U.S. adults annually. Table 2 shows the prevalence of specific types of mental disorder, including anxiety, mood, impulse control, and substance use disorders.

Major depressive disorder (MDD) is a serious mental disorder that can result in impairment and societal costs, including work disability and lost productivity (Katon, 2009). MDE indicates the presence of a 2-week period in the past year when a person experienced depressed mood, which is one of the components of the diagnostic criteria for MDD. In 2009, 6.5 percent of U.S. adults experienced MDE in the past year (Table 3). Table 4 shows annual prevalence estimates of MDE from 2005 to 2009.

In 2009, 3.2 percent of U.S. adults experienced SPD in the past 30 days (Table 5). Exhibit 2 and Table 6 show annual prevalence estimates for SPD over time. The estimates demonstrate that national levels of recent psychological distress in adults have remained relatively stable for more than a decade. Table 7 displays rates of past 30-day SPD for persons with selected physical health disorders (e.g., asthma, diabetes, cancer).

2.1.3 U.S. Population: Children

(Exhibit 4 and Tables 8 through 12)

Children experience emotional and behavioral problems that are specific to childhood (e.g., separation anxiety, enuresis). Furthermore, the prevalence of mental disorders seen in adulthood, such as major depression, is different in children. Prevalence data for children in the United States include estimates of emotional and behavioral difficulties (Table 8), mental disorders (Table 9), attention deficit hyperactivity disorder (ADHD) (Table 10), and MDE (Tables 11 and 12).

It is estimated that one out of eight U.S. children has had some form of an emotional or behavioral health disorder in the past year (Merikangas et al., 2010). Based on combined data from 2001 through 2004, prevalence of diagnosable mental disorders with severe impairment was 11.3 percent for children aged 8 to 15, and ADHD was the most common specific disorder (Exhibit 4 and Table 9). In 2009, ADHD was more than twice as prevalent among males as females (Table 10). Table 11 presents MDE prevalence rates for youth aged 12 to 17, broken out by demographic characteristics. In 2009, MDE was more prevalent among female youth (11.7 percent) than male youth (4.7 percent).

2.1.4 Substance Abuse

(Tables 13 and 14)

Persons with co-occurring mental and substance use disorders are an important subpopulation of interest. These individuals may experience treatment challenges and poorer outcomes (Najt, Fusar-Poli, & Brambilla, 2011) and may not receive integrated treatment that treats both disorders contemporaneously, as recommended (SAMHSA, 2007). Estimates are provided to illustrate the prevalence of substance dependence or abuse, including co-occurrence of substance dependence or abuse with AMI, SMI, and MDE for adults (Exhibit 3 and Table 13) and with MDE for youth aged 12 to 17 (Table 14).

In 2009, 19.7 percent of adults with AMI during the past year had a substance use disorder, with even higher prevalence among adults with SMI (25.7 percent) or MDE (22.4 percent). These are much higher rates of substance use disorders than experienced by persons without a mental disorder (6.5 percent) (Table 13). Past year co-occurring MDE and substance use disorder among youth also was common, occurring among 18.9 percent of youth with past year MDE (Table 14).

2.1.5 *Suicide*

(Exhibit 5 and Tables 15 and 16)

Suicide was the eleventh leading cause of death in the United States in 2007, accounting for more than 34,000 deaths (Xu, Kochanek, Murphy, & Tejada-Vera, 2010). Mental and substance use disorders are major risk factors for suicide (Goldsmith, Pellmar, Kleinman, & Bunney, 2002). In 2007, there were 11.3 suicides per 100,000 individuals in the U.S. population (Table 15). In that year, there were 0.5 suicides per 100,000 children aged 5 to 14 and 9.7 per 100,000 older adolescents and young adults aged 15 to 24 (Table 16). This subsection shows death rates for suicide by the most recent year (Table 15) as well as trends in death rates from 1985 to 2007 (Table 16). A limitation of these data is that they do not provide any information about suicide attempts.

Age-adjusted suicide rates are much lower for Hispanics (6.0 per 100,000 individuals in the U.S. population) than for non-Hispanics (12.0 per 100,000) (Table 15). The suicide rate for blacks is 5.0 per 100,000 in contrast with 12.5 per 100,000 for whites. As seen in Exhibit 5 and Table 16, suicide rates have decreased slightly from 12.5 per 100,000 individuals in the U.S. population in 1985 to 11.3 per 100,000 in 2007. The table also shows the much higher rates of suicide for men than for women (in 2007, 18.4 versus 4.7 per 100,000 population).

2.1.6 *Special Populations*

(Tables 17 through 22)

This subsection describes the prevalence of mental health disorders, behavioral and emotional problems, and symptoms within selected special populations. These special populations include persons aged 65 or older (Table 17), nursing home residents (Table 18), military personnel (Tables 19 and 20), inmates in State and Federal correctional facilities and local jails (Table 21), and children involved with the child welfare system (Table 22).

It is crucial to understand the extent of mental health needs of older adults, especially in an aging society. Projections indicate that almost one in five U.S. residents will be aged 65 or older in 2030 (Vincent & Velkoff, 2010). In 2009, 10.8 percent of persons aged 65 or older had past year AMI (Table 17). In 2004, nearly half (49.2 percent) of nursing home residents had a diagnosis of some type of mental illness (Table 18).

Active duty military personnel are another subpopulation of current interest. The length and nature of Operation Enduring Freedom (Afghanistan) and Operation Iraqi Freedom, and the multiple deployments that are often required, have put a spotlight on mental health issues, such as posttraumatic stress disorder (PTSD) and depression (Institute of

Medicine, 2010). In 2008, 10.6 percent of active duty military personnel (Army, Navy, Marine Corps, Air Force, and Coast Guard) reported having possible PTSD symptoms in the past 30 days that suggested a need for further evaluation (Table 19). Table 20 presents similar types of data for National Guard and Reserve military personnel.

Large numbers of persons with mental illness reside within the Nation's prisons and jails, raising concerns about access to adequate treatment and whether programs to divert persons from incarceration into community treatment would better serve many of these offenders (Kuehn, 2007). A large proportion of inmates report having mental health problems: 44.8 percent of Federal prison inmates (in 2004), 56.2 percent of State prison inmates (in 2004), and 64.2 percent of local jail inmates (in 2002) (Table 21).

Many children involved in the child welfare system for maltreatment have emotional or behavioral health needs. In 2008, 22.6 percent of children reported for maltreatment showed symptoms consistent with a behavior problem as assessed by a standardized instrument of emotional and behavioral health (Table 22).

2.2 Exhibits

Exhibits 1–5

Serious Mental Illness by Key Characteristics

In 2009, approximately 11 million U.S. adults had serious mental illness.

Serious mental illness (SMI) is defined as having a diagnosable mental, behavioral, or emotional disorder in the past year that results in serious functional impairment. These difficulties substantially interfere with a person's ability to carry out major life activities at home, at work, or in the community. Since 2008, the annual National Survey on Drug Use and Health (NSDUH) has included measures that permit the estimation of SMI in U.S. adults. NSDUH is a nationally representative survey of the civilian, noninstitutionalized population of the United States aged 12 or older and interviews approximately 67,500 persons each year.

Exhibit 1 shows rates of past year SMI by age, sex, Hispanic origin and race, poverty status, and health insurance status. The exhibit shows the following:

- In 2009, 4.8 percent of U.S. adults aged 18 or older had SMI in the past year (representing an estimated 11.0 million U.S. adults).
- The percentage of adults with past year SMI was highest among adults aged 18 to 25 (7.3 percent) and lowest among adults aged 50 or older (2.8 percent).
- Past year SMI was more likely among women aged 18 or older (6.4 percent) than among men in that age group (3.2 percent).
- SMI was particularly prevalent among adults living in poverty (9.1 percent) and among those covered by Medicaid/Children's Health Insurance Program (10.7 percent).

Exhibit 1. Percentage of persons aged 18 or older with past year serious mental illness (SMI), by selected characteristics, United States, 2009

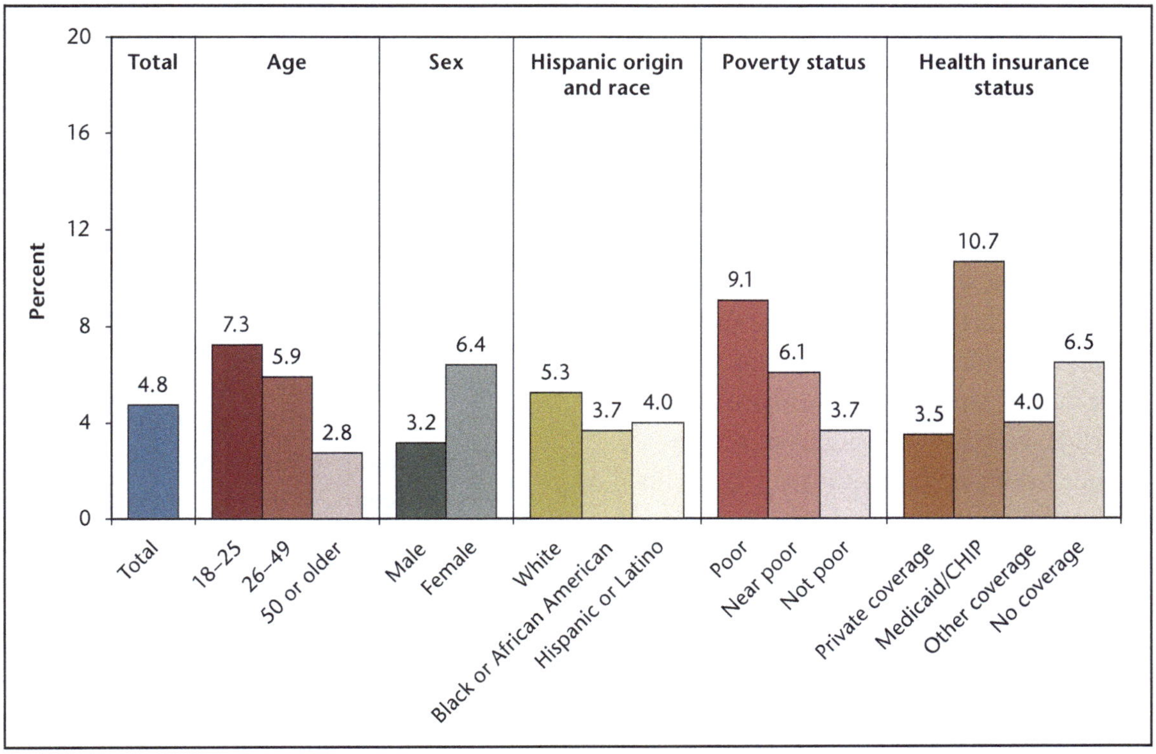

NOTES: Serious mental illness (SMI) among adults is defined as persons aged 18 or older who currently or at any time in the past year had a diagnosable mental, behavioral, or emotional disorder and resulting in substantial impairment in carrying out major life activities. Respondents could indicate multiple types of health insurance. CHIP is the Children's Health Insurance Program. Individuals aged 19 or younger are eligible for this plan. See Table 1 for more detail on the constructs included in this exhibit.

SOURCE: National Survey on Drug Use and Health, 2009, Substance Abuse and Mental Health Services Administration, Office of Applied Studies.

National Trends in Past 30-Day Incidence of Serious Psychological Distress among Adults

National levels of psychological distress in adults have remained relatively stable for more than a decade.

The National Health Interview Survey (NHIS) includes a measure to assess recent signs of adult mental health problems and is the only national survey that has provided an annual estimate of adult mental health status for more than a decade. NHIS is the leading survey to provide health estimates for the U.S. civilian noninstitutionalized population, including interviews in more than 33,000 households annually. The presence of the NHIS mental health indicator, serious psychological distress (SPD) in the past 30 days, allows for the examination of trends in U.S. adult mental health status over time. An indicator of recent SPD within NHIS also allows estimates that demonstrate the relationship of recent psychological distress to other health problems. SPD is not a diagnosis; rather, it refers to the presence of mental health symptoms in the past month that may negatively affect a person's ability to participate in family, community, and work life. Exhibit 2 examines rates of SPD in the past 30 days for adults from 1997 to 2009. The exhibit shows the following:

- In 2009, 3.2 percent of adults aged 18 or older experienced SPD during the past 30 days.
- National levels of past 30-day SPD among U.S. adults have remained relatively stable for more than a decade. The annual percentage of adults who experienced SPD during the past 30 days ranged from 2.4 percent in 1999 to 3.3 percent in 1997.
- Estimates of SPD in this exhibit should not be directly compared with the estimates of serious mental illness (SMI) in Exhibit 1. The two constructs, SPD and SMI, are measured differently. SPD is assessed by responses to a short screening measure focused on the presence of mental health symptoms in the *past 30 days*, whereas SMI is defined by measures to assess both symptoms and their resulting serious functional impairment *in the past year.*

Exhibit 2. National trends in past 30-day serious psychological distress (SPD) for persons aged 18 or older, United States, 1997–2009

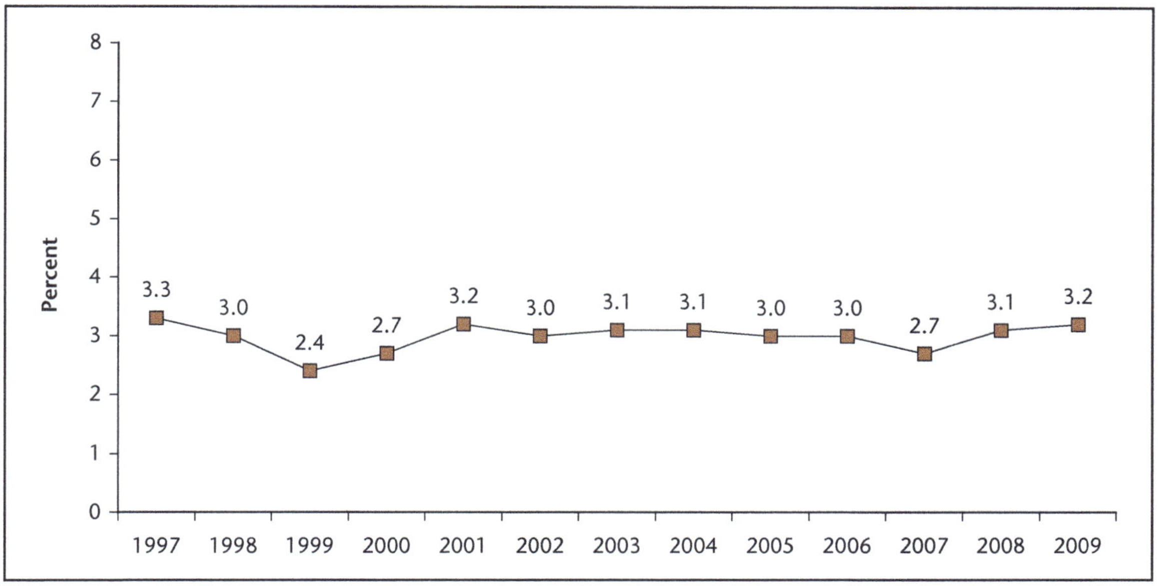

NOTES: Serious psychological distress (SPD) is defined as the presence of mental health symptoms in the past month that may negatively affect a person's ability to participate in family, community, and work life. See Table 6 for more detail on the constructs included in this exhibit.

SOURCE: National Health Interview Survey, 1997–2009, Centers for Disease Control and Prevention, National Center on Health Statistics.

Co-Occurring Serious Mental Illness and Substance Dependence or Abuse among U.S. Adults

In 2009, more than one quarter of adults with SMI had co-occurring substance dependence or abuse.

The association between mental illness and substance abuse or dependence is well established (SAMHSA, 2010). Co-occurrence of serious mental illness (SMI) with substance dependence or abuse is especially common. The National Survey on Drug Use and Health (NSDUH), a nationally representative survey of the civilian, noninstitutionalized population of the United States aged 12 or older, asks questions that assess the co-occurrence of mental illness and substance use disorders. Exhibit 3 examines the prevalence of co-occurring SMI and substance dependence or abuse in the past year. This exhibit shows the following:

- In 2009, more than one quarter (25.7 percent) of adults with SMI had co-occurring substance dependence or abuse, related to either illicit drugs or alcohol.
- Regardless of SMI status, alcohol dependence or abuse was more common than illicit drug dependence or abuse.
- Adults with SMI were more likely to have any substance dependence in the past year (25.7 percent) than those without any mental illness (6.5 percent).

Exhibit 3. Percentage of persons aged 18 or older with past year serious mental illness (SMI) or no mental illness, by past year substance dependence or abuse, United States, 2009

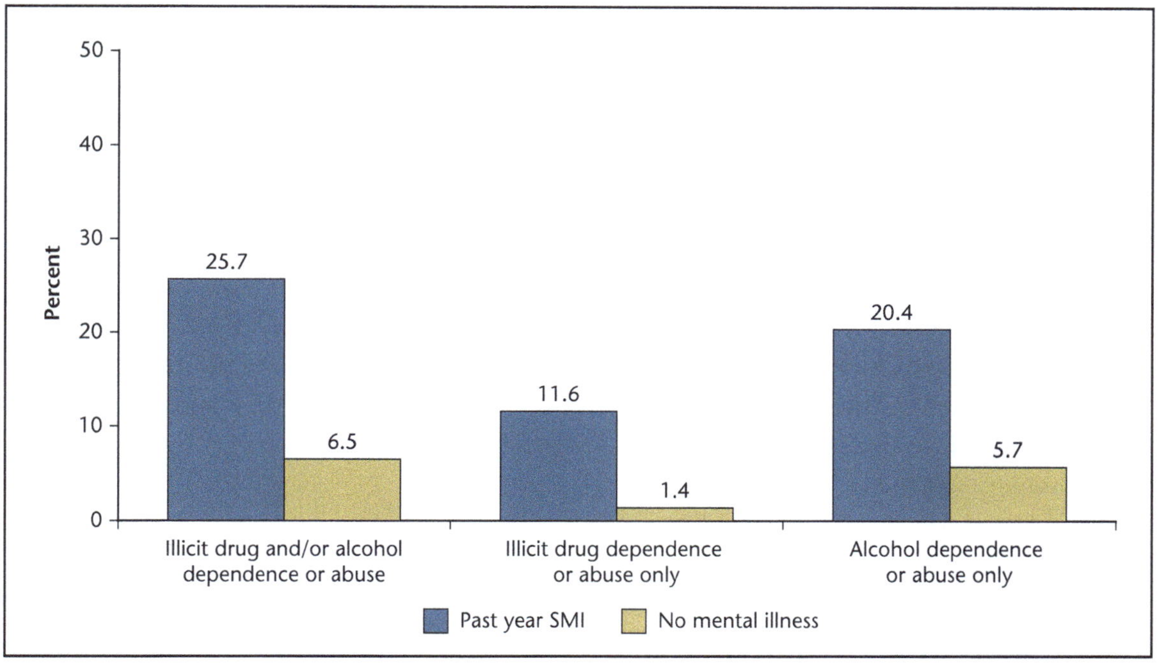

NOTES: Serious mental illness (SMI) among adults is defined as persons aged 18 or older who currently or at any time in the past year had a diagnosable mental, behavioral, or emotional disorder and resulting in substantial impairment in carrying out major life activities.

No mental illness includes adults who did not meet the criteria for any mental illness in the past year.

Substance abuse and dependence are broad categories associated with a pattern of substance use that leads to clinically significant impairment. Abuse may include symptoms such as failure to fulfill major role obligations, legal problems, use in situations that are physically hazardous, and continued use despite persistent social or interpersonal problems. Substance dependence symptoms may include drug taking in larger amounts than intended, inability to cut down on drug use, a great deal of time spent on activities necessary to obtain the drug, and continued use despite knowledge of health or social problems caused by the drug. See Table 13 for more details on the constructs in this exhibit.

SOURCE: National Survey on Drug Use and Health, 2009, Substance Abuse and Mental Health Services Administration, Office of Applied Studies.

Mental Health Disorders among Children

One out of eight U.S. children has a mental health disorder.

Many U.S. children experienced some form of mental health disorder in the past year. Using a sample drawn from several years of the National Health and Nutrition Examination Surveys (NHANES), a recently published study by Merikangas et al. (2010) reported results of parent and child mental health diagnostic interviews. NHANES is a nationally representative probability sample of noninstitutionalized U.S. children aged 8 to 15 who were evaluated in person at mobile examination survey centers. This particular study included 3,042 participants aged 8 to 15 who had participated in one of the NHANES surveys between 2001 and 2004. Select mental health disorders were assessed, including generalized anxiety disorder, panic disorder, eating disorders, depressive disorders, attention deficit hyperactivity disorder (ADHD), and conduct disorders. The study provides aggregate annual estimates of any childhood mental health disorder in the past year as well as the subset of these disorders that caused severe impairment to a child's ability to function at home, at school, in the community, or with peers. This study provides the most up-to-date national prevalence estimates of specific childhood mental health disorders within a sample that includes both school-age children and youth.

According to recent findings from Merikangas et al. (2010), approximately one out of eight U.S. children (13.1 percent) had one of the assessed mental health disorders in the past year. The most common are ADHD, mood disorders, and conduct disorders. Exhibit 4 provides national estimates of mental health disorders in the general population of U.S. children aged 8 to 15. The study found the following:

- One of eight children aged 8 to 15 (13.1 percent) met the criteria for any mental health disorder in the past year; 11.3 percent met the criteria for a mental health disorder with severe impairment in the past year.
- Boys had a higher rate of any past year disorder than girls. This was primarily driven by the high rate of ADHD in boys. Girls, on the other hand, had higher rates of mood disorders than boys.
- For most disorders, there was only a minimal difference between the prevalence of any mental health disorder and the prevalence of any mental health disorder with severe impairment.

Exhibit 4. Percentage of persons aged 8 to 15 with any mental disorder and any disorder with severe impairment in the past year, by sex and age group, United States, 2001–2004

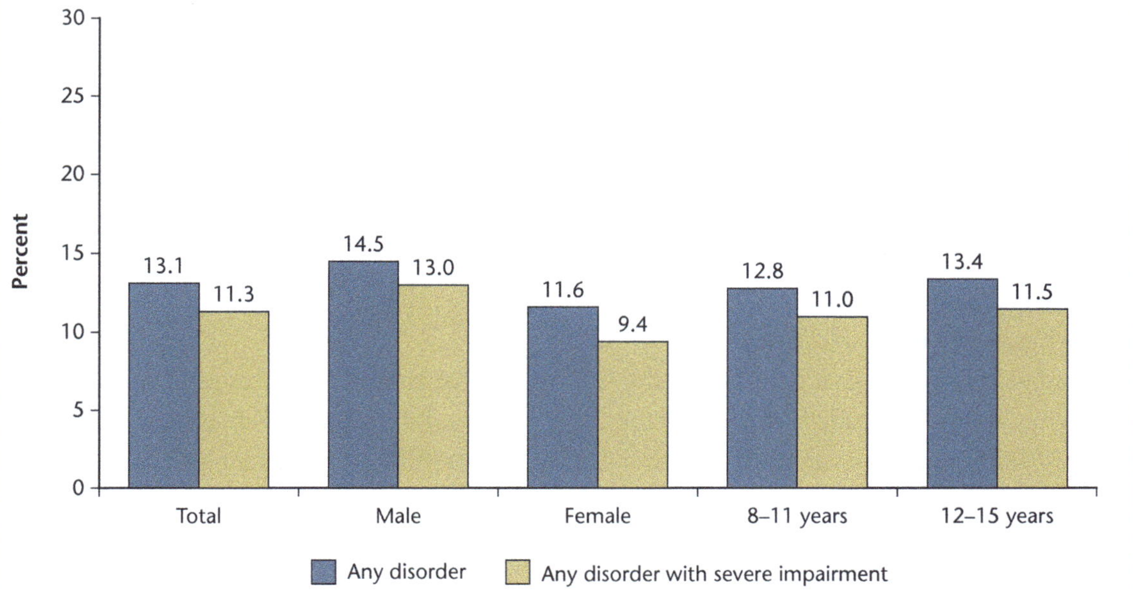

NOTES: Mental disorders were assessed using a structured diagnostic interview that contained modules. Disorder with severe impairment indicates two intermediate ratings or one severe rating on the six impairment questions within a diagnostic module. See Table 9 for more details on the constructs in this exhibit.

SOURCE: Merikangas, K. R., He, J.-P., Brody, D., Fisher, P. W., Bourdon, K., & Koretz, D. S. (2010). Prevalence and treatment of mental disorders among US children in the 2001–2004 NHANES. *Pediatrics, 125*(1), 75–81.

Suicide Rates among Children and Adults by Sex

In 2007, more than 34,000 deaths in the United States resulted from suicide. Males were much more likely than females to die from suicide.

For more than two decades, the National Vital Statistics System has included detailed data on deaths and death rates for the U.S. population aged 5 to 85 or older. From 2000 to 2007, the age-adjusted death rate for suicide increased by 8.6 percent (Xu, Kochanek, Murphy, & Tejada-Vera, 2010). Exhibit 5 shows the number of deaths resulting from suicide for every 100,000 people in the United States by sex from 1985 to 2007. This exhibit shows the following:

- In 2007, there were 11.3 suicides per 100,000 individuals in the U.S. population.
- Of the 2,423,712 deaths reported in the United States in 2007, 34,598 deaths resulted from suicide.
- The annual estimates of U.S. death rates resulting from suicide ranged from 10.4 per 100,000 individuals in 2000 to 12.5 per 100,000 in 1985.
- Suicide death rates are consistently higher among males than females. In 2007, 18.4 deaths per 100,000 U.S. males were due to suicide, compared with 4.7 deaths per 100,000 U.S. females.

Exhibit 5. Age-adjusted death rates for suicide, by sex, United States, selected years 1985–2007

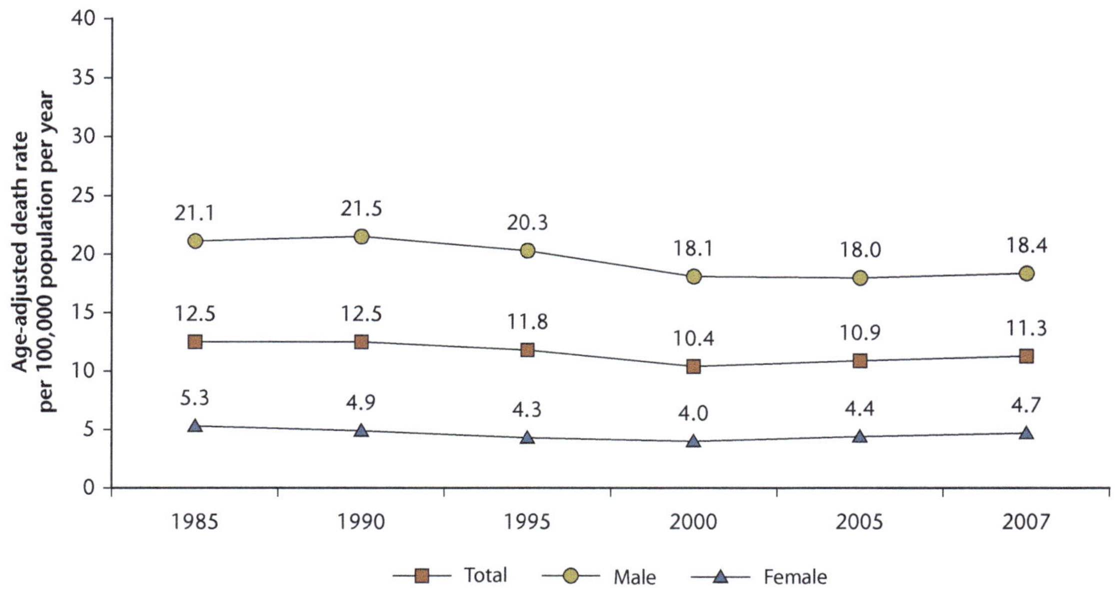

NOTE: Age-adjusted rates per 100,000 U.S. standard population. See Table 16 for more details on the constructs in this exhibit.

SOURCES: 1985–1995 data with age-adjusted rates obtained from National Vital Statistics System, Centers for Disease Control and Prevention, National Center for Health Statistics.

Xu, J. Q., Kochanek, K. D., Murphy, S. L., & Tejada-Vera, B. (2010). Deaths: Final data for 2007. *National Vital Statistics Reports, 58*(19). Hyattsville, MD: National Center for Health Statistics.

2.3 References

Goldsmith, S. K., Pellmar, T. C., Kleinman, A. M., & Bunney, W. E. (Ed.). (2002). *Reducing suicide: A national imperative.* Washington, DC: The National Academies Press.

Institute of Medicine. (2010). *Returning home from Iraq and Afghanistan: Preliminary assessment of readjustment needs of veterans, service members, and their families.* Washington, DC: The National Academies Press.

Katon, W. (2009). The impact of depression on workplace functioning and disability costs. *American Journal of Managed Care, 15*(11 Suppl), S322–S327.

Kuehn, B. M. (2007). Mental health courts show promise. *Journal of the American Medical Association, 297*(15), 1641–1643.

Merikangas, K. R., He, J.-P., Brody, D., Fisher, P. W., Bourdon, K., & Koretz, D. S. (2010). Prevalence and treatment of mental disorders among US children in the 2001–2004 NHANES. *Pediatrics, 125*(1), 75–81.

Najt, P., Fusar-Poli, P., & Brambilla, P. (2011, April 30). Co-occurring mental and substance abuse disorders: A review of the potential predictors and clinical outcomes. *Psychiatry Research, 186*(2–3), 159–164.

Substance Abuse and Mental Health Services Administration (SAMHSA). (2007). *Services integration, overview paper 6.* SAMHSA Co-Occurring Center for Excellence. Rockville, MD: SAMHSA. Retrieved from http://store.samhsa.gov/shin/content//SMA07-4294/SMA07-4294.pdf

Substance Abuse and Mental Health Services Administration (SAMHSA). (2010). *Results from the 2009 National Survey on Drug Use and Health: Volume I. Summary of national findings* (DHHS Publication No. SMA 10-4856, NSDUH Series H-38A). Rockville, MD: SAMHSA, Office of Applied Studies.

Substance Abuse and Mental Health Services Administration (SAMHSA). (2011). *Leading change: A plan for SAMHSA's roles and actions 2011–2014* (DHHS Publication No. SMA 11-4629). Rockville, MD: SAMHSA. Retrieved from http://store.samhsa.gov/product/SMA11-4629

Vincent, G. K., & Velkoff, V. A. (2010). *The next four decades. The older population in the United States: 2010 to 2050* (P25-1138). Current Population Reports. Washington, DC: U.S. Census Bureau. Retrieved from http://www.census.gov/prod/2010pubs/p25-1138.pdf

Xu, J. Q., Kochanek, K. D., Murphy, S. L., & Tejada-Vera, B. (2010). Deaths: Final data for 2007. *National Vital Statistics Reports, 58*(19). Hyattsville, MD: National Center for Health Statistics.

3. PROVIDERS AND SETTINGS FOR MENTAL HEALTH SERVICES

3.1 Narrative

3.1.1 Overview

As documented previously, mental illness and its associated impairment may impose substantial burdens on individuals and families that could be reduced by effective treatment. This section provides information on mental health treatments available to adults and children in the United States and the extent to which these treatments are being used. Among the populations examined are those addressed by the Substance Abuse and Mental Health Services Administration's (SAMHSA's) strategic initiatives, such as military personnel and people involved in or at risk of involvement in the criminal justice system. Many diverse data sources were used to produce the estimates, including sources that examine service use at the national level, such as the National Survey on Drug Use and Health (NSDUH) and the National Comorbidity Survey Replication, and sources that examine service use within specific specialty and nonspecialty treatment settings, such as the National Nursing Home Survey or the Nationwide Emergency Department Sample of the Healthcare Cost and Utilization Project.

This section also reports on the capacity of the mental health treatment system; that is, the number of institutions and professionals in both specialty and nonspecialty treatment settings. Service capacity is important to address in light of the recently passed health reform and mental health parity laws. Once fully implemented, these laws are likely to remove some barriers to behavioral health care, in which case it will be important that treatment capacity is adequate to meet the additional demand. For example, this volume includes estimates of specialty mental health treatment capacity from the National Survey of Mental Health Treatment Facilities.

3.1.2 Adult Mental Health Services

(Exhibits 6 through 9 and Tables 23 through 55)

Mental Health Services

People receive mental health treatment in a variety of ways, including specialty outpatient and inpatient care settings; general medical providers; nonspecialty settings, such as schools, nursing homes, or correctional facilities; and through prescription medication. Nationwide rates of mental health service utilization among adults by treatment setting are provided by self-reported mental health need (Tables 23,

24, and 26) and by individual characteristics (Tables 25, 27, and 28). Approximately one in eight adults in the United States received some type of specialty mental health treatment in the past year. More specifically, in 2009, 13.3 percent of all U.S. adults (or over 30 million) used outpatient, inpatient, or prescription medication treatment for a mental health problem in the past year (Exhibit 7 and Table 25). Over 11 percent—about 85 percent of the 13 percent—used prescription medication (Table 25). Among adults with any mental illness (AMI), 21.2 percent received outpatient mental health treatment, 3.1 percent received inpatient treatment, and 32.4 percent received a prescription medication for mental health (Table 24). For adults with serious mental illness (SMI), the corresponding proportions were 38.0 percent (outpatient), 6.8 percent (inpatient), and 54.0 percent (medication). However, a high proportion of adults with AMI (62.1 percent) or SMI (39.8 percent) did not receive any mental health services (Exhibit 6 and Table 24). Since 2002, adults' use of specialty outpatient mental health treatment has declined slightly, while inpatient treatment use has remained fairly stable (Exhibit 8 and Table 26).

Prescription medication has become an increasingly important component of behavioral health treatment in recent years, accounting for a growing share of spending (Mark, Levit, Vandivort-Warren, Buck, & Coffey, 2011). This is illustrated by information on trends in mental health/substance abuse (MH/SA) prescription medication fills among adults from 1996 to 2008 (Exhibit 9 and Tables 30 and 31). The data indicate that the number of prescription fills for these medications more than doubled between 1996 and 2008, which corresponds to 7 percent annual growth. However, this growth was general to all pharmaceuticals and not unique to MH/SA medications. Within the MH/SA category, three of the four medication classes reported (antidepressant, antipsychotic, and antimanic) increased at faster rates, with only antianxiety medications experiencing slower than average growth in prescribing (Exhibit 9 and Tables 30 and 31).

Nonspecialty Mental Health Services

Nonspecialty mental health services are a key part of mental health treatment for adults in the United States. This volume provides information on services used by individuals in several important nonspecialty sectors, including emergency departments (Tables 32, 33, 34, 35, 36, and 37); physicians' offices (Tables 38, 39, and 40); nursing homes, home health care agencies, and hospice facilities (Table 41); and clubhouses (Tables 42, 43, and 44). Clubhouses follow a model of service provision that focuses on the nonclinical aspects of helping people with severe and persistent mental illness. Clubhouses often provide, for example, employment services.

Emergency departments are intended to serve people with acute need, such as those with an acute mental health episode. However, this setting also serves many people who do not have insurance because the uninsured cannot be refused care at a hospital. Moreover, because a disproportionate share of people with mental illness are uninsured (Hazlett, McCarthy, Londner, & Onyike, 2004), emergency departments serve a disproportionate number of people with mental illness. In 2008, mental health was the primary diagnosis for 4.5 percent of emergency department visits by youth aged 10 to 17 (see Table 34) and 5 percent of visits by adults aged 18 to 64, but for only 2 percent of visits by adults aged 65 or older (see Table 33). Also, among those with a primary mental health diagnosis, diagnosis categories differed by age group. For youth with a primary mental health diagnosis, the most common categories were mood disorders (34.6 percent); anxiety disorders (14.9 percent); and attention deficit, conduct, and disruptive behavior disorders (12.7 percent). For adults, attention deficit, conduct, and disruptive behavior disorders accounted for less than 1 percent of visits, but other categories were much more important, such as alcohol and substance-related disorders, particularly for those aged 18 to 64 (see Table 33).

Physicians' offices also are commonly used for mental health problems. Indeed, general practice physicians write the majority of prescriptions for psychotropic medication (Mark, Levit, & Buck, 2009). Given the prominence of medication in treating mental health conditions (see Table 25), data are needed on treating mental health in physicians' offices. In 2008, more than 6 percent of all office visits involved any mental diagnosis, and 3.9 percent involved a primary diagnosis (Table 38). Nonspecialty care physicians also play an important role, with specialties other than psychiatry accounting for 44 percent of visits with a primary mental diagnosis (Table 39) and 63.3 percent of visits with any mental diagnosis (Table 40).

Mental Health Service Capacity

In presenting data on the capacity of mental health treatment specialty and nonspecialty systems, the demographic characteristics of the behavioral health workforce are important to consider because they may affect some patients' experience of treatment. Estimates portray characteristics of clinically trained mental health personnel in terms of their age, sex, and Hispanic origin and race, by provider type (Table 45). Prior research has identified a demographic mismatch between patients and providers that is larger for behavioral health care than for general medical care (Miranda, McGuire, Williams, & Wang, 2008). This section also illustrates time trends from 1986 to 2004 in the number of mental health organizations with 24-hour hospital/residential treatment settings and the corresponding number of beds relative to the population (Tables 46 and 47).

Evidence on the capacity of nonspecialty service settings includes data on the service capacity of jails, prisons, and correctional facilities (Tables 48 and 49); community health centers (CHCs) (Tables 50, 51, 52, and 53); and clubhouses (Table 54). These service locations often play an important role in mental health treatment. For instance, CHCs are an important part of the safety net for mental health care, and their role is likely to be enhanced under health reform (Lo Sasso & Byck, 2010). Estimates show the growth over time in the proportion of CHCs providing behavioral health services (Table 51) and in the number of specialty mental health and substance abuse encounters at CHCs (Table 53) for the period 1998 through 2007. Many psychiatric patients continue to be seen in general hospital beds ("scatter beds") that are not part of psychiatric units. These discharges are compared with psychiatric unit discharges in terms of various patient, facility, and treatment characteristics. Comparisons are also made between discharges from scatter beds in hospitals with and without psychiatric units (Table 55).

3.1.3 Child Mental Health Services

(Exhibits 10 though 13 and Tables 56 through 66)

Because youth populations differ in important ways from adults, their service patterns are presented separately (Tables 56 to 66). Children and youth may receive mental health treatment across a variety of settings, including education and juvenile justice settings. In 2009, youth were most likely to have received mental health services in either specialty mental health outpatient or education settings. Specifically, 12.0 percent of youth aged 12 to 17 received specialty mental health treatment, with the most common source being outpatient care from a private therapist, psychologist, psychiatrist, social worker, or counselor (9.3 percent) (Exhibit 12 and Table 56). Also, 12.1 percent received mental health treatment from the education system, and 0.4 percent received treatment from the juvenile justice system (Exhibit 12 and Table 56).

Specialty Mental Health Services

More than half of children aged 8 to 15 with a mental disorder received some form of mental health treatment in the past year (Exhibit 10 and Table 57). Table 57 presents the proportion of children aged 8 to 15 with various mental disorders who saw someone at a hospital, clinic, or office because of a mental health problem. Children with anxiety disorders were less likely to receive treatment than children with mood or disruptive behavior disorders. Because attention deficit hyperactivity disorder (ADHD) is much more prevalent among youth, this section presents data on the use of prescription medicine for ADHD among youth aged 2 to 17. In 2007, 4.2 percent of U.S. children were taking prescription medication for ADHD (Table 58).

Patterns of mental health services for children with emotional disturbance have changed substantially over time, in particular the use of residential treatment centers (Table 61) and MH/SA medications (Tables 62 and 63). For instance, time trends from 1996 to 2008 in MH/SA prescription medication fills among youth aged 17 or younger are reported by selected medication classes (Exhibit 13 and Tables 62 and 63). MH/SA prescription medication fills for children have increased notably since 1996. The rise is driven largely by an increase in the use of stimulant medication, which is likely prescribed for ADHD.

Mental Health Service Capacity for Children

Information on mental health service capacity for children is presented for two specific service systems: residential treatment centers (Tables 64 and 65) and schools (Table 66). Information is provided on the number of residential treatment centers for children with emotional disturbance and the number of inpatient beds in State and county psychiatric hospitals among children aged 17 or younger (Tables 64 and 65). Data are also shown on the percentage of schools that provided various mental health, social, or prevention services in 2006 and the methods they used to deliver those services (Table 66). The table indicates, for example, that more than 95 percent of schools provided crisis intervention for personal problems. Other common services provided by schools include identification of abuse, identification of family problems, and counseling for emotional or behavioral disorders (Table 66).

3.1.4 Special Populations

(Tables 67 through 69)

SAMHSA's strategic initiatives highlight the importance of providing support and treatment to America's service men and women, together with their families and communities, and of meeting the behavioral health needs of incarcerated adults and children (SAMHSA, 2011). The final set of tables on providers and settings of care contains estimates on service use in military populations (Tables 67 and 68) and youth in the juvenile justice system (Table 69). Among active duty military in 2008, 8.5 percent reported receiving prescribed medication for depression, anxiety, or sleeping problems; nearly 20 percent received mental health counseling (Table 67). In 2003, 52.7 percent of youth in the juvenile justice system received some form of counseling (Table 69).

3.2 Exhibits

Exhibits 6–13

Receipt of Mental Health Treatment by Adults with Any Mental Illness and Serious Mental Illness

A significant proportion of adults with serious mental illness do not report receiving treatment.

People with serious mental illness (SMI) are of particular concern to providers and policy makers. SMI impairs functioning in everyday life and can cause great distress. Treatment for people with SMI is particularly important in aiding recovery. The National Survey on Drug Use and Health (NSDUH) includes questions that assess types of mental health treatment received by U.S. adults. Exhibit 6 describes the types of mental health treatment received by people with any mental illness (AMI), as well as treatment received specifically by people with SMI. Individuals may receive more than one type of treatment. The exhibit shows the following:

- In 2009, individuals with SMI were more likely to receive mental health treatment than individuals with AMI, but both groups were often unlikely to receive any treatment. Among those with AMI in the past year, 62.1 percent (or an estimated 27.9 million people) did not receive treatment. Among those with SMI, 39.8 percent (or an estimated 4.3 million people) did not receive treatment.
- The most common form of mental health treatment for individuals with either AMI or SMI was prescription medication.

Exhibit 6. Percentage of persons aged 18 or older who received mental health treatment in the past year, by mental illness status, United States, 2009

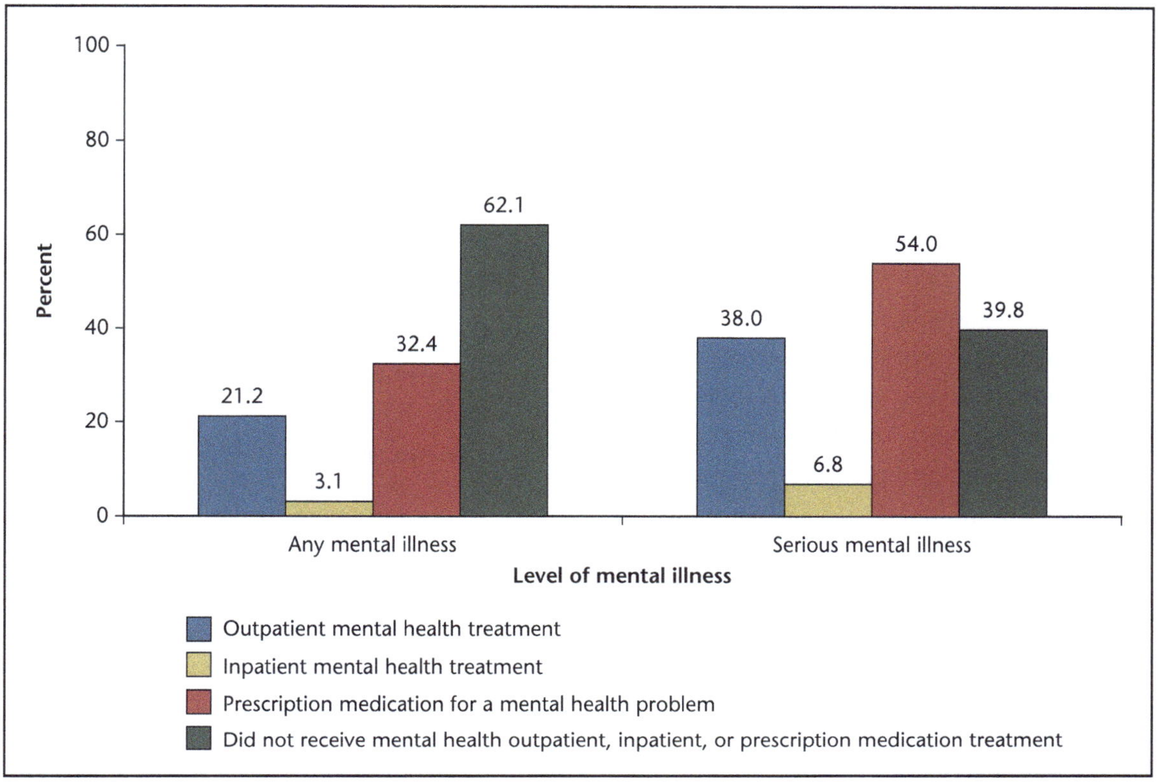

NOTES: Any mental illness (AMI) among adults is defined as persons aged 18 or older who currently or at any time in the past year had a diagnosable mental, behavioral, or emotional disorder, regardless of the level of impairment in carrying out major life activities. AMI includes persons with mental illness having serious, moderate, or mild functional impairment. Serious mental illness (SMI) is a subset of the AMI group. SMI among adults is defined as persons aged 18 or older who currently or at any time in the past year had a diagnosable mental, behavioral, or emotional disorder and resulting in substantial impairment in carrying out major life activities. See Table 24 for more details on the constructs in this exhibit.

Respondents with unknown treatment/counseling information were excluded. Respondents could indicate multiple service sources; thus, these response categories are not mutually exclusive.

SOURCE: National Survey on Drug Use and Health, 2009, Substance Abuse and Mental Health Services Administration, Office of Applied Studies.

Mental Health Service Use by Key Characteristics

Approximately one in eight adults in the United States received some type of mental health specialty outpatient, inpatient, or prescription medication treatment in the past year.

The receipt of mental health treatment varies by key characteristics of the recipients. Exhibit 7 uses the 2009 National Survey on Drug Use and Health (NSDUH) to show how mental health treatment use for adults varied by important demographic and socioeconomic factors. This exhibit shows adults' report of mental health treatment receipt and provides population estimates not limited to individuals with mental health problems. The exhibit shows the following:

- A higher proportion of women than men received mental health treatment in the past year (17.1 versus 9.2 percent, respectively).
- Among the three Hispanic origin and race groups examined, non-Hispanic whites had the highest proportion of treatment receipt (16.0 percent).
- Adults who were covered by Medicaid or the Children's Health Insurance Program (CHIP) had particularly high rates of mental health treatment receipt (23.6 percent) compared with adults covered by other types of insurance (14.0 percent for some other form of coverage).

Exhibit 7. Percentage of persons aged 18 or older who received mental health treatment or counseling in the past year, by selected characteristics, United States, 2009

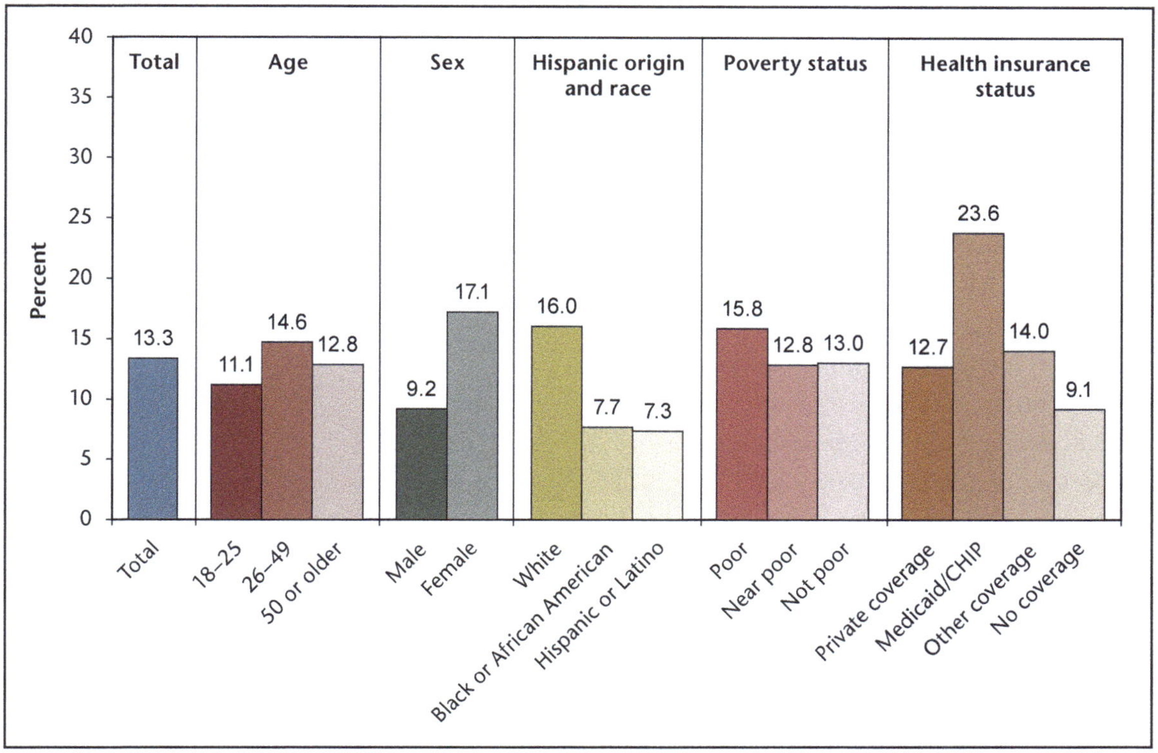

NOTES: Mental health treatment or counseling is defined as having received outpatient care or inpatient care or having used prescription medication for problems with emotions, nerves, or mental health. Respondents with unknown treatment/counseling information were excluded.

Poverty status is based on respondent age, family income, family size, and composition using the U.S. Census Bureau's poverty thresholds. "Poor" persons are defined as living in households where the family income is less than 100 percent of the U.S. Census poverty threshold. "Near poor" persons have incomes of 100 percent to less than 200 percent of the poverty threshold. "Not poor" persons have incomes that are 200 percent of the poverty threshold or greater.

CHIP is the Children's Health Insurance Program. Respondents could indicate multiple types of health insurance; thus, these response categories are not mutually exclusive. See Table 25 for more details on the constructs in this exhibit.

SOURCE: National Survey on Drug Use and Health, 2009, Substance Abuse and Mental Health Services Administration, Office of Applied Studies.

Adults Using Outpatient and Inpatient Mental Health Treatment

Since 2002, adult use of outpatient mental health treatment has declined slightly, while inpatient treatment use has remained stable.

Mental health treatment may include outpatient and inpatient care. It is important to understand the degree to which both types of treatment have changed over time. The National Survey on Drug Use and Health (NSDUH) includes questions that assess the types of mental health treatment received by U.S. adults. Exhibit 8 describes the proportion of adults between 2002 and 2009 using outpatient or inpatient mental health treatment. This exhibit does not include estimates of adults' self-reported use of prescription medication for a mental health problem. The exhibit shows the following:

- Over the 8-year period studied, the proportion of adults using outpatient treatment declined from 7.4 percent in 2002 to 6.3 percent in 2009.
- Use of inpatient treatment remained stable at 1 percent or less of the U.S. adult population.

Exhibit 8. Percentage of persons aged 18 or older who received mental health treatment or counseling in the past year, United States, 2002–2009

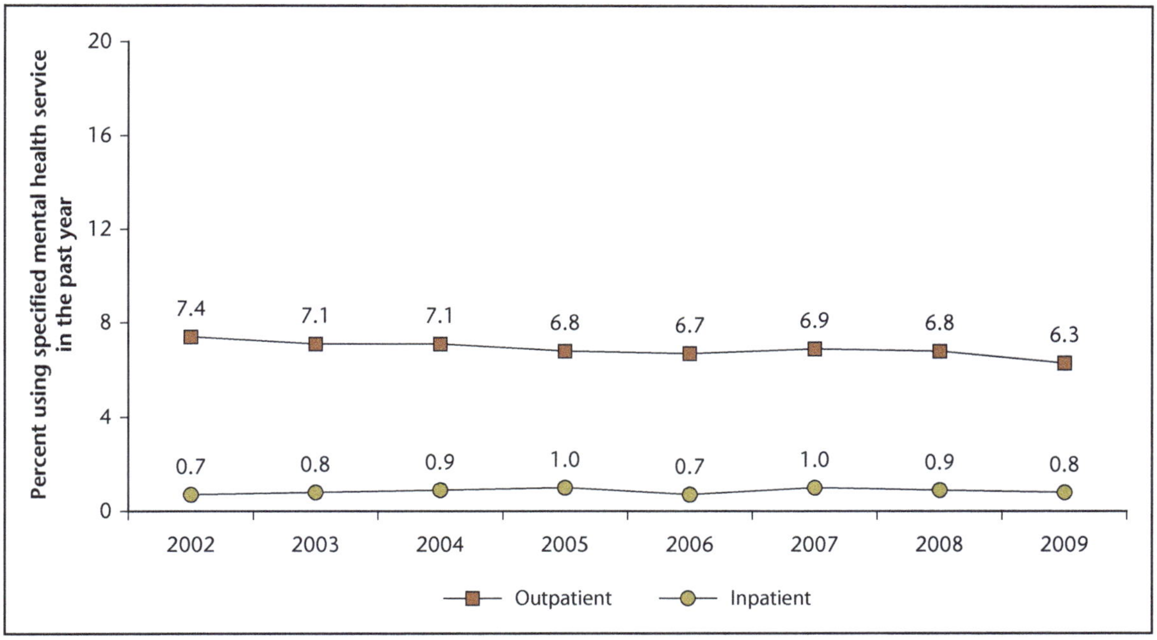

NOTES: Respondents could indicate multiple service sources; thus, these response categories are not mutually exclusive. Outpatient treatment includes any mental health treatment or counseling received at an outpatient mental health clinic or center; the office of a private therapist, psychologist, psychiatrist, social worker, or counselor that was not part of a clinic; a doctor's office that was not part of a clinic; an outpatient medical clinic; a partial day hospital or day treatment program; or some other place. Inpatient treatment includes a stay of overnight or longer in a hospital or other facility for mental health problems. See Tables 25 and 26 for more details on the constructs in this exhibit.

SOURCE: National Survey on Drug Use and Health, 2002–2009, Substance Abuse and Mental Health Services Administration, Office of Applied Studies.

Mental Health/Substance Abuse Medication Fills among Adults

The rise from 1996 to 2008 in mental health/substance abuse medication fills for adults was driven largely by antidepressant medication.

In the past decade, medication has become an increasingly prominent part of treatment for behavioral health problems. One way to measure the use of medication is to examine data from pharmacies on the number of prescriptions being purchased or filled. The Medical Expenditure Panel Survey (MEPS) includes a component that gathers data about prescription medication fills directly from pharmacies across the United States. This data collection method makes MEPS a particularly reliable source of information for assessing trends in psychotropic medication. Exhibit 9 shows, for four major classes of psychotropic medication, the extent of the increase in prescription fills from 1996 to 2008. The measure includes first-time purchases and refills. The exhibit shows the following:

- Throughout the period studied, antidepressant medication was the most common class of medication filled, and antianxiety medication was the second most common.
- The increase in medication fills over the period was driven largely by antidepressant medication. This class of medication had the largest increase in medication fills over the period, from 55.9 million fills in 1996 to 154.7 million fills in 2008.
- Fills for other classes of medications also increased over the period studied. For example, antianxiety medications—the second most common psychotropic medication—rose from 32.6 million in 1996 to 54.3 million in 2008. In 1996, the number of antianxiety medication fills was about 60 percent of the number of antidepressant fills; by 2008, that proportion fell to about 30 percent.

Exhibit 9. Mental health/substance abuse medication fills among persons aged 18 or older, United States, 1996–2008

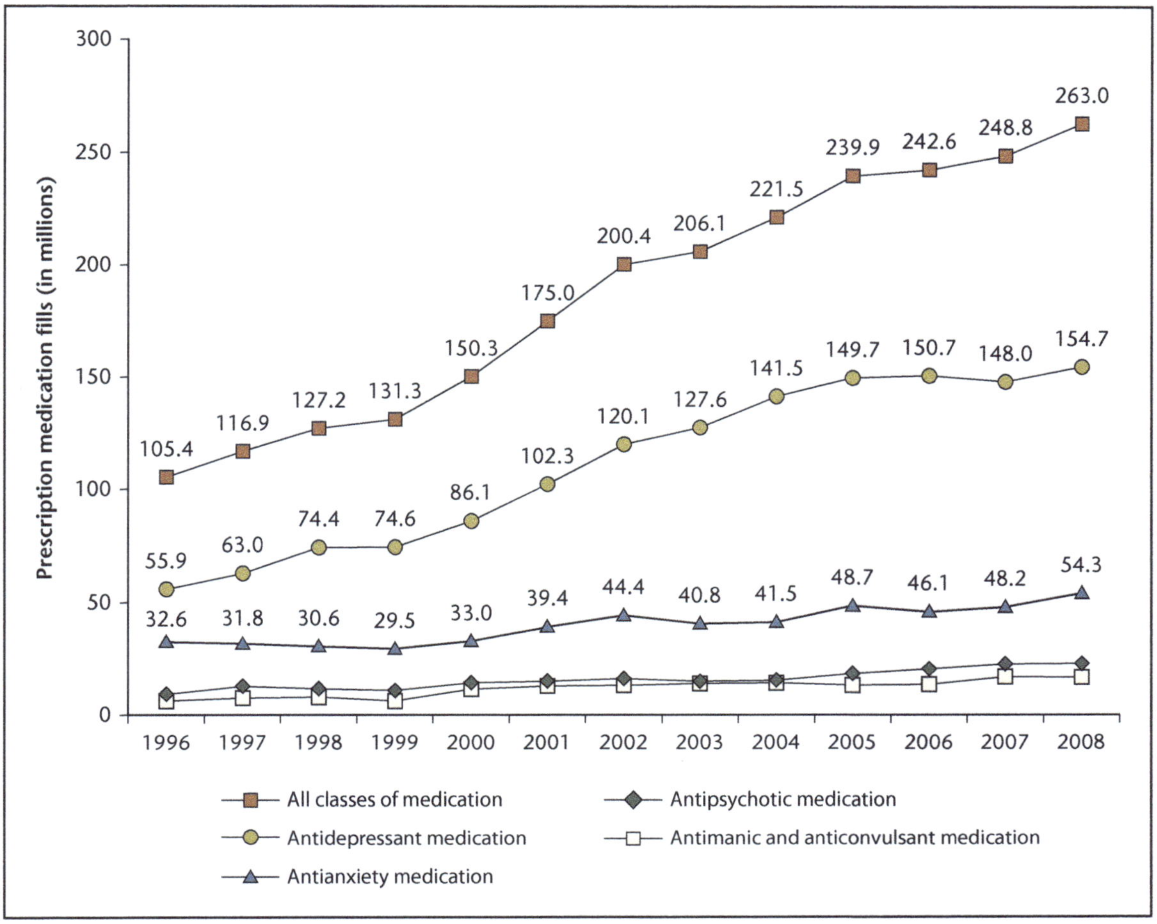

NOTES: For legibility, data labels for antipsychotic and antimanic medications are suppressed.

Antianxiety medications include sedative and hypnotic medications.

See Appendix C for complete list of medications. Categorization of medications follows that of the National Institute of Mental Health (http://www.nimh.nih.gov/health/publications/mental-health-medications/alphabetical-list-of-medications.shtml). See Tables 30 and 31 for more details on the constructs in this exhibit.

SOURCE: Medical Expenditure Panel Survey, 1998–2008, Center for Financing, Access, and Cost Trends, Agency for Healthcare Research and Quality.

Zuvekas, S. H. (2005). Prescription drugs and the changing patterns of treatment for mental disorders, 1996–2001. *Health Affairs, 24*(1), 195–205.

Mental Health Service Receipt by Children and Youth Aged 8 to 15 with Selected Mental Disorders

More than half of children aged 8 to 15 with a selected mental disorder received any mental health treatment in the past year.

Children and youth with mental disorders are vulnerable to experiencing problems at home, with peers, and in school. Having friends, academic achievement, and strong family relationships are critical to positive child development and the successful transition to early adulthood. This makes early mental health treatment engagement for children with emotional and behavioral disorders particularly important, especially among children also experiencing severe functional impairment. Findings from the National Health and Nutrition Examination Survey (NHANES) as reported in Merikangas et al. (2010) show the percentage of children aged 8 to 15 with particular past year emotional or behavioral disorders who received mental health treatment. This NHANES-based study included 3,042 participants aged 8 to 15 who had participated in one of the NHANES surveys between 2001 and 2004. This study showed the following:

- About half of children aged 8 to 15 with at least one of the mental disorders assessed received mental health services in the past year.
- Children with mental disorders with severe impairment were no more likely to have received a mental health service in the past year than children with any emotional or behavioral disorder (with or without severe impairment).
- Children with anxiety disorders were the least likely to have received treatment. Only one in three children with anxiety disorders, with or without severe impairment (32.2 percent and 33.9 percent, respectively), reported receiving treatment in the past year.

Exhibit 10. Percentage of persons aged 8 to 15 with selected mental disorders who received mental health treatment in the past year, by level of impairment, United States, 2001–2004

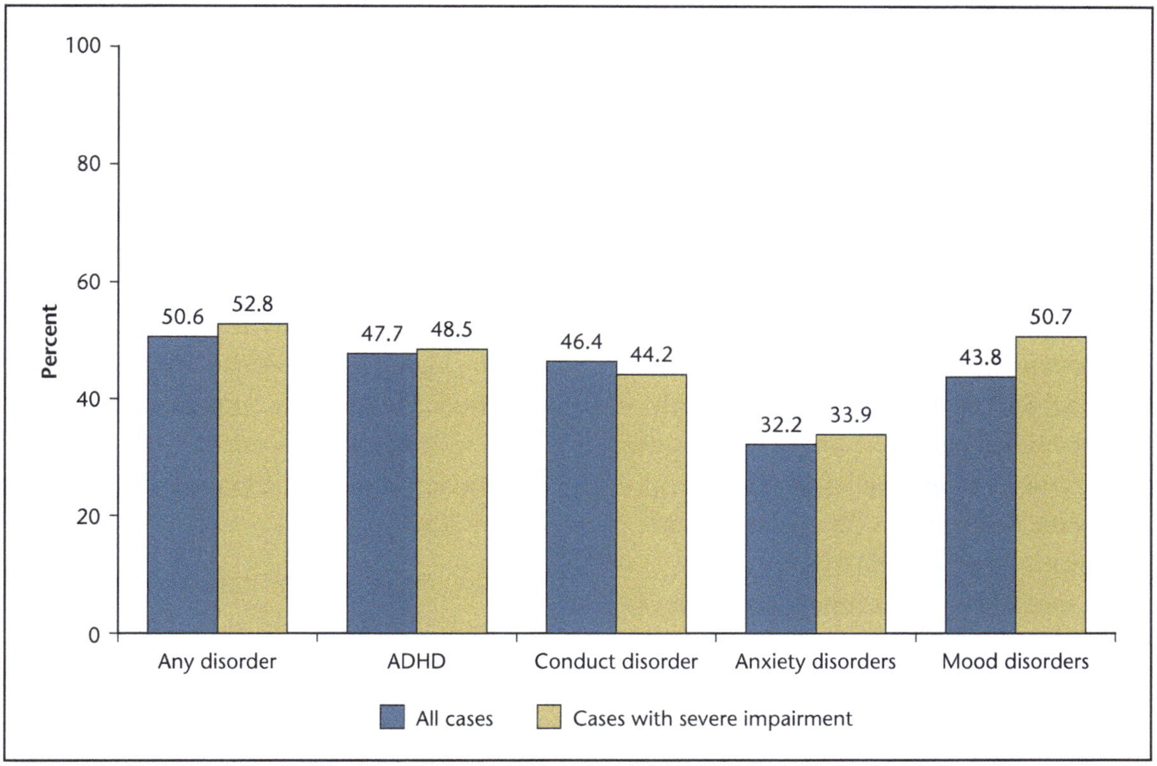

NOTES: Mental disorders were assessed using a structured diagnostic interview that contained modules. Disorder with severe impairment indicates two intermediate ratings or one severe rating on the six impairment questions within a diagnostic module. See Table 57 for more details on the constructs in this exhibit.

ADHD = attention deficit hyperactivity disorder.

SOURCE: Merikangas, K. R., He, J.-P., Brody, D., Fisher, P. W., Bourdon, K., & Koretz, D. S. (2010). Prevalence and treatment of mental disorders among US children in the 2001–2004 NHANES. *Pediatrics, 125*(1), 75–81.

Youth Receiving Specialty Mental Health Treatment in the Past Year by Key Characteristics

Female youth were more likely to have received specialty mental health treatment than male youth.

Use of mental health treatment among youth varies according to some key characteristics, particularly sex. Use of mental health treatment among youth, however, does not vary significantly by other characteristics, such as age and poverty. The National Survey on Drug Use and Health (NSDUH) includes questions that ask youth aged 12 to 17 to self-report on their receipt of specific types of specialty mental health treatment. Based on NSDUH data from 2009, mental health treatment use among youth aged 12 to 17 varied by important demographic and socioeconomic factors (Exhibit 11). The exhibit shows the following:

- Female youth were more likely to have received specialty mental health treatment in the past year than male youth (14.0 percent versus 10.1 percent). This difference was driven largely by the higher likelihood for female youth to receive specialty outpatient services. Use of specialty inpatient mental health treatment did not differ significantly by sex.
- Use of specialty mental health treatment by youth did not differ significantly by age, Hispanic origin and race, or poverty status.

Exhibit 11. Percentage of persons aged 12 to 17 who received any specialty mental health treatment in the past year, by selected characteristics, United States, 2009

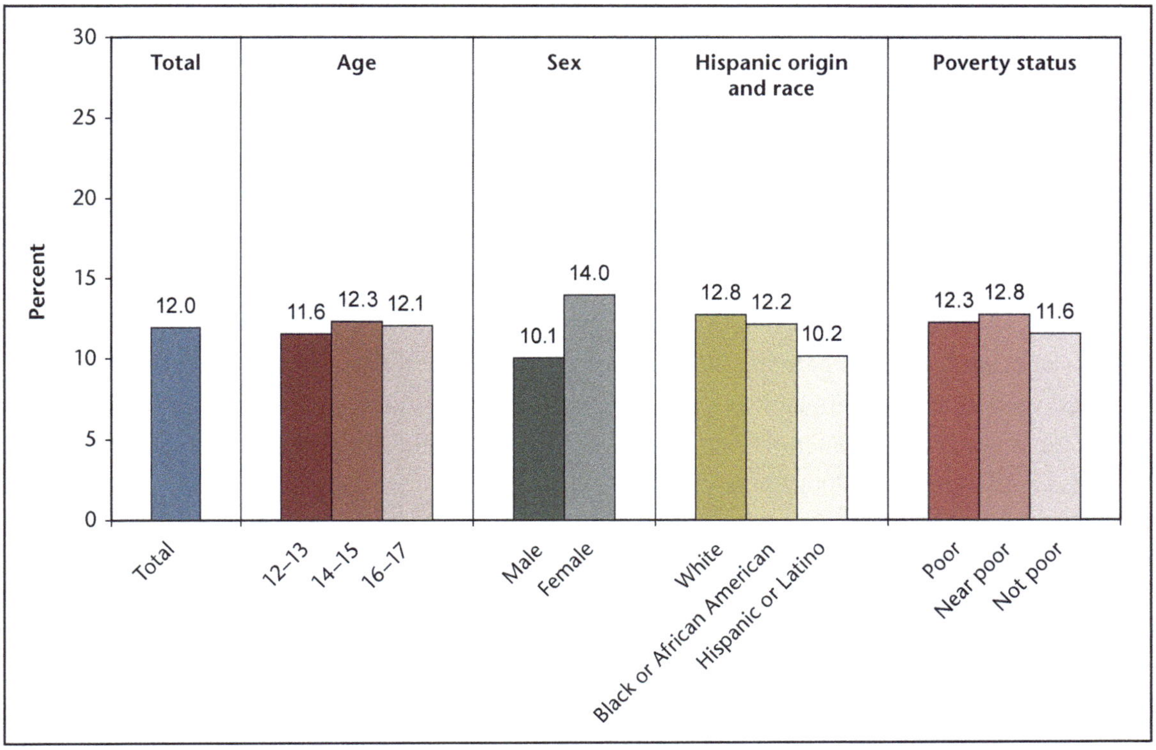

NOTES: Specialty mental health treatment includes outpatient mental health treatment or inpatient or residential care.

Poverty status is based on respondent age, family income, family size, and composition using the U.S. Census Bureau's poverty thresholds. "Poor" persons are defined as living in households where the family income is less than 100 percent of the U.S. Census poverty threshold. "Near poor" persons have incomes of 100 percent to less than 200 percent of the poverty threshold. "Not poor" persons have incomes that are 200 percent of the poverty threshold or greater.

Respondents with unknown receipt of mental health service information were excluded. Respondents could indicate multiple service sources; thus, the response categories are not mutually exclusive. See Table 59 for more details on the constructs in this exhibit.

SOURCE: National Survey on Drug Use and Health, 2009, Substance Abuse and Mental Health Services Administration, Office of Applied Studies.

Mental Health Service Use by Youth Aged 12 to 17 by Type of Treatment and Treatment Setting

Youth are most likely to have received mental health services in either specialty mental health outpatient or education settings.

Children and youth with emotional or behavioral health disorders receive mental health treatment in a variety of settings, including specialty mental health and nonspecialty settings. Nonspecialty settings, such as schools or primary care, are particularly important service settings to both identify emotional and behavioral health problems in childhood and provide services to children and youth with emotional or behavioral health disorders. The National Survey on Drug Use and Health (NSDUH) includes questions that assess the types of specialty and nonspecialty mental health treatment received by U.S. youth aged 12 to 17. Youth are asked to self-report on each type of treatment received in the past year and can indicate more than one type of treatment. Exhibit 12 presents data on mental health treatment for youth aged 12 to 17:

- In 2009, 12.0 percent of U.S. youth aged 12 to 17 reported using specialty mental health services in the past year, including services in inpatient (including residential treatment and treatment through therapeutic foster care) and outpatient mental health treatment locations.
- Approximately the same percentage of youth (12.1 percent) reported receiving some mental health–related service in an education setting. This included talking with a school social worker, psychologist, or counselor; receiving special education services; or being placed in a special school or program for students with emotional or behavioral problems.
- Of the 2.9 million youth who received any specialty mental health services in the past year, the majority (10.8 percent or 2.6 million) received outpatient treatment services and 2.3 percent (0.6 million) received inpatient services with some of these youth receiving both outpatient and inpatient treatment services.

Exhibit 12. Percentage of persons aged 12 to 17 who received mental health treatment in the past year, by type of treatment and treatment setting, United States, 2009

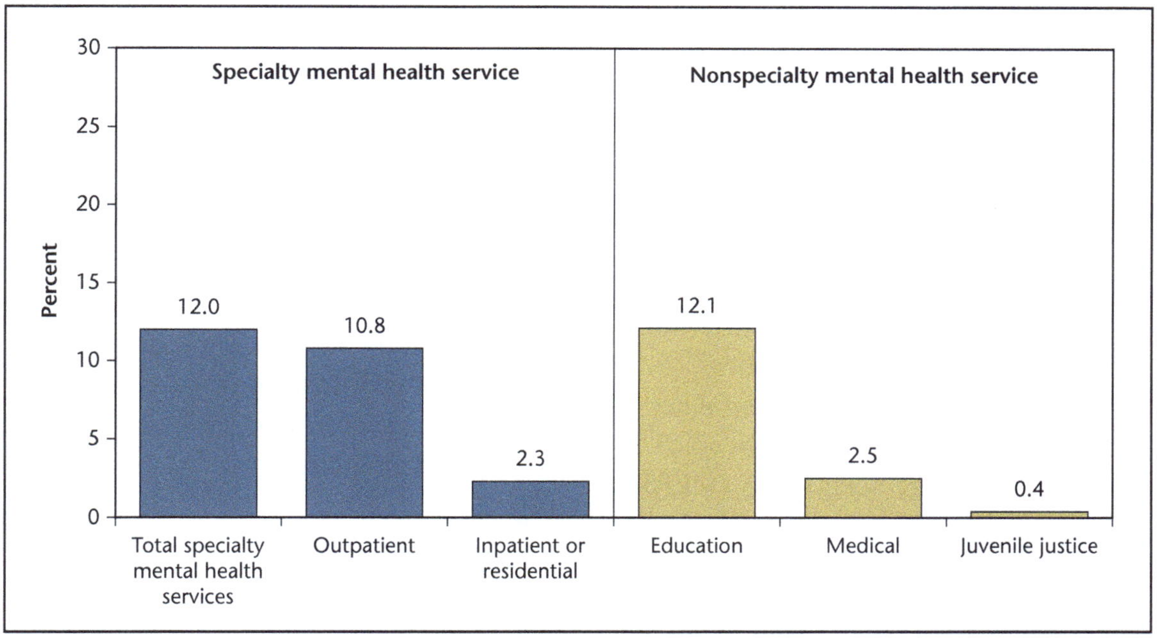

NOTES: Receipt of mental health services for persons aged 12 to 17 is defined as having received treatment/counseling for emotional or behavioral problems not caused by drug or alcohol use. Respondents with unknown receipt of mental health service information were excluded. Respondents could indicate multiple service sources; thus, the response categories are not mutually exclusive. See Table 59 for more details on the constructs in this exhibit.

SOURCE: National Survey on Drug Use and Health, 2009, Substance Abuse and Mental Health Services Administration, Office of Applied Studies.

Mental Health/Substance Abuse Medication Fills among Children

The increase from 1996 to 2008 in psychotropic medication fills for children was driven largely by an increase in the use of stimulant medication.

Psychotropic medication is an important part of mental health treatment for children, and the role of medication in treatment has become more prominent in recent years. Data from pharmacy records on the number of prescriptions being purchased or filled provide one useful metric to monitor prescription medication use. The Medical Expenditure Panel Survey (MEPS) includes a component that gathers data about prescription medication fills directly from pharmacies across the United States. This data collection method makes MEPS a particularly reliable source of information for assessing trends in psychotropic medication. Exhibit 13 illustrates the increase in psychotropic prescription medication fills for three major classes of psychotropic medication from 1996 to 2008: antidepressant, antipsychotic, and stimulant. These prescription fills were specifically for the treatment of a childhood emotional or behavioral health problem. The measure includes first-time purchases and refills. The exhibit shows the following:

- The number of psychotropic medication fills for children nearly doubled between 1996 and 2008.
- Consistently over time, stimulant medication was the most common class of examined psychotropic medication filled. Antidepressant medication was the second most common.
- The increase in psychotropic medication fills from 1996 to 2008 was driven largely by stimulant medications.
- Over time, the number of antidepressant medication fills has been about one quarter of the number of stimulant fills.
- Antipsychotic medication use appears to have become more prominent over time. Before 2001, data on these fills did not include a sufficient number to be reported reliably for children. In 2001, the first year for which reliable estimates could be obtained, the number of fills was 1.4 million. By 2005, that number had risen to 4 million, and the number remained about or just below that level until 2008. Evidence elsewhere in this volume (see Exhibit 20) suggests that changes in fills for antipsychotic medication are driven by the number of people being prescribed medication, rather than the number of fills being prescribed per person.

Exhibit 13. Trends in mental health/substance abuse medication fills for persons aged 17 or younger, by medication class, United States, 1996–2008

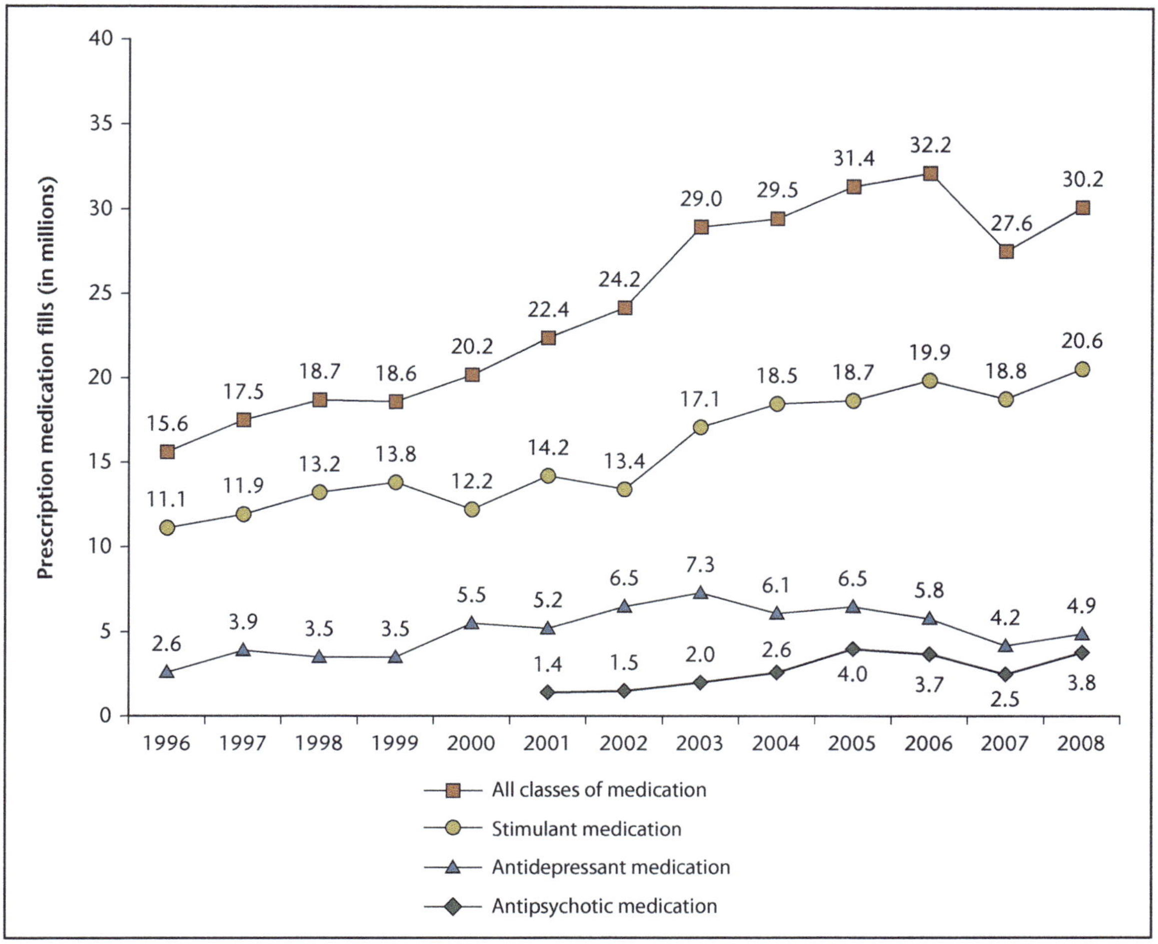

NOTES: Estimates for antipsychotic medication before 2001 are considered unreliable.

Antianxiety medications include sedative and hypnotic medications.

See Appendix C for complete list of medications. Categorization of medications follows that of the National Institute of Mental Health (http://www.nimh.nih.gov/health/publications/mental-health-medications/alphabetical-list-of-medications.shtml). See Tables 62 and 63 for more details on the constructs in this exhibit.

SOURCES: Medical Expenditure Panel Survey, 1996–2008, Center for Financing, Access, and Cost Trends, Agency for Healthcare Research and Quality.

Zuvekas, S. H. (2005). Prescription drugs and the changing patterns of treatment for mental disorders, 1996–2001. *Health Affairs, 24*(1), 195–205.

3.3 References

Hazlett, S. B., McCarthy, M. L., Londner, M. S., & Onyike C. U. (2004, February). Epidemiology of adult psychiatric visits to US emergency departments. *Academic Emergency Medicine, 11*(2), 193–195.

Lo Sasso, A. T., & Byck, G. R. (2010). Funding growth drives community health center services. *Health Affairs, 29*(2), 289–296.

Mark, T. L., Levit, K. R., Vandivort-Warren, R., Buck, J. A., & Coffey, R. M. (2011). Changes in US spending on mental health and substance abuse treatment, 1986–2005, and implications for policy. *Health Affairs, 30*(2), 284–292.

Mark, T. L., Levit, K. R., & Buck, J. A. (2009). Datapoints: Psychotropic drug prescriptions by medical specialty. *Psychiatric Services, 60*(9), 1167.

Merikangas, K. R., He, J.-P., Brody, D., Fisher, P. W., Bourdon, K., & Koretz, D. S. (2010). Prevalence and treatment of mental disorders among US children in the 2001–2004 NHANES. *Pediatrics, 125*(1), 75–81.

Miranda, J., McGuire, T. G., Williams, D. R., & Wang, P. (2008). Mental health in the context of health disparities. *American Journal of Psychiatry, 165*(9), 1102–1108.

Substance Abuse and Mental Health Services Administration (SAMHSA). (2011). *Leading change: A plan for SAMHSA's roles and actions 2011–2014* (DHHS Publication No. SMA 11-4629). Rockville, MD: SAMHSA. Retrieved from http://store.samhsa.gov/product/SMA11-4629

Zuvekas, S. H. (2005). Prescription drugs and the changing patterns of treatment for mental disorders, 1996–2001. *Health Affairs, 24*(1), 195–205.

4. PAYERS AND PAYMENT MECHANISMS

4.1 Narrative

4.1.1 Overview

Funding for mental health care has changed considerably in the past decade, and change seems likely to continue. Ongoing budget crises in many States threaten the availability of some services for many vulnerable populations. For people with third-party coverage—such as private insurance, Medicare, and Medicaid—recent parity legislation is part of a series of legislative attempts to make the coverage for behavioral health care equivalent to that for general medical care. Forthcoming health care reform is likely to provide third-party coverage for behavioral health services for millions of people who were not covered previously. In the face of such changes, decision makers who must budget and plan the provision of care need access to data that monitor how much is spent on mental health services, from what sources, and on what services.

This section provides national information on mental health expenditures and how these expenditures relate to expenditures on all health care, as well as information on the major funders, including private insurance, Medicare, Medicaid, the U.S. Department of Veterans Affairs (VA), and State Mental Health Agencies (SMHAs). The data directly address the Substance Abuse and Mental Health Services Administration's (SAMHSA's) strategic initiative Data, Outcomes, and Quality, which is intended to improve the accessibility of mental health information for staff, stakeholders, funders, and policy makers (SAMHSA, 2011).

4.1.2 Mental Health Expenditures: Overview

(Exhibits 14 through 18 and Tables 70 through 77)

The exhibits and tables on mental health expenditures begin with a broad overview of mental health expenditures at the national level from 1986 to 2005. Data on U.S. mental health and all health expenditures are from the SAMHSA Spending Estimates Project (SAMHSA, 2010). The estimates are developed to mirror the National Health Expenditure products of the Centers for Medicare & Medicaid Services (CMS) and thus are developed using many of the same data sources, methods, and definitions (CMS, 2011). In keeping with previous volumes of *Mental Health, United States,* dollar estimates are expressed in nominal terms, unless otherwise stated. That is, no adjustment is made for inflation in general prices.

Overall, expenditures on mental health treatment in the United States were about $113 billion in 2005, which is about 6.1 percent of the total U.S. expenditures on all types of health care (Tables 70 and 71). Mental health expenditures by all types of payer sources increased from 1986 to 2005, but as a share of all health expenditures, mental health expenditures declined or remained relatively stable across all types of payers (Tables 70 and 71).

From 1986 to 2005, there were substantial changes in the distribution of mental health expenditures across provider type and by payer. More was spent on specialty mental health providers than nonspecialty providers from 1986 through 2005 (Exhibit 15 and Table 72). However, specialty care as a percentage of all mental health expenditures decreased over this period. During this same period, the share of mental health expenditures accounted for by prescription medications increased from 7.4 percent in 1986 to 26.6 percent in 2005. The main changes in the distribution of expenditures for mental health care by payer included the increase in the share of expenditures by private insurance and Medicaid and the decrease in the share of expenditures by other State and local sources (Exhibit 18 and Table 75). Finally, the share of total mental health expenditures on inpatient mental health services decreased from 1986 to 2005, while the share of outpatient mental health services increased steadily (Tables 76 and 77).

4.1.3 Revenues and Expenditures by Public Funding Source

(Tables 78 through 88)

Nearly 60 percent of all mental health spending is from public funding sources (SAMHSA, 2010). Thus, sources such as Medicare, Medicaid, VA, and SMHAs play a very important role in providing access to mental health treatment. Medicaid alone—which covers qualifying people with lower incomes and with disabilities—accounts for nearly 30 percent of mental health spending. Tables 78 through 81 present estimates based on claims data from Medicaid beneficiaries with fee-for-service coverage in 13 States for the year 2003. These estimates reveal how the use of mental health services under Medicaid varies across population characteristics such as age, sex, Hispanic origin and race, eligibility status, diagnoses, and use of service type. For example, in 2003, 26.8 percent of beneficiaries who were eligible for Medicaid because of a disability used mental health services, compared with only 8.6 percent of adults and 8.2 percent of children (Table 78).

Medicare provides coverage to two vulnerable groups: those who qualify by disability and those aged 65 or older. Although Medicare accounted for 18.3 percent of spending on all medical conditions in 2005 (see Table 75), it accounted for much less (7.7 percent) of mental health spending. Nevertheless, because of the aging U.S. population, data are needed to track spending on mental health conditions. Tables 82 through 84 present estimates on use of mental health services among Medicare beneficiaries.

VA is an important provider of services to veterans, and estimates of VA behavioral health spending are presented in Table 85. From fiscal year (FY) 2008 to FY 2009, the number of specialty mental health encounters increased for inpatient stays and outpatient visits and decreased for residential days.

SMHAs have a particularly important role in funding mental health services. For example, when examining all sources of spending on mental health (e.g., Exhibit 17 and Table 74), nearly 20 percent of all mental health spending in 2005 was through other State and local sources, which includes funds controlled by SMHAs. Because their funding sources are from State funds, such as general funds, SMHA funds are at risk with the ongoing State budget crises. Tables 86 through 88 illustrate the impact that the recession is having on State financing for behavioral health services. Many States are reporting budget cuts for FY 2010 and FY 2011.

4.1.4 *Private Employer-Sponsored Mental Health Benefits*

(Tables 89 through 94)

Tables 89 through 91 present information on mental health benefits offered by private employers. Approximately 30 percent of mental health expenditures are funded through private insurance (see Table 75). Private insurance policies can have a significant impact on the amount and types of services that persons with mental health conditions receive.

Information from private employers provides an important baseline against which to evaluate the Mental Health Parity and Addiction Equity Act (MHPAEA). The data in this section come from a variety of sources, including the Bureau of Labor Statistics (Table 89); the Brandeis Health Plan Survey on Alcohol, Drug Abuse, and Mental Health Services (Tables 90 and 91); the Mercer National Survey of Employer-Sponsored Health Plans (Table 92); and the Kaiser Family Foundation/Health Research & Educational Trust Employer Health Benefits Survey (Tables 93 and 94). Data from all sources are consistent in showing that before the MHPAEA, the majority of plans offered by private employers had separate limits on mental health outpatient and inpatient services, such as limits on the number of outpatient visits and inpatient days.

4.1.5 *Mental Health Prescription Medication Use*

(Exhibits 19 and 20 and Tables 95 and 96)

For the past decade, psychotropic medications have been used increasingly to treat mental health conditions. The final set of exhibits and tables (Exhibits 19 and 20 and Tables 95 and 96) presents separate estimates on the use of and spending on psychotropic medication for adults and children. In 2008, about 27 million U.S. adults and 3.5 million children used psychotropic medications (Exhibits 19 and 20 and Tables 95 and 96). Antidepressant medications had the most users and highest expenditures for adults, whereas stimulants had the most users and highest expenditures for children.

4.2 Exhibits

Exhibits 14–20

Trends in Expenditures on Mental Health Care by Type of Service

Prescription medication spending has increased faster than any other type of mental health care.

Mental health care is provided by different providers in a number of settings: physicians; other professionals, such as psychologists, counselors, and social workers; hospitals; specialty facilities that are not hospitals, such as residential treatment centers for children; and retail prescription medication. An ongoing Substance Abuse and Mental Health Services Administration (SAMHSA) project provides estimates for mental health and substance use that are similar to the National Health Expenditure estimates (SAMHSA, 2010), which measure spending on health in the United States by type of service delivered and source of funding. Because the estimates used methods that have been consistent and comprehensive for nearly 20 years, they are the most reliable means of examining spending on mental health care over time. Exhibit 14 uses these data to show the following:

- From 1986 to 2005, mental health expenditures increased for all types of providers. In 1986, about $31 billion was spent on mental health, and in 2005, about $113 billion was spent on mental health (not shown; see Table 70).
- Hospitals was one of the categories with the largest amount of expenditures over the period studied. From 1986 to 2005, it was the largest category; in 2005, it was approximately the same as retail prescription medication spending.
- Prescription medication spending increased more rapidly than any other category from 1986 to 2005.
- For each year examined, the amount of mental health spending on physicians has been similar to the amount of spending on all specialty facilities that are not part of a hospital, which include organizations providing outpatient and/or residential services or a combination of services to individuals with mental illness or substance use diagnoses. In 2005, about $15 billion was spent on each of these categories.

Exhibit 14. Mental health expenditures, by type of provider, United States, selected years 1986–2005

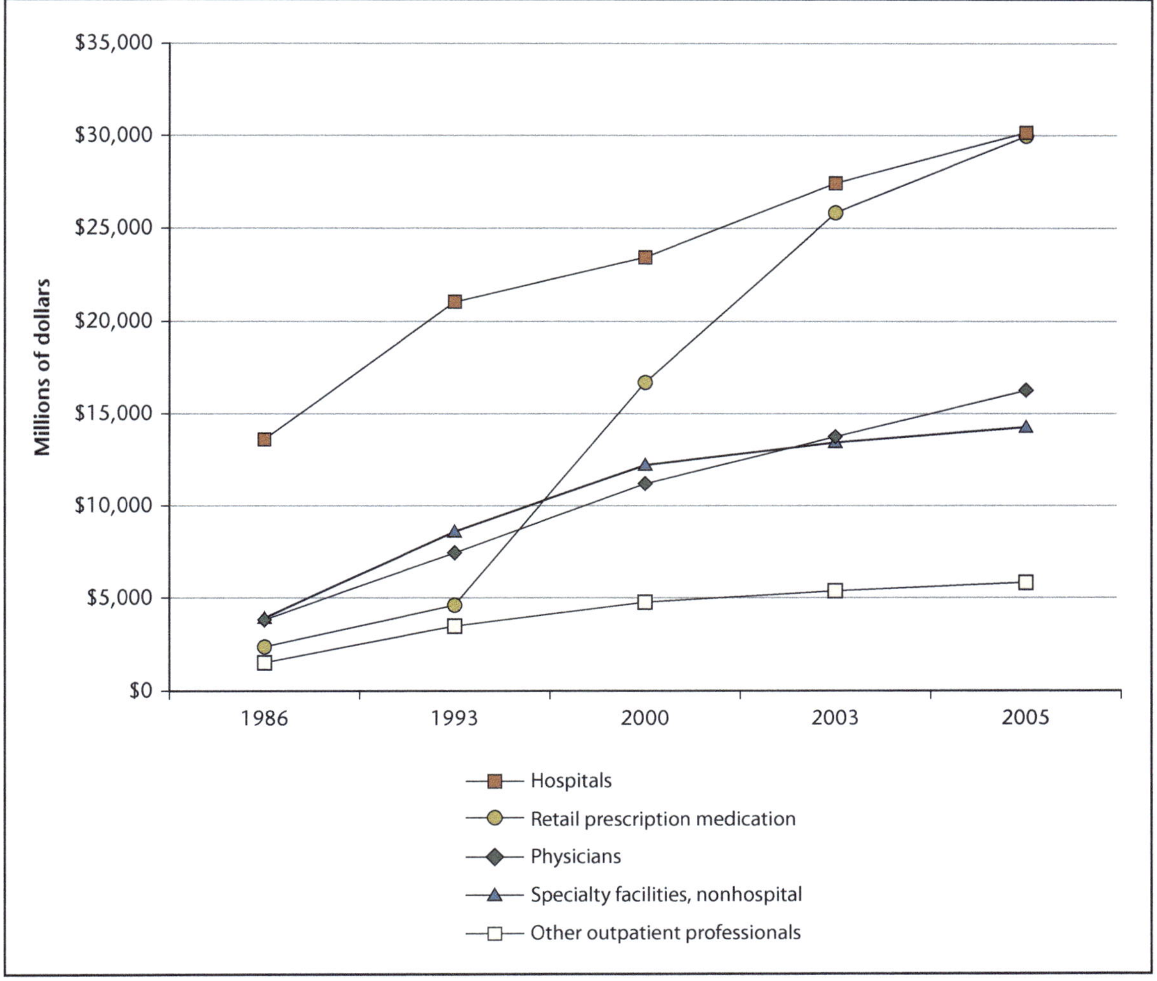

NOTES: The data include revisions and may differ from previously published data. Data are based on estimates of national expenditures for mental health services. For the sake of clarity, the exhibit omits data labels and two provider types: freestanding nursing homes and freestanding home health. Estimates are presented in nominal dollars. See Tables 70 and 71 for more details on the constructs in this exhibit.

SOURCE: Substance Abuse and Mental Health Services Administration (SAMHSA). (2010). *National expenditures for mental health services and substance abuse treatment, 1986–2005* (DHHS Publication No. SMA 10-4612). Rockville, MD: Center for Mental Health Services and Center for Substance Abuse Treatment, SAMHSA.

Distribution of Mental Health Care Expenditures by Type of Service

Specialty care and prescription medication accounted for most mental health expenditures in 2005.

In addition to the total dollar amount over time, it is also instructive to examine how the share of broad categories of services has changed over time. Exhibit 15 presents the distribution of mental health expenditures across the main types of services in 1986 and 2005. The data come from an ongoing Substance Abuse and Mental Health Services Administration (SAMHSA) project that provides estimates for mental health and substance use similar to the National Health Expenditure estimates (SAMHSA, 2010). The exhibit shows the following:

- In 2005, specialty services accounted for the largest share (50.0 percent) of spending on mental health.
- However, between 1986 and 2005, the share of mental health spending on specialty services diminished proportionately. In 1986, specialty services accounted for 61.3 percent of mental health spending.
- The share of expenditures for prescription medication increased proportionately from 7.4 percent in 1986 to 26.6 percent in 2005.
- The share of expenditures for insurance administration remained relatively stable over the period studied (between 4.9 and 7.4 percent).

Exhibit 15. Distribution of mental health expenditures, by type of service, United States, 1986 and 2005

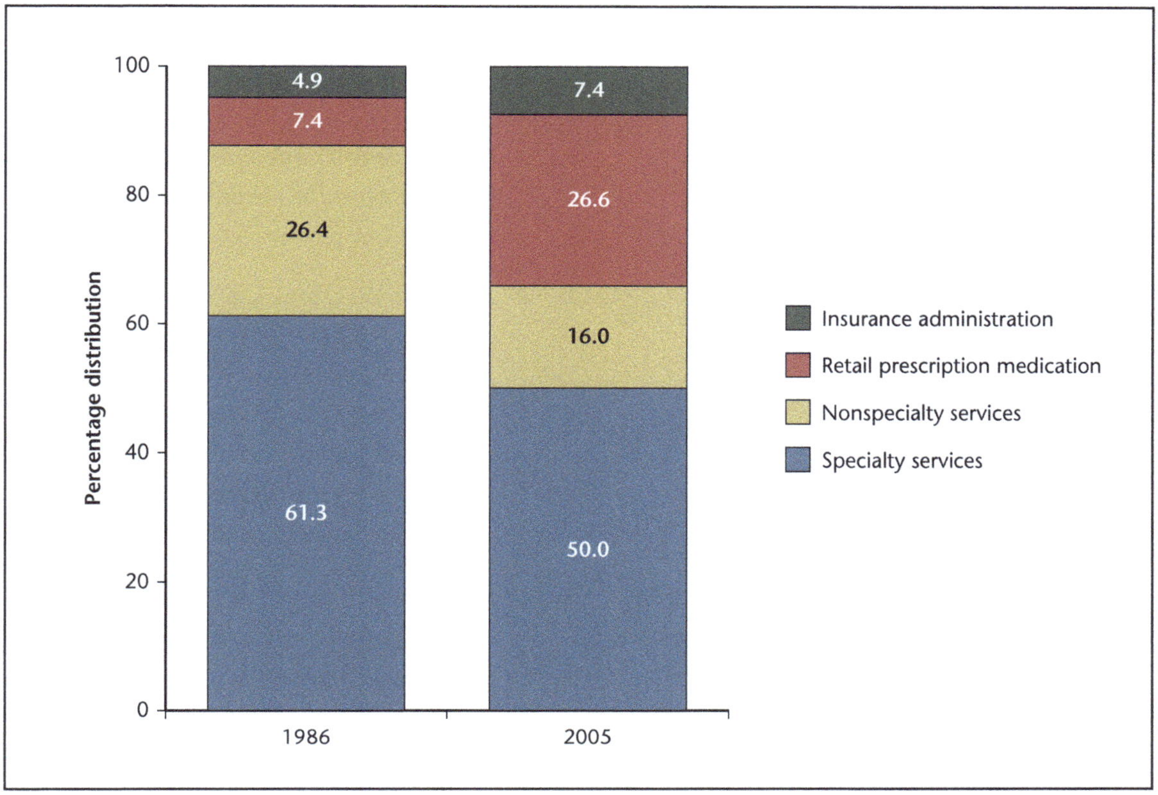

NOTES: The data include revisions and may differ from previously published data. Data are based on national expenditures for mental health services. See Table 72 for more details on the constructs in this exhibit.

SOURCE: Substance Abuse and Mental Health Services Administration (SAMHSA). (2010). *National expenditures for mental health services and substance abuse treatment, 1986–2005* (DHHS Publication No. SMA 10-4612). Rockville, MD: Center for Mental Health Services and Center for Substance Abuse Treatment, SAMHSA.

Trends in Mental Health Expenditures by Payer

Between 1986 and 2005, there were particularly large increases in spending on private insurance and Medicaid.

Mental health care is financed through a variety of private and public sources. Exhibit 16 describes mental health expenditures by payer, including private insurance and several types of public funding sources. Private payers include insurance, usually through an employer, and out-of-pocket payments. Public payers include Medicare, Medicaid, other Federal, and other State and local sources. The data come from a Substance Abuse and Mental Health Services Administration (SAMHSA) project that provides estimates for mental health and substance use similar to the National Health Expenditure estimates (SAMHSA, 2010). The exhibit shows the following:

- Mental health expenditures increased for every category of payer between 1986 and 2005.
- Between 1986 and 2005, there were particularly large increases in spending for private insurance and Medicaid. These two sources of payment each accounted for about $30 billion in mental health expenditures in 2005 compared with about $6 billion in 1986.
- In the 1980s and 1990s, other State and local government spending was the largest single source of spending on mental health care. By 2005, this source was the third largest, behind private insurance and Medicaid.
- Medicare spending on mental health services has been lower than out-of-pocket spending. Out-of-pocket spending refers to direct spending by consumers for health care services that is not covered by insurance, such as a co-payment. In 2005, Medicare spending was about $9 billion and out-of-pocket spending was about $14 billion.

Exhibit 16. Mental health expenditures, by payer, United States, selected years 1986–2005

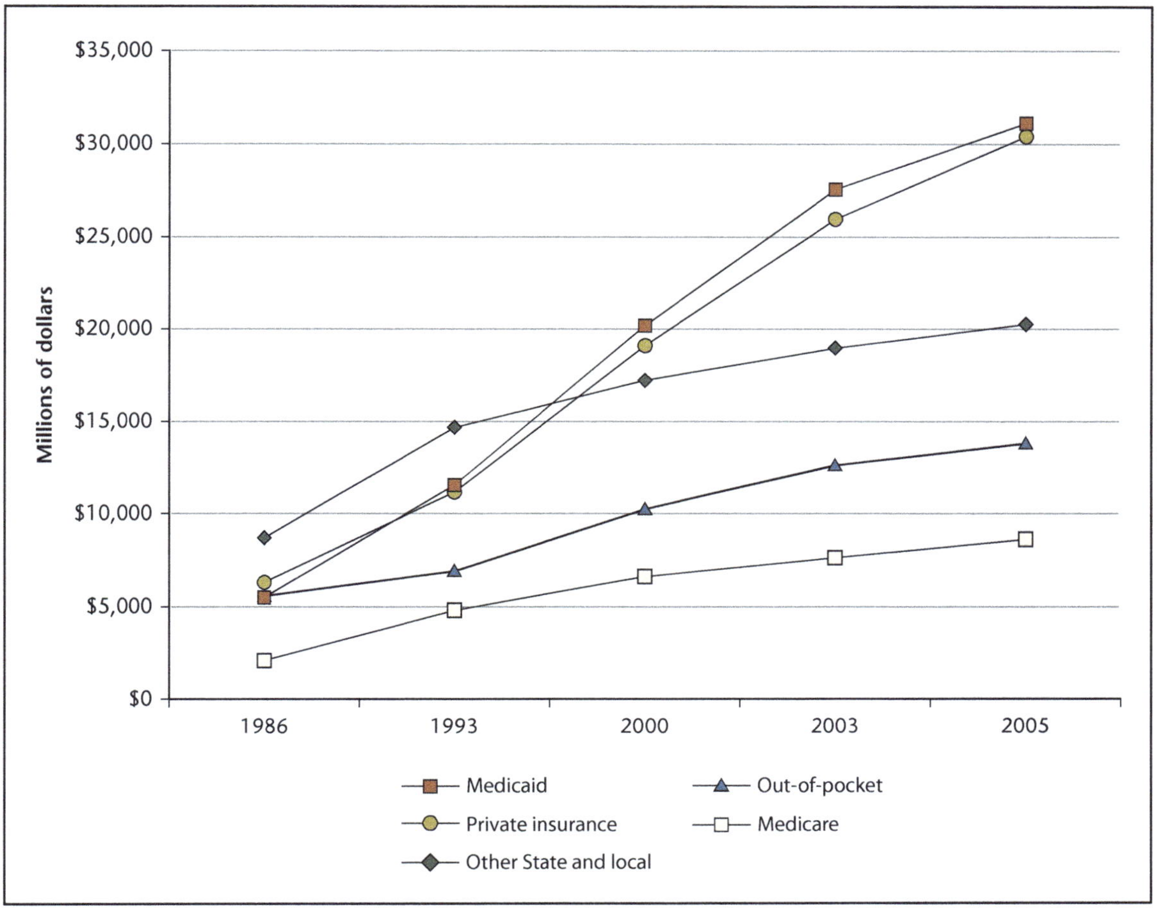

NOTES: The data include revisions and may differ from previously published data. Data are based on national expenditures for mental health services. For the sake of clarity, the exhibit omits data labels and two sources of expenditures: other private and other Federal (which includes SAMHSA block grants). Estimates are presented in nominal dollars. See Table 73 for more details on the constructs in this exhibit.

SOURCE: Substance Abuse and Mental Health Services Administration (SAMHSA). (2010). *National expenditures for mental health services and substance abuse treatment, 1986–2005* (DHHS Publication No. SMA 10-4612). Rockville, MD: Center for Mental Health Services and Center for Substance Abuse Treatment, SAMHSA.

Trends in Mental Health Expenditures as a Percentage of All Health Expenditures by Payer

Between 1986 and 2005, total mental health expenditures declined as a share of all health expenditures.

Previous exhibits have used Substance Abuse and Mental Health Services Administration (SAMHSA) data to show how mental health expenditures have increased between 1986 and 2005 (Exhibits 14 and 15). The data come from a SAMHSA project that provides estimates for mental health and substance use similar to the National Health Expenditure estimates (SAMHSA, 2010), which is one of the most reliable sources for examining spending on mental health care over time. The exhibit shows the following:

- As a share of all health expenditures, mental health expenditures declined or remained relatively stable from 1986 to 2005 across all types of payers.
- Between 1986 and 2005, the proportion of all health expenditures accounted for by mental health remained the same for three categories of payer: out-of-pocket, private insurance, and Medicare.
- The share of all health expenditures accounted for by mental health decreased for Medicaid expenditures from 12.1 percent in 1986 to 10.0 percent in 2005.
- The share of all health expenditures accounted for by mental health decreased the most in the other State and local category from 24.2 percent in 1986 to 18.7 percent in 2005.

Exhibit 17. Mental health expenditures as a share of all health expenditures, by payer, United States, 1986 and 2005

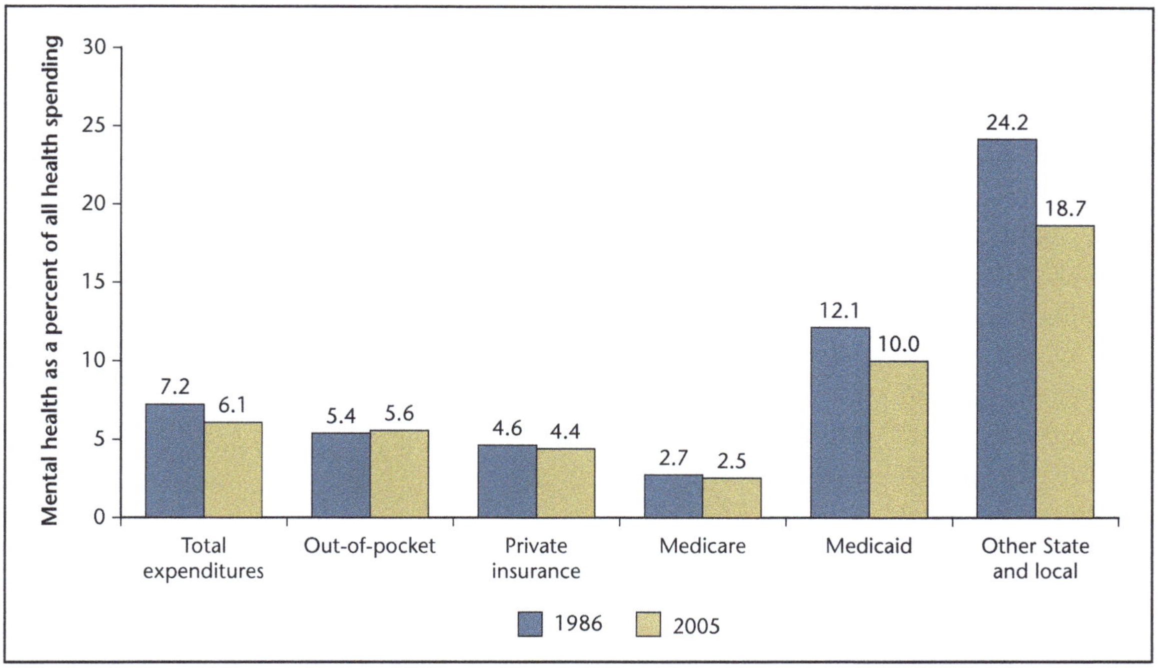

NOTES: The data include revisions and may differ from previously published data. Data are based on national expenditures for mental health services. See Table 74 for more details on the constructs in this exhibit.

SOURCE: Substance Abuse and Mental Health Services Administration (SAMHSA). (2010). *National expenditures for mental health services and substance abuse treatment, 1986–2005* (DHHS Publication No. SMA 10-4612). Rockville, MD: Center for Mental Health Services and Center for Substance Abuse Treatment, SAMHSA.

Distribution of Mental Health Expenditures by Payer

Medicaid and private insurance accounted for the largest share of mental health expenditures in 2005.

The role that different payers play in financing mental health spending has changed over time. Exhibit 18 displays the percentage distribution of mental health expenditures accounted for by payer type. The data come from an ongoing Substance Abuse and Mental Health Services Administration (SAMHSA) project to produce estimates on national spending on mental health (SAMHSA, 2010). The exhibit shows the following:

- In 2005, Medicaid and private insurance accounted for the largest share of mental health expenditures—just under 30 percent of total mental health expenditures.
- Between 1986 and 2005, the share of mental health expenditures accounted for by Medicaid and private insurance grew proportionately.
- In the 1980s, State and local government sources accounted for the largest proportion of mental health expenditures, but the share diminished proportionately over time.

Exhibit 18. Distribution of mental health expenditures, by payer, United States, 1986 and 2005

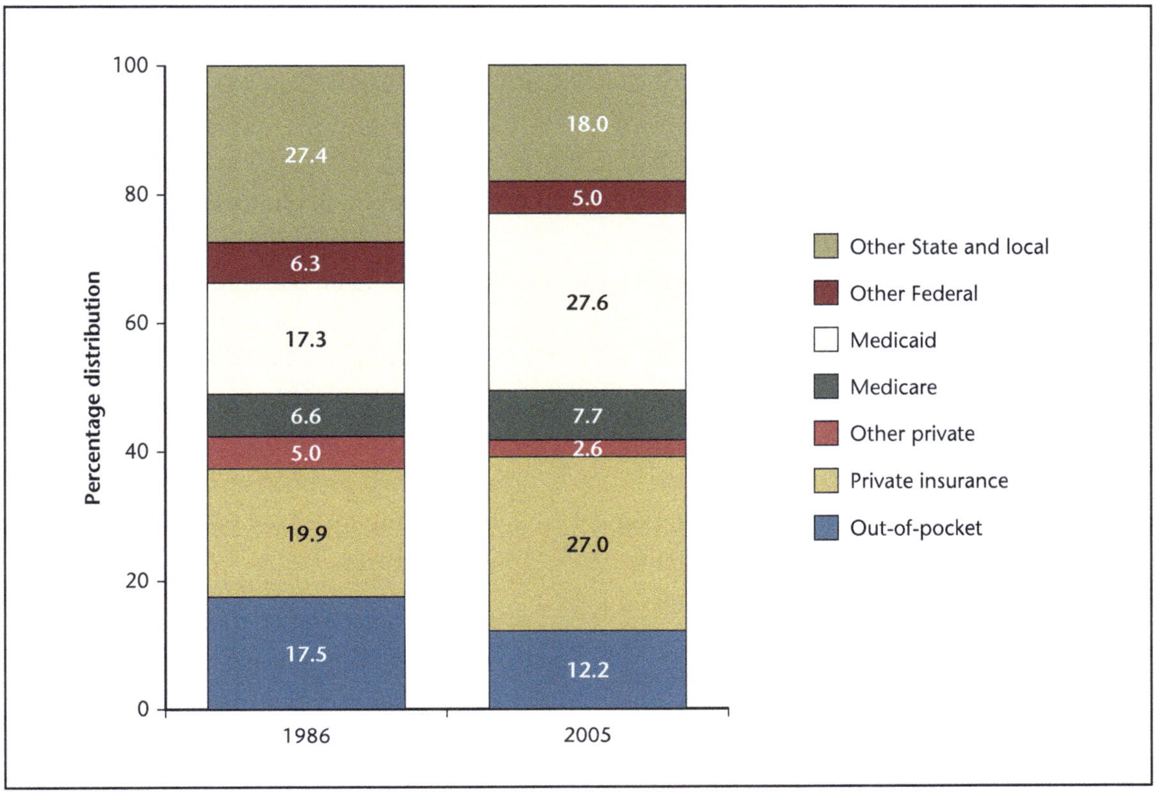

NOTES: The data include revisions and may differ from previously published data. Data are based on national expenditures for mental health services. See Table 75 for more details on the constructs in this exhibit.

SOURCE: Substance Abuse and Mental Health Services Administration (SAMHSA). (2010). *National expenditures for mental health services and substance abuse treatment, 1986–2005* (DHHS Publication No. SMA 10-4612). Rockville, MD: Center for Mental Health Services and Center for Substance Abuse Treatment, SAMHSA.

Trends in Adult Utilization of and Expenditures on Mental Health/Substance Abuse Medication

In 1998, 2003, and 2008, antidepressant medications were the most utilized medication class and also had the highest expenditures.

Expenditures on prescription medication accounted for more than one quarter of all expenditures on mental health treatment in recent years. The Medical Expenditure Panel Survey (MEPS) includes a component that gathers data about adult use of and expenditures on psychotropic medications from pharmacies across the United States. This data collection method makes MEPS a particularly reliable source of information for assessing trends in psychotropic medication. Exhibit 19 shows trends in the use of and expenditures on psychotropic medications for adults by class of medication. The exhibit shows the following:

- The number of adult users and the amount of expenditures on psychotropic medications increased over time. In 2008, about 27 million adults used psychotropic medications, accounting for about $25 billion in expenditures. In comparison, in 1998, about 15 million adults used psychotropic medications, accounting for about $10 billion in expenditures.
- Of the four classes detailed, antidepressant medications had the most adult users and the highest expenditures. The number of adult users of antidepressants grew rapidly during this period. In 2008, about 22 million adults used antidepressant medications, accounting for about $12 billion in expenditures on this class of medication.
- Antidepressant medication expenditures grew rapidly from 1998 to 2003, but then leveled off from 2003 to 2008. Antipsychotic medication expenditures increased somewhat from 1998 to 2003 and increased greatly from 2003 to 2008.

Exhibit 19. Number of users of and expenditures on selected mental health/ substance abuse (MH/SA) medications for an MH/SA condition among persons aged 18 or older, by selected therapeutic categories, United States, 1998, 2003, and 2008

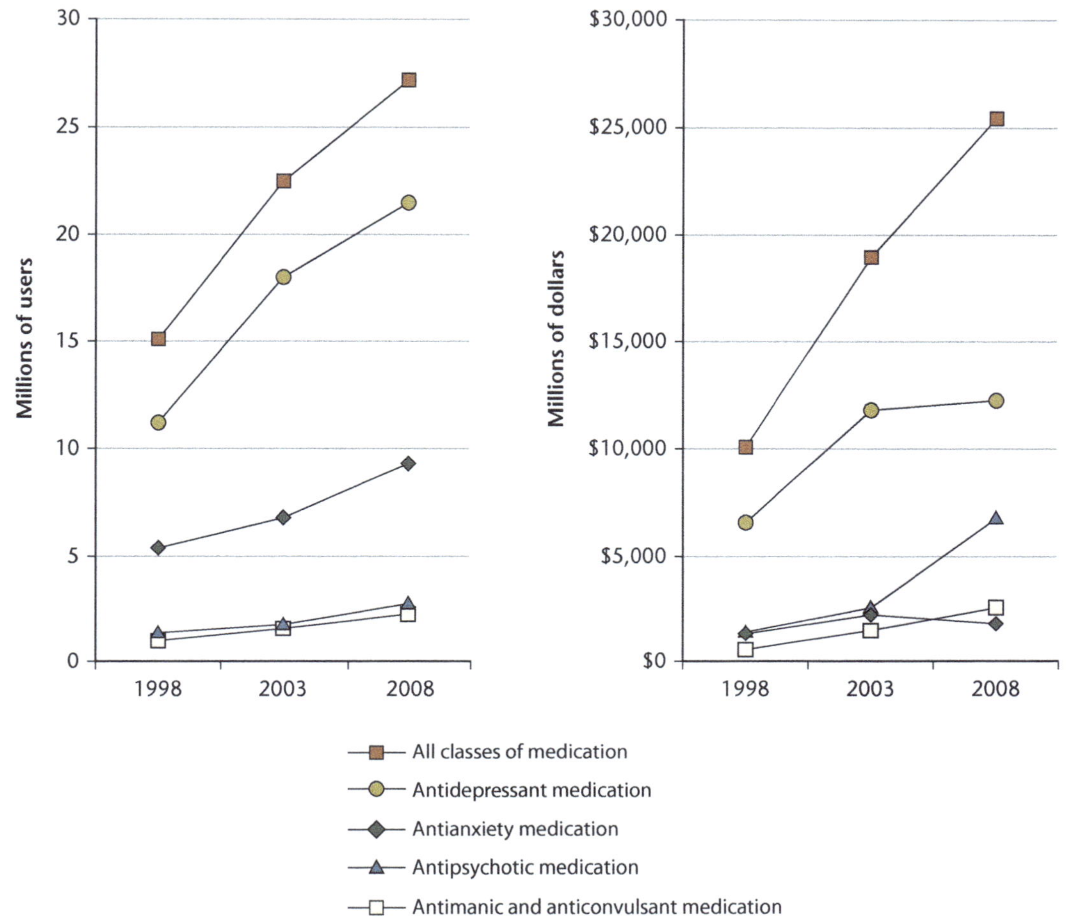

NOTES: For the sake of clarity, data labels have been omitted from this chart. Antianxiety medications include sedative and hypnotic medications. See Appendix C for complete list of medications. Categorization of medications follows that of the National Institute of Mental Health (http://www.nimh.nih.gov/health/publications/mental-health-medications/alphabetical-list-of-medications.shtml). See Table 95 for more details on the constructs in this exhibit.

SOURCES: Medical Expenditure Panel Survey, 1998–2008, Center for Financing, Access, and Cost Trends, Agency for Healthcare Research and Quality.

Zuvekas, S. H. (2005). Prescription drugs and the changing patterns of treatment for mental disorders, 1996–2001. *Health Affairs, 24*(1), 195–205.

Trends in Utilization of and Expenditures on Psychotropic Medication for Children and Youth

By 2008, stimulant medications—such as medications for attention deficit hyperactivity disorder—had the most users and accounted for the highest expenditures.

Because the mental illnesses that are most prevalent among children and youth are quite different from the mental illnesses that are most prevalent among adults, the classes of psychotropic medication used to treat children and youth are also quite different. The Medical Expenditure Panel Survey (MEPS) includes a component that gathers data from pharmacies across the United States about use of and expenditures on psychotropic medications for children and youth. This data collection method makes MEPS a particularly reliable source of information for assessing trends in psychotropic medication. Exhibit 20 describes the trend in use of and expenditures on these medications for children and youth in 1998, 2003, and 2008. The exhibit shows the following:

- Between 1998 and 2008, the number of children using psychotropic medications and the associated expenditures increased. In 2008, about 3.5 million children used psychotropic medications, accounting for about $4 billion in expenditures. In comparison, in 1998, about 2.6 million children used psychotropic medications, accounting for about $1 billion in expenditures.
- Of the three medication classes detailed, stimulant medications—such as medications for attention deficit hyperactivity disorder—had the most users and expenditures. In 2008, 2.8 million children used stimulant medication, accounting for about $2.6 billion in expenditures.
- The number of children using antidepressant medications and the associated expenditures increased between 1998 and 2003, but decreased between 2003 and 2008.
- Expenditures on antipsychotic medications for children overtook expenditures on antidepressants between 2003 and 2008.

Exhibit 20. Number of users of and expenditures on psychotropic medications for a mental health condition among persons aged 17 or younger, by selected therapeutic categories, United States, 1998, 2003, and 2008

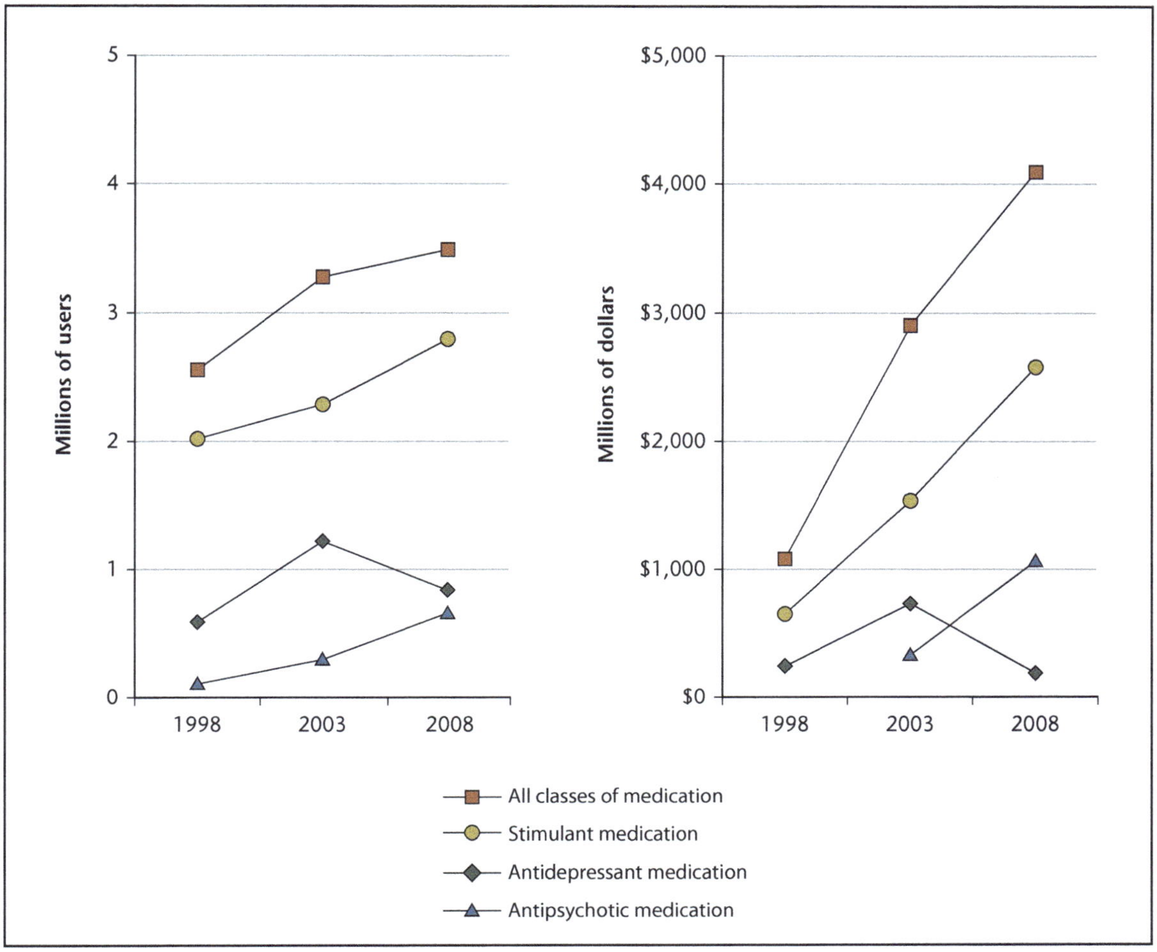

NOTES: Antianxiety medication and antipsychotic medication expenditures in 1998 were suppressed from this chart because the estimates are considered unreliable. For the sake of clarity, data labels have been omitted from this chart. See Appendix C for complete list of medications. Categorization of medications follows that of the National Institute of Mental Health (http://www.nimh.nih.gov/health/publications/mental-health-medications/alphabetical-list-of-medications.shtml). See Table 96 for more details on the constructs in this exhibit.

SOURCES: Medical Expenditure Panel Survey, 1998–2008, Center for Financing, Access, and Cost Trends, Agency for Healthcare Research and Quality.

Zuvekas, S. H. (2005). Prescription drugs and the changing patterns of treatment for mental disorders, 1996–2001. *Health Affairs, 24*(1), 195–205.

4.3 References

Centers for Medicare & Medicaid Services (CMS). (2011). National health expenditure data: Overview. Retrieved from http://www.cms.gov/NationalHealthExpendData/

Substance Abuse and Mental Health Services Administration (SAMHSA). (2010). *National expenditures for mental health services and substance abuse treatment, 1986–2005* (DHHS Publication No. SMA 10-4612). Rockville, MD: Center for Mental Health Services and Center for Substance Abuse Treatment, SAMHSA.

Substance Abuse and Mental Health Services Administration (SAMHSA). (2011). *Leading change: A plan for SAMHSA's roles and actions 2011–2014* (DHHS Publication No. SMA 11-4629). Rockville, MD: SAMHSA.

Zuvekas, S. H. (2005). Prescription drugs and the changing patterns of treatment for mental disorders, 1996–2001. *Health Affairs, 24*(1), 195–205.

5. STATES: PEOPLE, PROVIDERS, AND PAYERS

5.1 Narrative

5.1.1 Overview

States play an important role in helping monitor mental health indicators and prioritizing and providing treatment. In 2005, public sources funded $66 billion in mental health spending, which was 58 percent of all mental health care spending. About half of that public spending—nearly $34 billion—was spent by States (see Tables 73 and 75 in Section 7). These findings, together with the fact that much of the legislation on mental health treatment is written by State governments, indicates that State-level estimates are critical to a comprehensive view of mental health in the United States.

This section is organized similarly to the three previous sections and includes, in the following order, the number and characteristics of people with mental illness (people), the number and types of mental health facilities and practitioners (providers), and expenditures for mental health services (payers). The data presented support the Substance Abuse and Mental Health Services Administration (SAMHSA) in one of its eight strategic initiatives, Data, Outcomes, and Quality, by improving the accessibility of mental health prevalence, capacity, and expenditures data for provider staff, stakeholders, funders, and policy makers in need of State-level estimates (SAMHSA, 2011).

5.1.2 Mental Health of States' Populations

(Exhibits 21, 22, and 23 and Tables 98 through 102)

The exhibits in this subsection map State-level estimates of key mental health–related indicators. For each exhibit, the corresponding data table in Section 7 (indicated in the exhibit note) was used to place each State into one of five ranked categories from highest to lowest. Although the text describes and summarizes each exhibit, further study may be needed to interpret any State-to-State variation in the estimates.

Data on the mental health of State populations describe the number of people with any mental illness (AMI), the subgroup with serious mental illness (SMI), and the number of people with major depressive episode (MDE). Data on adults are presented in Exhibits 21 and 22 and Tables 98 and 99, and data on youth are presented in Exhibit 23 and Table 100. Monitoring the number of people with SMI is important because SMI is particularly debilitating and interferes with a person's ability to cope in everyday situations. MDE is defined as a 2-week period during the year when a person experiences depressed mood. Monitoring MDE is important because MDE is one of the components of major depression, which is one of the most common mental illness diagnoses.

The main findings for the exhibits and tables indicate that there was little variation across States in the rates of past year SMI (a range of 3.7 percentage points) or MDE (a range of 4.3 percentage points) for adults or in the rate of past year MDE for youth (a range of 3.5 percentage points). To obtain statistically accurate estimates at the State level for these data, two years of data were combined. Thus, the estimates for SMI and MDE span the years 2008 to 2009.

Suicide prevention remains an important concern for State policy makers. Key to supporting this prevention activity is monitoring the rate of death by suicide. In 2006, suicide was the 11th leading cause of death in the United States (Heron, Hoyert, Murphy, Xu, Kochanek, & Tejada-Vera, 2009). As seen in Table 101, national death rates by suicide have increased slightly from 2005 to 2007 (from 10.9 percent to 11.3 percent). In 2007, the rates across States ranged from 5.8 percent to 22.1 percent.

Receipt of mental health treatment is more common among certain subpopulations. Rates of mental illness in the inmate population are understood to be particularly high, and in a time of tight State budgets, this is of particular concern to State policy makers who must find a way to fund treatment. In 2000, 12.8 percent of total inmates (over 137,000 inmates) received therapy and counseling, which was the most common form of mental health service received (Table 102). There is a large range, between 2.7 percent and 37.3 percent, for the receipt of this service across States in 2000.

5.1.3 Providers and Settings for Mental Health Services at the State Level

(Exhibits 24, 25, 26, and 27 and Tables 103 through 118)

Mental health treatment relies on specialist care (from psychiatrists, for example) and nonspecialist care (from primary care providers, for example); much of the care is delivered in an outpatient setting. Tables 103 and 104 present estimates on adults receiving outpatient specialty and nonspecialty mental health treatment. To provide statistically reliable estimates at the State level, data from 5 years (2005–2009) are combined. Over those years, the percentage of adults receiving treatment from outpatient specialty providers ranged from 3.0 to 9.5 percent. The percentage of adults receiving mental health treatment from outpatient nonspecialty providers ranged from 1.1 to 3.7 percent.

Table 106 presents treatment receipt estimates for youth aged 12 to 17 for the period 2005 to 2009 combined. Data from 5 years are combined to provide statistically reliable estimates at the State level. Nationwide, 11.4 percent of youth (2.9 million youth) received treatment from outpatient specialty providers, and rates across States ranged from 8.0 to 16.9 percent. Nationally, 2.8 percent of youth aged 12 to 17 (over 700,000 youth) received treatment from providers who were not mental health specialists (a medical pediatrician or other family doctor), and State-level estimates ranged from 1.5 to 4.5 percent.

State-level estimates for the number of mental health organizations and service capacity vary considerably, with States that have a greater proportion of the population living in rural areas often having lower capacity. Table 109 presents estimates of the number of mental health professionals across disciplines. The District of Columbia and Maryland—with relatively high proportions of the population living in urban areas—have the highest rates of mental health professionals. States with large proportions of the population living in rural areas, such as Mississippi and Nevada, often have the lowest rates, although the rates vary by discipline. An important limitation of these data is that they do not distinguish between adult and child service providers.

Exhibit 26 and Table 111 present estimates on the shortage of mental health professionals in the adult household population across all States. Overall, many northeast States (Connecticut, the District of Columbia, Maryland, Massachusetts, New Hampshire, and New York) do not appear to be facing a shortage of professionals. States facing a shortage, such as Alabama, Idaho, Mississippi, Nevada, and Wyoming, have a relatively large proportion of the population living in rural areas. The supply of inpatient psychiatric beds in U.S. hospitals also varies across States, as illustrated in Tables 113, 114, and 115, and in Exhibit 27. The most populated States in the country (California, New York, and Texas) had the most inpatient psychiatric beds (Federal and non-Federal) relative to all States, whereas the District of Columbia, Mississippi, and Wyoming had the highest number of these beds per 100,000 adults (Exhibit 27 and Table 115). The total number of mental health organizations within States varies widely, with less populated States and States with a relatively large proportion of the population living in rural areas having fewer facilities, as seen in Tables 116, 117, and 118. Nationwide, the most common forms of mental health organizations are outpatient clinics and general hospitals that treat psychiatric patients.

5.1.4 States' Payers and Payment Mechanisms

(Tables 119 through 132)

Mental health spending from all public and private sources totaled almost $113 billion in 2005 (see Table 70). Thirty percent of that spending comes from State sources (see Table 75). State Mental Health Agencies (SMHAs) have considerable authority in directing State mental health treatment resources. SMHA revenues are derived from State general funds, followed by Medicaid and the State block grant programs, as seen in Table 119. In fiscal year (FY) 2008, 44 of 51 SMHAs devoted at least half of their funding to community mental health programs (Table 120).

The recent recession has particularly affected State budgets, leading to concern about how States can support people with mental health conditions. Approximately two thirds of States have cut mental health care funding in the past 3 years, with total cuts reaching nearly $1.6 billion (Honberg, Diehl, Kimball, Gruttadaro, & Fitzpatrick, 2011). Furthermore, mental health spending grew at a slower rate than the national gross domestic product in 2004 and 2005, and it continued to shrink as a share of all health spending (Mark et al., 2011; SAMHSA, 2011). Tables 121 and 122 describe the impact for SMHAs across the Nation in terms of funding and the decline in the number of inpatient State psychiatric beds. The South Atlantic region experienced the largest percentage of budget cuts in FY 2009, FY 2010, and FY 2011 (Table 121). Nationwide, approximately 2,200 inpatient State psychiatric beds were closed in 2010 (Table 122). Further study may be needed to determine the potential impact of closing psychiatric beds on the provision of care.

One of the main sources of funding for mental health treatment in States is Medicaid, a program funded by the Federal and State governments and administered by the States. It provides funding for low-income individuals and others in certain defined eligibility categories to receive health coverage, including treatment for mental health conditions. Of the $113 billion spent on mental health nationwide, 28 percent of the spending was through Medicaid (see Table 64). Spending by Medicaid programs across 13 States can be seen in Tables 123 through 127. The most common diagnostic category covered by Medicaid across all 13 States in 2003 was neurotic and other depressive disorders (over 280,000 beneficiaries), followed by major depression (over 254,000 beneficiaries), and all other diagnoses (over 234,000 beneficiaries) (Table 124).

Another source of funding for mental health treatment is the Federal Medicare program, which provides coverage to people aged 65 or older or those who qualify because of a disability. Medicare has received considerable attention from policy makers because it accounts for 23 percent of all health care spending and about half of health spending paid for by the government (National Center for Health Statistics, 2011). For mental health, Medicare is an important but relatively small share of spending at about 8 percent (see Exhibit 18 and Table 75). Tables 128 through 132 provide data on Medicare spending. In 2007, more than $8 billion of Medicare funds were spent on mental health and substance abuse treatment units in community hospitals nationwide. Medicare mental health expenditures per claimant were on average $1,500 but also varied across the States (Table 129).

5.2 Exhibits

Exhibits 21–27

Adults with Serious Mental Illness

In the 2008–2009 period, State-specific prevalence of adults with past year serious mental illness ranged from 3.5 percent to 7.2 percent.

Serious mental illness (SMI) is of particular concern to policy makers and providers because having this kind of diagnosable mental illness involves serious functional impairment that can greatly diminish a person's quality of life. Since 2008, the annual National Survey on Drug Use and Health (NSDUH) has included measures that permit the estimation of SMI in adults across the United States. Exhibit 21 uses two years of data combined (2008 and 2009) to display geographic variation across the States in the proportion of adults with past year SMI. The two years of data were combined to achieve statistically precise estimates. The exhibit shows the following patterns:

- During the 2008–2009 period, State-specific variation in the proportion of people with SMI ranged from 3.47 percent to 7.20 percent. Because State-to-State variation in the rate of SMI was low, the five categories have a small range of values, of about 0.7 of a percentage point. Two States were in the category corresponding with the highest State-specific prevalence of SMI (6.45 to 7.20 percent): Arkansas and Rhode Island.
- Four States were in the second highest category (5.71 to 6.44 percent): Idaho, Indiana, Utah, and West Virginia.
- The remaining 44 States and the District of Columbia were fairly evenly spread across the third highest (4.96 to 5.70 percent), fourth highest (4.21 to 4.95 percent), and lowest (3.47 to 4.20 percent) categories.
- The States in the lowest category of State-specific prevalence (3.47 to 4.20 percent) are along the East Coast, as well as Alaska, Hawaii, Mississippi, North Dakota, and South Dakota.

Exhibit 21. Percentage of persons aged 18 or older with past year serious mental illness (SMI), by State, 2008–2009

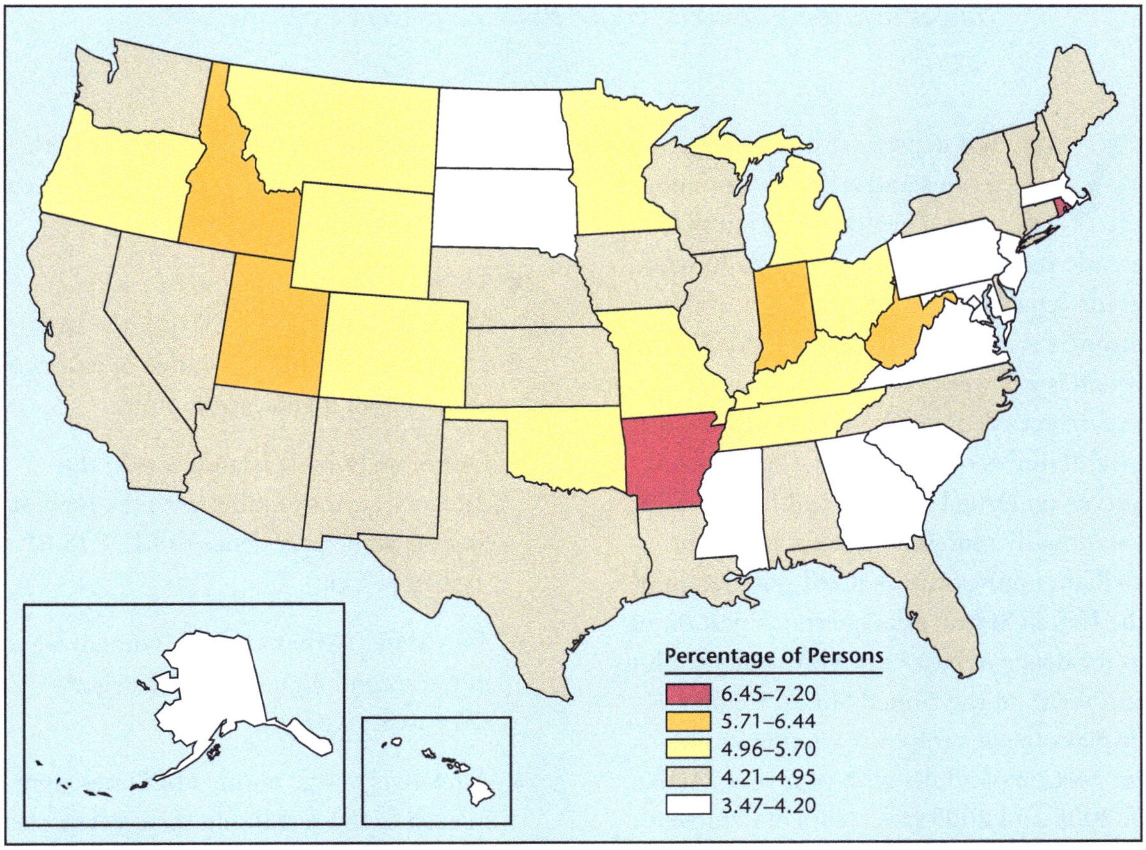

NOTES: Serious mental illness (SMI) is defined as having a diagnosable mental, behavioral, or emotional disorder, other than a substance use disorder, that met the criteria in the *Diagnostic and Statistical Manual of Mental Disorders, Fourth Edition* (DSM-IV) (APA, 1994) and resulted in serious functional impairment. Each State was placed into one of five categories that range from highest to lowest SMI. Category cutoffs were created by taking the difference between the values for the highest and lowest ranked States and then dividing that difference by five. See Table 98 for more details on the constructs in this exhibit.

SOURCE: National Survey on Drug Use and Health, 2008 and 2009, Substance Abuse and Mental Health Services Administration, Office of Applied Studies.

Adults with Past Year Major Depressive Episode

In the 2008–2009 period, State-level prevalence rates of adults with a past year major depressive episode ranged from 5.2 percent to 9.5 percent.

Major depressive disorder is a serious and relatively common mental health condition that can greatly reduce a person's ability to function in life. One important component of this disorder is major depressive episode (MDE), which is a 2-week period over which a person experiences depressed mood. To assess the mental illness of the Nation, the National Survey on Drug Use and Health (NSDUH), a nationally representative survey of the civilian, noninstitutionalized population of the United States, asks questions pertaining to incidence of past year MDE among adults and youth in the United States. Exhibit 22 displays the geographic variation in the proportion of adults with past year MDE in 2008 and 2009 (two years of data were combined to obtain statistically precise estimates). The exhibit shows the following:

- State-specific prevalence of adults with past year MDE ranged from 5.20 percent to 9.46 percent.
- There was little variation in past year MDE across the States. Thus, the five categories have a small range of values of about 0.9 of a percentage point.
- One State (Rhode Island) was in the category corresponding with the highest State-specific prevalence of MDE (8.61 to 9.46 percent).
- Two States (Arkansas and Indiana) were in the second highest MDE category (7.76 to 8.60 percent).
- A relatively large number of States were in each of the remaining three categories; 15 States were in the third highest category (6.91 to 7.75 percent); 21 States were in the fourth highest category (6.05 to 6.90 percent); and 11 States, plus the District of Columbia, were in the lowest category (5.20 to 6.04 percent).

Exhibit 22. Percentage of persons aged 18 or older with past year major depressive episode (MDE), by State, 2008–2009

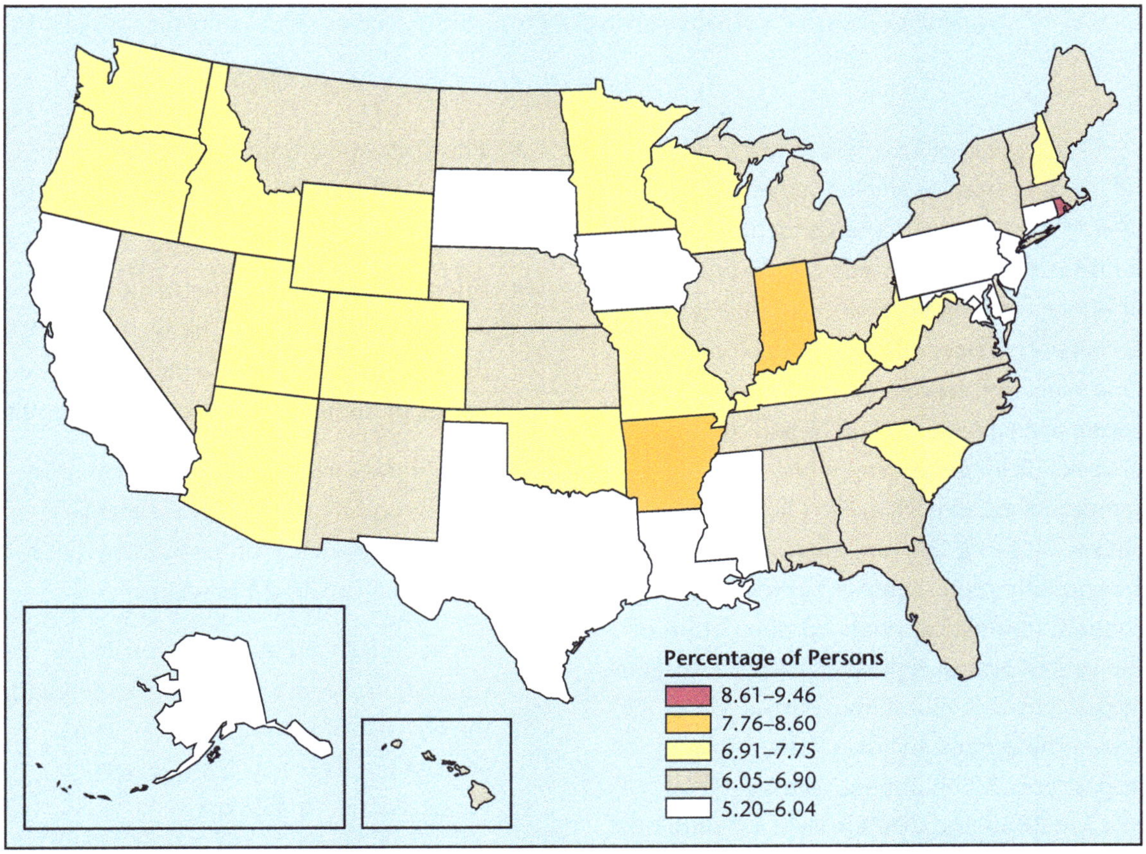

NOTES: Major depressive episode (MDE) is defined as a period of at least 2 weeks when a person experienced a depressed mood or loss of interest or pleasure in daily activities and had a majority of specified depression symptoms. Each State was placed into one of five categories that range from highest to lowest MDE. Category cutoffs were created by taking the difference between the values for the highest and lowest ranked States and then dividing that difference by five. See Table 99 for more details on the constructs in this exhibit.

SOURCE: National Survey on Drug Use and Health, 2008 and 2009, Substance Abuse and Mental Health Services Administration, Office of Applied Studies.

Youth with Past Year Major Depressive Episode

In the 2008–2009 period, State-level prevalence rates of youth with a past year major depressive episode ranged from 6.8 percent to 10.3 percent.

Depression involves many troubling symptoms, including persistent sadness, discouragement, diminished feelings of self-worth, and loss of interest in usual activities. Each year, depression affects millions of adolescents. One aspect of depression is having a major depressive episode (MDE), a period of 2 weeks or longer during which certain symptoms are experienced. The National Survey on Drug Use and Health (NSDUH), a nationally representative survey of the civilian, noninstitutionalized population of the United States, reports State-level estimates of past year MDE among youth. Exhibit 23 shows the geographic dispersion by State of past year MDE among youth aged 12 to 17 in 2008 and 2009 (two years of data were combined to ensure statistically precise estimates). The exhibit shows the following:

- The State-specific prevalence of youth with MDE ranged from 6.75 percent to 10.28 percent.
- There was relatively little variation in past year MDE across the States. Thus, the five categories have a small range of values of about 0.7 of a percentage point.
- One State (Oregon) was in the category corresponding to the highest State-specific prevalence of past year MDE for youth (9.57 to 10.28 percent).
- Seven States were in the lowest MDE category for youth (6.75 to 7.45 percent): the District of Columbia, Maryland, Mississippi, Nevada, New Jersey, Pennsylvania, and Texas.
- The middle three categories of past year MDE prevalence among youth had roughly equivalent numbers (14 to 15) of States in each category.

Exhibit 23. Percentage of persons aged 12 to 17 with a past year major depressive episode (MDE), by State, 2008–2009

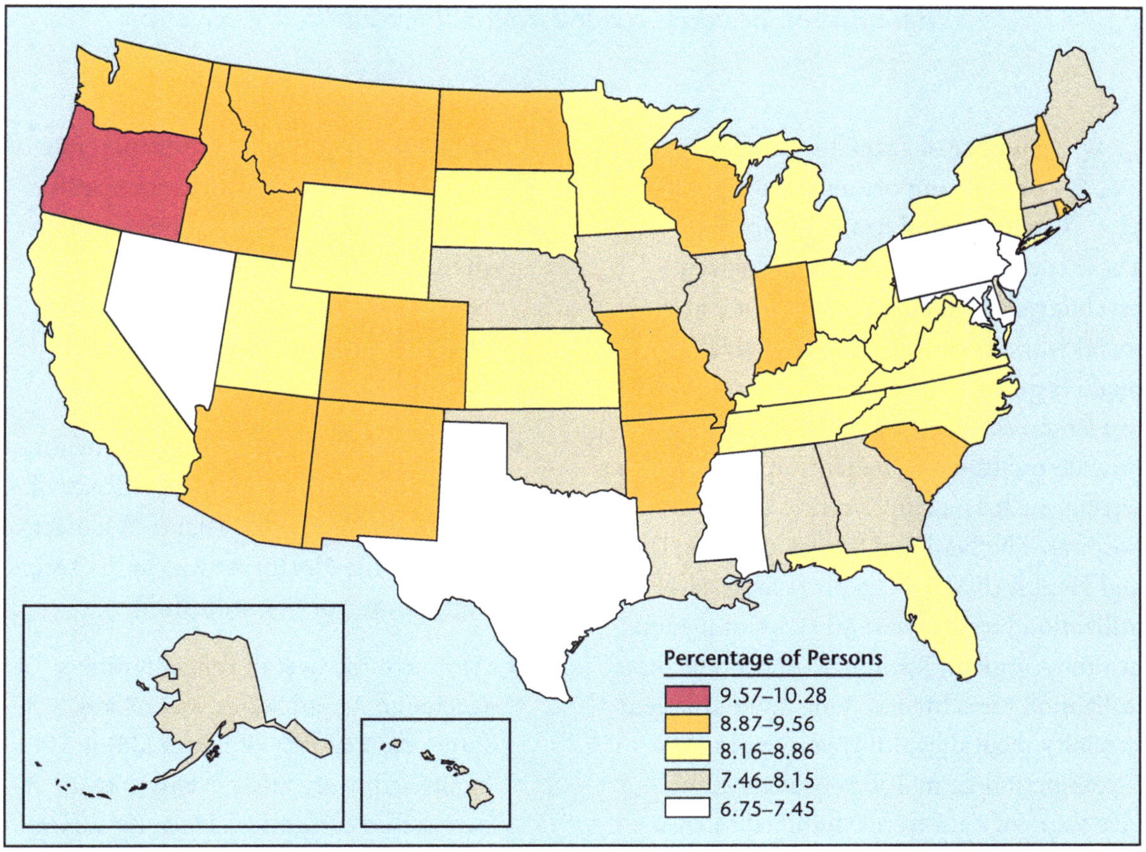

NOTES: Major depressive episode (MDE) is defined as a period of at least 2 weeks when a person experienced a depressed mood or loss of interest or pleasure in daily activities and had a majority of specified depression symptoms. Each State was placed into one of five categories that range from highest to lowest MDE. Category cutoffs were created by taking the difference between the values for the highest and lowest ranked States and then dividing that difference by five. See Table 100 for more details on the constructs in this exhibit.

SOURCE: National Survey on Drug Use and Health, 2008 and 2009, Substance Abuse and Mental Health Services Administration, Office of Applied Studies.

Adults Using Outpatient Specialty Mental Health Treatment

In the 2005–2009 period, State-level utilization rates of outpatient specialty mental health treatment for adults ranged from 3.0 percent to 9.5 percent.

A number of specialist professionals provide important services to people with mental health symptoms. These specialists include psychologists, psychiatrists, therapists, counselors, and social workers. Except for when treatment requires an overnight stay in inpatient or residential settings, specialists typically provide treatment to patients in an outpatient setting, such as a clinic, office, or day hospital. The National Survey on Drug Use and Health (NSDUH) reports State-level utilization rates for several types of mental health treatment. Exhibit 24 shows the State utilization rates for receiving any outpatient specialty mental health treatment in the 5-year period from 2005 through 2009. Five years of data were combined to ensure statistically precise estimates. The exhibit shows the following:

- The highest State-level utilization rate of outpatient mental health treatment for adults was 9.5 percent, which was more than three times the lowest rate of 3.0 percent. This range is high compared with the variation in mental health prevalence across States.
- Two States were in the highest category of treatment utilization: the District of Columbia and Rhode Island. A cluster of States in the Northeast was in the second highest category of utilization.
- Although the overall range in rate of receipt across all States was relatively large, the majority of States (36 of 51 examined) were fairly evenly spread across two categories. Thus, for a large subset of States, the range of estimates was low.
- Twenty-four States were in the second lowest category, for which the utilization rate was between 4.32 and 5.62 percent. These States were spread across the country, excluding the Northeast and much of the Southeast.
- Twelve States were in the lowest category. These States were all in the South and Southeast, plus Hawaii and South Dakota.

Exhibit 24. Percentage of persons aged 18 or older who received outpatient specialty mental health treatment, by State, 2005–2009

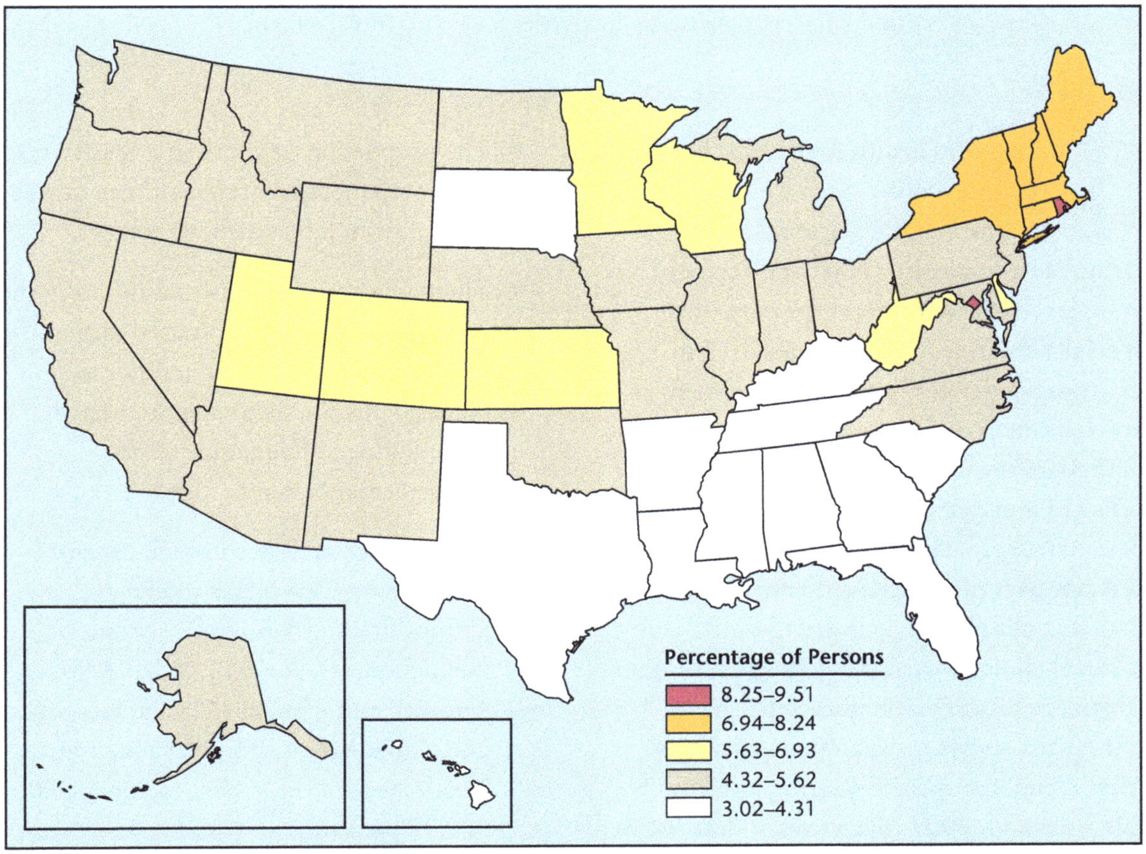

NOTES: Each State was placed into one of five categories that range from highest to lowest proportion of the population who received treatment. Category cutoffs were created by taking the difference between the values for the highest and lowest ranked States and then dividing that difference by five. See Table 103 for more details on the constructs in this exhibit.

SOURCE: National Survey on Drug Use and Health, 2005–2009, Substance Abuse and Mental Health Services Administration, Office of Applied Studies.

Youth Using Outpatient Specialty Mental Health Treatment

In the period 2005–2009, the State-level rates of youth using past outpatient mental health treatment was between 8.0 and 16.9 percent.

The mental health treatment that youth use most often is outpatient treatment. The National Survey on Drug Use and Health (NSDUH) reports State-level utilization rates for outpatient specialty treatment by youth aged 12 to 17. This survey defines outpatient treatment as any treatment or counseling received at an outpatient mental health clinic or center; the office of a private therapist, psychologist, psychiatrist, social worker, or counselor that was not part of a clinic; a doctor's office that was not part of a clinic; an outpatient medical clinic; a partial day hospital or day treatment program; or some other place. Exhibit 25 shows geographic variation of these estimates in the 5-year period from 2005 through 2009 (five years of data were combined to ensure statistically precise estimates). The exhibit shows the following:

- The proportion of youth in a State who used outpatient mental health treatment ranged from 8.00 to 16.90 percent.
- There was relatively little variation in the proportion of youth who used outpatient mental health treatment across the States. Thus, the five categories have a small range of values, of about 1.8 percentage points.
- The number of States in each category was uneven. Two States (New Hampshire and Vermont) were in the highest category (15.12 to 16.90 percent), and 6 States (Alaska, Georgia, Louisiana, Mississippi, Nevada, and Texas) were in the lowest category (8.00 to 9.77 percent).
- Nine States were in the second highest category (13.34 to 15.11 percent), 18 States were in the middle category (11.56 to 13.33 percent), and 16 States were in the second lowest category (9.78 to 11.55 percent).

Exhibit 25. Percentage of persons aged 12 to 17 who received outpatient specialty mental health treatment, by State, 2005–2009

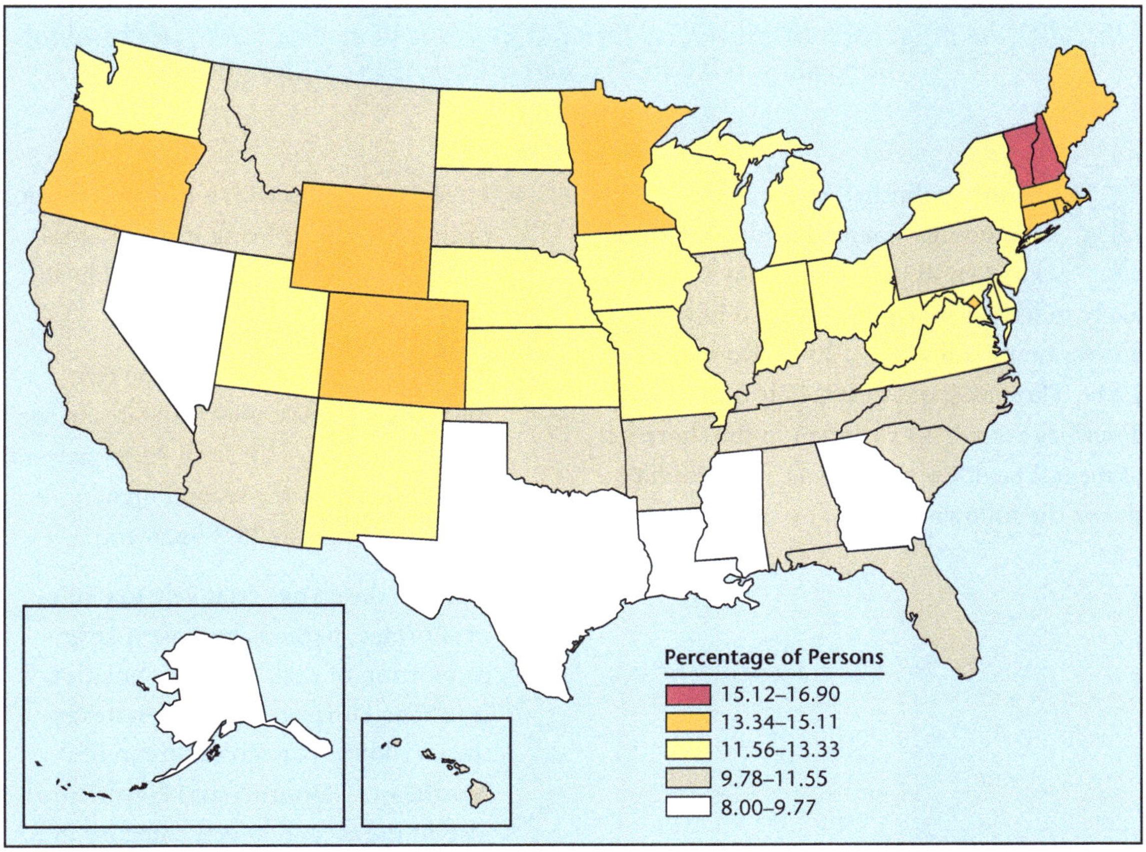

NOTES: Each State was placed into one of five categories that range from highest to lowest proportion of the population who received treatment. Category cutoffs were created by taking the difference between the values for the highest and lowest ranked States and then dividing that difference by five. See Table 106 for more details on the constructs in this exhibit.

SOURCE: National Survey on Drug Use and Health, 2005–2009, Substance Abuse and Mental Health Services Administration, Office of Applied Studies.

Shortage of Mental Health Professionals in the United States, 2006

In 2006, the proportion of individuals facing a shortage of mental health professionals ranged from 0.0 to 31.6 percent across the States.

Recently published research has shown that counties with a relatively large rural population may be more likely to have a shortage of mental health professionals (Ellis et al., 2009; Konrad et al., 2009; Thomas et al., 2009, 2010). Exhibit 26 describes State-level variation in the shortage of mental health professionals. The exhibit shows the following:

- In general, States with a large proportion of the population living in rural areas had a greater shortage of mental health professionals.
- Thirty-three States were in the two highest categories, with 18 States in the highest category (25.28 to 31.59 percent) and 15 States in the second highest category (18.96 to 25.27 percent).
- The Northeast has relatively low rates of shortage, perhaps because a large proportion of each State's population is urban. Thirteen of the 15 States in the two lowest categories are in the Northeast. California and Hawaii are also in the second lowest category (6.32 to 12.63 percent).

Exhibit 26. Estimated shortage of mental health professionals in the United States, by State, 2006

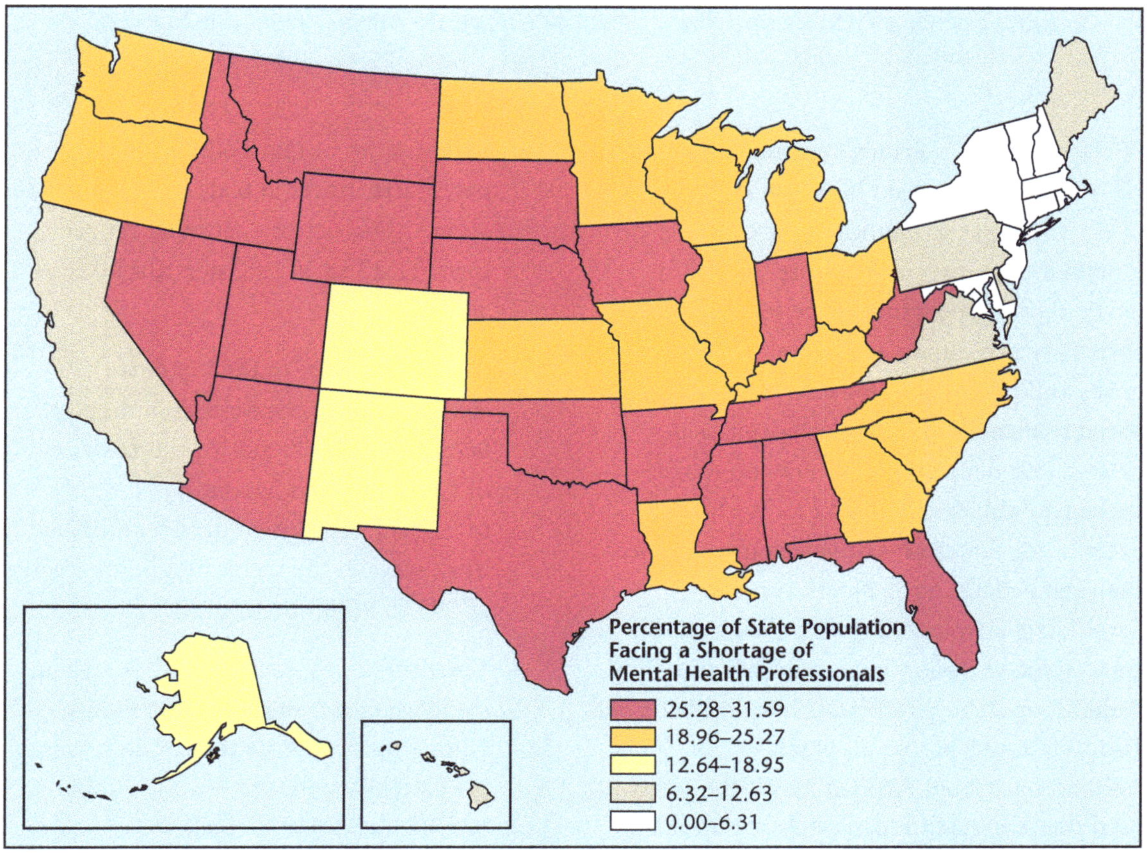

NOTES: Each State was placed into one of five categories that range from highest to lowest proportion of the population facing a shortage of mental health professionals. Category cutoffs were created by taking the difference between the values for the highest and lowest ranked States and then dividing that difference by five. See Table 111 for details of how the shortage measures were developed.

SOURCES: Ellis, A. R., Konrad, T. R., Thomas, K. C., & Morrissey, J. P. (2009). County-level estimates of mental health professional supply in the United States. *Psychiatric Services, 60*(10), 1315–1322.

Konrad, T. R., Ellis, A. R., Thomas, K. C., Holzer, C. E., & Morrissey, J. P. (2009). County-level estimates of need for mental health professionals in the United States. *Psychiatric Services, 60*(10), 1307–1314.

Thomas, K. C., Ellis, A. R., Konrad, T. R., Holzer, C. E., & Morrissey, J. P. (2009). County-level estimates of mental health professional shortage in the United States. *Psychiatric Services, 60*(10), 1323–1328.

Thomas, K. C., Ellis, A. R., & Morrissey, J. P. (2010). Where are the psychiatric physician assistants? Reply. *Psychiatric Services, 61*(1), 95–96.

Non-Federal Inpatient Psychiatric Hospital Beds

In 2007, the number of non-Federal inpatient psychiatric hospital beds (per 100,000 adults) across all States and the District of Columbia ranged from 21.2 to 222.7.

People with serious symptoms of mental illness may need inpatient care. Among the types of facilities that can provide inpatient care, psychiatric hospitals are a particularly important source for specialist care. However, in an era of State budget crises and preferences for community-based treatment, psychiatric hospitals are closing and dedicated beds may no longer be as available (see Table 122). With a few exceptions, States and private sources rather than the Federal government fund most psychiatric hospitals. Exhibit 27 shows the geographic variation in the number of non-Federal inpatient psychiatric hospital beds per 100,000 adults across all States in 2007. The estimates are from Aron et al. (2009), who used the American Hospital Association's annual survey database for fiscal year 2007. That database has been maintained since 1946 to provide estimates on the structure, facilities, and services of the Nation's hospitals and health care providers. The exhibit shows the following:

- The number of non-Federal inpatient psychiatric hospital beds across all States and the District of Columbia ranged from 21.22 to 222.72 per 100,000 adults.
- Two States were in the top two categories with the highest number of beds per 100,000 adults: the District of Columbia and Mississippi (96.84 to 222.72 beds). New Jersey and New York were in the second highest category (77.93 to 96.83 beds).
- Thirteen States, including all States on the West Coast of the United States, among others across the country, were in the category with the fewest number of beds (21.22 to 40.12 beds).

Exhibit 27. Inpatient psychiatric hospital beds in non-Federal hospitals, per 100,000 adults, by State, 2007

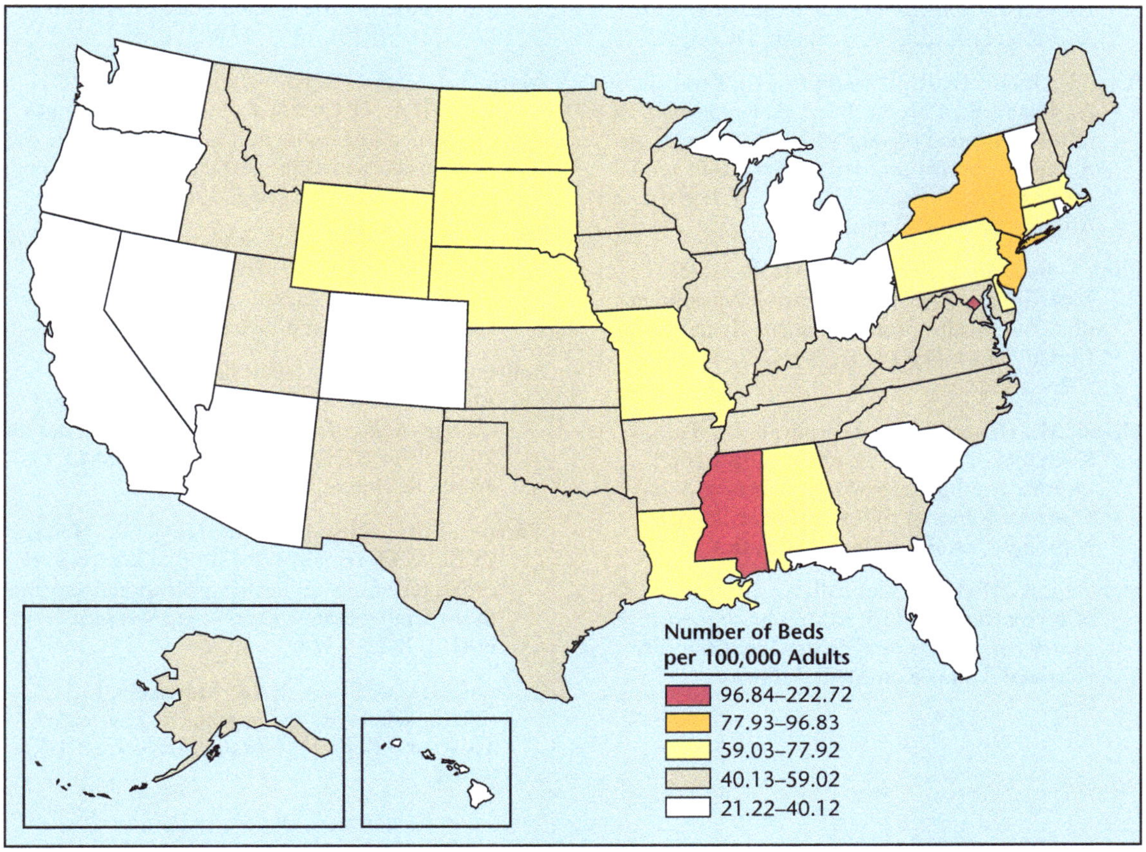

NOTES: Each State was placed into one of five categories that range from highest to lowest number of beds per 100,000 adults. Category cutoffs were created by taking the difference between the values for the highest and lowest ranked States and then dividing that difference by five. Because the District of Columbia had an outlier value, it was excluded from the threshold calculations but included in the exhibit. See Table 115 for more details on the constructs in this exhibit.

SOURCES: Aron, L., Honberg, R., Duckworth, K., Kimball, A., Edgar, E., Carolla, B., ... & Fitzpatrick, M. (2009). *Grading the States 2009: A report on America's health care system for adults with serious mental illness*. Arlington, VA: National Alliance on Mental Illness.

State Single Year of Age and Sex Resident Population Estimates: April 1, 2000 to July 1, 2009, U.S. Census Bureau.

5.3 References

American Psychiatric Association (APA). (1994). *Diagnostic and statistical manual of mental disorders* (4th ed.). Washington, DC: APA.

Aron, L., Honberg, R., Duckworth, K., Kimball, A., Edgar, E., Carolla, B., ... & Fitzpatrick, M. (2009). *Grading the States 2009: A report on America's health care system for adults with serious mental illness.* Arlington, VA: National Alliance on Mental Illness.

Ellis, A. R., Konrad, T. R., Thomas, K. C., & Morrissey, J. P. (2009). County-level estimates of mental health professional supply in the United States. *Psychiatric Services, 60*(10), 1315–1322.

Heron, M., Hoyert, D. L., Murphy, S. L., Xu, J., Kochanek, K. D., & Tejada-Vera, B. (2009). Deaths: Final data for 2006. *National Vital Statistics Reports, 57*(14). Hyattsville, MD: National Center for Health Statistics.

Honberg, R., Diehl, S., Kimball, A., Gruttadaro, D., & Fitzpatrick, M. (2011, March). *State mental health cuts: A national crisis.* Arlington, VA: National Alliance on Mental Illness.

Konrad, T. R., Ellis, A. R., Thomas, K. C., Holzer, C. E., & Morrissey, J. P. (2009). County-level estimates of need for mental health professionals in the United States. *Psychiatric Services, 60*(10), 1307–1314.

Mark, T. L., Levit, K. R., Vandivort-Warren, R., Buck, J. A., & Coffey, R. M. (2011). Changes in US spending on mental health and substance abuse treatment, 1986–2005, and implications for policy. *Health Affairs, 30*(2), 284–292.

National Center for Health Statistics. (2011). *Health, United States, 2010: With special feature on death and dying.* Hyattsville, MD: Centers for Disease Control and Prevention.

Substance Abuse and Mental Health Services Administration (SAMHSA). (2011). *Leading change: A plan for SAMHSA's roles and actions 2011–2014* (DHHS Publication No. SMA 11-4629). Rockville, MD: SAMHSA.

Thomas, K. C., Ellis, A. R., Konrad, T. R., Holzer, C. E., & Morrissey, J. P. (2009). County-level estimates of mental health professional shortage in the United States. *Psychiatric Services, 60*(10), 1323–1328.

Thomas, K. C., Ellis, A. R., & Morrissey, J. P. (2010). Where are the psychiatric physician assistants? Reply. *Psychiatric Services, 61*(1), 95–96.

6. DATA GAPS

Mental Health, United States, 2010 compiles estimates from multiple and disparate data sources to serve as a comprehensive, up-to-date reference source on the Nation's mental health. This section notes the key gaps in the estimates that may help delineate potential areas for further study.

Despite the strengths of the data sources in this volume, they are limited in their ability to serve as a **public health surveillance system** that can track over time the U.S. population's overall mental health status; capacity of, access to, and receipt of treatment; and the degree to which the need for treatment is met. At its best, a robust mental health surveillance system would provide information within subregions (States, counties, or rural/metropolitan area) of the United States. Such data could be used, for example, to track the impact of natural disasters on populations' mental health status, as well as the ongoing mental health of particular subpopulations, such as children and older adults. Public health surveillance systems that exist for other diseases, such as HIV/AIDS, could serve as examples for mental health.

As part of, or in addition to, performing a mental health surveillance function, data are needed over the course of peoples' lives to help monitor **recovery from and the course of mental illness.** Mental health conditions often are long-lasting and have symptoms that greatly impair a person's ability to function in daily life. Studies that compare, for example, depression to other long-lasting and recurrent chronic diseases, such as arthritis, asthma, and diabetes, show that depression is associated with one of the greatest decrements to health (Moussavi, Chatterji, Verdes, Tandon, Patel, & Ustun, 2007). Data are needed to monitor and track mental illness from the onset of a person's symptoms through the period of recovery. Severity, acuity, and functioning are critical determinants of what resources would be needed to address mental health conditions. Thus, data would ideally contain measures of diagnosis or class of disease and reliable indicators of disease severity and acuity and/or a person's functioning. Were such surveillance data available, they could help the Substance Abuse and Mental Health Services Administration (SAMHSA) achieve one of its eight strategic initiatives: to support recovery from mental illness.

Surveillance data are particularly needed for people in **vulnerable subpopulations**, many of which have higher rates of mental health conditions. No reliable national- or subnational-level data are available to monitor the mental health of children, people who are homeless, and military families. Data for other subgroups may be old and infrequently available. This is compounded by the fact that data on people in institutional settings—such as those who are incarcerated or in nursing homes—are often excluded from the sampling frame of large-scale surveys, such as the National Survey on Drug Use and Health (NSDUH). Ongoing efforts, such as a forthcoming survey of inmates, seek to rectify this.

Data on **gaps in treatment capacity** for specific mental health services and supports, as well as for specific population groups (e.g., children, older adults, returning military, persons in jails and prisons, persons with major depression), are important for ensuring that the appropriate mix and level of services and supports are available where they are needed. Assessing gaps in capacity entails collecting data on treatment need and treatment receipt and then combining these data. Over the next several years, health care reform will greatly expand health insurance coverage for many currently uninsured individuals. However, expanding insurance eligibility for individuals with mental illnesses may have limited impact if Federal, State, and local mental health systems are unable to estimate future demand appropriately and identify and expand capacity to eliminate gaps in treatment capacity.

The increase in demand for the mental health treatment system that will arise from health care reform also raises questions about the degree to which the **mental health workforce** can meet the increased demand. No single data source exists for such workforce data. Rather, separate data sets are available for each provider type that vary by the measures they contain, the frequency of data collection, and the methods of data collection. Some use membership surveys (thereby missing nonmembers and nonresponders), whereas others use licensure data (which may include professionals who are working part time or not clinically active). Despite occasional comprehensive analyses that unify these various data sets, there is no program to systematically collect data over time, as would be required for consistent monitoring.

In 2005, Medicaid accounted for 28 percent of all mental health spending (SAMHSA, 2010). The expanded demand for mental health services from health care reform means that Medicaid will take an even greater role in underwriting mental health treatment. However, **national and regularly updated estimates of detailed Medicaid mental health spending** using these data are not available. The preferred data for tracking spending and health care use in Medicaid are on claims filed for reimbursement. The Centers for Medicare & Medicaid Services makes these data available for analysis. But there are several challenges to obtaining reliable estimates from these available data. Chief among them is that most States place the majority of Medicaid beneficiaries in managed care, and reliable estimates on utilization and spending are typically not available for Medicaid managed care beneficiaries.

Another issue concerning obtaining reliable estimates from existing data is that estimates of the amount of **mental health care being provided by nonspecialty physicians**, such as primary care physicians, typically depend on a mental health diagnosis being recorded in the medical chart or billing record. However, analyses have shown that even though primary care physicians write the majority of prescriptions for psychotropic medications, these prescriptions are not accompanied by a mental health diagnosis. Thus, spending on mental health treatment provided by primary care physicians may be underestimated in current estimates. Better data are needed on how to allocate expenditures to primary care physician visits when a psychotropic medication is provided.

Addressing any one of the above data gaps may require considerable coordination among data providers, such as Federal agencies. For example, data on military families' behavioral health needs may require collaboration among SAMHSA, the U.S. Department of Veterans Affairs (VA), and the Department of Defense. The gaps may need to be addressed so that policy and treatment provision can keep pace with the changing face of the U.S. mental health service delivery system. In a period of considerable financial strain on taxpayer-supported services and system-wide health care reform, good data are critical to making informed and timely decisions on the provision of scarce mental health resources.

6.1 References

Moussavi, S., Chatterji, S., Verdes, E., Tandon, A., Patel, V., & Ustun, B. (2007, September). Depression, chronic diseases, and decrements in health: Results from the World Health Surveys. *The Lancet, 370*(9590), 851–858. doi: 10.1016/S0140-6736(07)61415-9

Substance Abuse and Mental Health Services Administration (SAMHSA). (2010). *National expenditures for mental health services and substance abuse treatment, 1986–2005* (DHHS Publication No. SMA 10-4612). Rockville, MD: Center for Mental Health Services and Center for Substance Abuse Treatment, SAMHSA.

This page intentionally left blank

7. TABLES

7.1 Mental Health of the Population

7.1.1 ***U.S. Population: Adults***
Tables 1–7

7.1.2 U.S. Population: Children

7.1.3 Substance Abuse

7.1.4 Suicide

7.1.5 Special Populations

Table 1. Number and percentage of persons aged 18 or older with past year any mental illness (AMI) and serious mental illness (SMI), by selected characteristics, United States, 2009

[Data are based on a survey of a representative sample of the national population]

Characteristic	Past year AMI		Past year SMI	
	Number (1,000s)	Percent	Number (1,000s)	Percent
Total	**45,132**	**19.9**	**10,950**	**4.8**
Age				
18–25	10,068	30.0	2,456	7.3
26–49	22,113	22.3	5,859	5.9
50 or older	12,952	13.7	2,636	2.8
Sex				
Male	17,137	15.6	3,484	3.2
Female	27,995	23.8	7,466	6.4
Hispanic origin and race				
Not Hispanic or Latino	39,593	20.2	9,708	5.0
White	32,158	20.7	8,204	5.3
Black or African American	4,726	17.9	971	3.7
American Indian or Alaska Native	237	21.6	63	5.8
Native Hawaiian or Other Pacific Islander	123	16.7	*	*
Asian	1,556	15.5	203	2.0
Two or more races	793	32.7	235	9.7
Hispanic or Latino	5,539	17.8	1,242	4.0
Poverty status[1]				
Poor	8,291	30.0	2,526	9.1
Near poor	9,837	22.4	2,674	6.1
Not poor	26,567	17.2	5,664	3.7
Health insurance status[2]				
Private coverage	26,689	17.3	5,431	3.5
Medicaid/CHIP[3]	6,417	33.4	2,063	10.7
Other coverage[4]	8,505	16.1	2,098	4.0
No coverage	9,006	24.9	2,336	6.5
Geographic region				
Northeast	8,045	19.1	1,773	4.2
Midwest	10,094	20.3	2,708	5.4
South	16,257	19.6	4,032	4.9
West	10,736	20.5	2,436	4.7
County type				
Large metro	23,595	19.5	5,263	4.4
Small metro	13,935	20.2	3,565	5.2
Nonmetro	7,602	20.3	2,122	5.7
Current employment				
Full-time	19,628	17.1	4,118	3.6
Part-time	7,429	23.4	1,765	5.6
Unemployed	4,083	27.7	1,046	7.1
Other[5]	13,992	21.2	4,021	6.1

See notes on 87.

Table 1 notes

*Estimates are considered unreliable because of low precision.

[1] Poverty status is based on respondent age, family income, family size, and composition using the U.S. Census Bureau's poverty thresholds. "Poor" persons are defined as living in households where the family income is less than 100 percent of the U.S. Census poverty threshold. "Near poor" persons have incomes of 100 percent to less than 200 percent of the poverty threshold. "Not poor" persons have incomes that are 200 percent of the poverty threshold or greater.

[2] Respondents could indicate multiple types of health insurance; thus, these response categories are not mutually exclusive.

[3] CHIP is the Children's Health Insurance Program (formerly State Children's Health Insurance Program [SCHIP]). Individuals aged 19 or younger are eligible for this plan.

[4] Other health insurance is defined as having Medicare, Civilian Health and Medical Program of the Uniformed Services (CHAMPUS), TRICARE, Civilian Health and Medical Program of the Department of Veterans Affairs (CHAMPVA), Veterans Administration (VA), military health care, or any other type of health insurance.

[5] The other employment category includes retired persons, disabled persons, homemakers, students, or other persons not in the labor force.

NOTES: The National Survey on Drug Use and Health (NSDUH) is a nationally representative survey of the civilian, noninstitutionalized population of the United States aged 12 or older. The survey interviews approximately 67,500 persons each year.

Mental illness among persons aged 18 or older is defined according to two dimensions: (1) the presence of a diagnosable mental, behavioral, or emotional disorder in the past year (excluding developmental and substance use disorders) of sufficient duration to meet diagnostic criteria specified in the *Diagnostic and Statistical Manual of Mental Disorders, Fourth Edition* (DSM-IV) (APA, 1994); and (2) the level of interference with or limitation of one or more major life activities resulting from a disorder (functional impairment). Adult NSDUH respondents' mental illness was determined based on modeling their responses to questions on distress (K6 scale) and impairment (truncated version of the World Health Organization Disability Assessment Schedule). Serious mental illness (SMI) among adults is defined as persons aged 18 or older who currently or at any time in the past year had a diagnosable mental, behavioral, or emotional disorder as defined above and resulting in substantial impairment in carrying out major life activities, based on Global Assessment of Functioning (GAF) scores of 50 or less. Any mental illness (AMI) among adults is defined as persons aged 18 or older who currently or at any time in the past year had a diagnosable mental, behavioral, or emotional disorder as defined above, regardless of the level of impairment in carrying out major life activities. AMI includes persons with mental illness having serious, moderate, or mild functional impairment; SMI is a subset of the AMI group.

SOURCE: National Survey on Drug Use and Health, 2009, Substance Abuse and Mental Health Services Administration, Office of Applied Studies.

Table 2. Percentage of persons aged 18 or older with a mental disorder, by severity, United States, 2001–2002

[Data are based on household interviews of a sample of the national population]

Disorder by disorder group	12-month prevalence (percent)	Serious severity[1] (percent)	Moderate severity[2] (percent)	Mild severity[3] (percent)
Anxiety disorder				
Panic disorder	2.7	42.6	36.7	20.7
Generalized anxiety disorder	2.7	35.7	46.5	17.7
Social phobia	7.1	37.7	44.5	17.7
Specific phobia	9.1	24.2	38.6	37.2
Agoraphobia without panic	0.9	42.9	36.4	20.7
Posttraumatic stress disorder	3.6	42.7	32.7	24.7
Adult separation anxiety disorder	1.9	51.7	31.6	16.6
Any anxiety disorder	19.0	27.3	40.0	32.6
Mood disorder				
Dysthymia	1.5	55.5	36.0	8.4
Major depressive disorder	6.8	41.5	47.5	11.0
Bipolar disorder	2.8	56.6	38.9	4.5
Any mood disorder	9.7	46.0	44.4	9.6
Impulse disorder				
Oppositional defiant disorder	1.0	60.7	20.0	19.3
Conduct disorder	1.0	34.7	20.1	45.2
Attention deficit hyperactivity disorder	4.1	37.8	26.5	35.8
Intermittent explosive disorder	4.1	32.9	44.6	22.5
Any impulse control disorder	10.5	32.9	36.8	30.3
Substance disorder				
Alcohol abuse	3.1	50.6	16.7	32.7
Alcohol dependence	1.3	98.3	1.7	0.0
Drug abuse	1.3	47.6	18.0	34.5
Drug dependence	0.4	100.0	0.0	0.0
Any substance use disorder	3.8	47.9	18.8	33.3
Any disorder				
Any	26.9	25.5	39.7	34.7
1 disorder	14.2	8.0	38.8	53.2
2 disorders	6.2	26.9	48.5	24.5
3+ disorders	6.6	61.6	33.4	5.0

[1] Twelve-month cases were classified as "serious severity" if they had any of the following: a suicide attempt in the past 12 months, work disability or substantial limitation due to a mental or substance disorder, positive screen results for nonaffective psychosis, bipolar I or II disorder, substance dependence with serious role impairment (as defined by disorder-specific impairment questions), an impulse control disorder with repeated serious violence, or any disorder that resulted in 30 or more days out of role in the year.

[2] Cases were defined as "moderate severity" if they had any of the following: suicide gesture, plan, or ideation; substance dependence without serious role impairment; at least moderate work limitation due to a mental or substance disorder; or any disorder with at least moderate role impairment in two or more domains of the Sheehan Disability Scale.

[3] All other cases meeting the criteria for a 12-month disorder were defined as "mild severity."

Table 2 notes *(continued)*

NOTES: The National Comorbidity Survey Replication is a nationally representative household survey of 9,282 English speakers aged 18 or older in the United States.

Percentages in the three severity columns are reported as proportions of all cases meeting the criteria for a 12-month mental disorder and sum to 100 percent across each row. Table originally published in Substance Abuse and Mental Health Services Administration (SAMHSA). (2010). *Mental Health, United States, 2008* (DHHS Publication No. SMA 10-4590). Rockville, MD: Center for Mental Health Services, SAMHSA.

Diagnostic and Statistical Manual of Mental Disorders, Fourth Edition (DSM-IV) (APA, 1994) diagnoses were based on the *World Mental Health Composite International Diagnostic Interview* (Kessler & Ustun, 2004), a fully structured lay interview that generates diagnoses according to *International Classification of Diseases, 10th Revision* (ICD-10) (WHO, 1991) and DSM-IV criteria. DSM-IV criteria are used herein. Twelve-month disorders considered in this study included anxiety disorders (panic disorder, generalized anxiety disorder, social phobia, specific phobia, agoraphobia without panic disorder, posttraumatic stress disorder, separation anxiety disorder), mood disorders (dysthymia, major depressive disorder, bipolar disorder I or II), impulse control disorders (oppositional defiant disorder, conduct disorder, attention deficit hyperactivity disorder, intermittent explosive disorder), and substance use disorders (alcohol and drug abuse and dependence). See Kessler et al. (2005) for additional detail on the disorders presented.

SOURCES: National Comorbidity Survey Replication, 2001/2002, National Institute of Mental Health.

Kessler, R. C., Chiu, W. T., Demler, O., Merikangas, K. R., & Walters, E. E. (2005). Prevalence, severity, and comorbidity of 12-month DSM-IV disorders in the National Comorbidity Survey Replication. *Archives of General Psychiatry, 62*(6), 617–627.

Table 3. Number and percentage of persons aged 18 or older with a past year major depressive episode (MDE), by selected characteristics, United States, 2009

[Data are based on a survey of a representative sample of the national population]

Characteristic	Number (1,000s)	Percent
Total	**14,766**	**6.5**
Age		
18–25	2,656	8.0
26–49	7,514	7.6
50 or older	4,595	4.9
Sex		
Male	5,209	4.8
Female	9,557	8.2
Hispanic origin and race		
Not Hispanic or Latino	12,960	6.7
White	10,854	7.0
Black or African American	1,424	5.4
American Indian or Alaska Native	70	6.5
Native Hawaiian or Other Pacific Islander	*	*
Asian	320	3.2
Two or more races	251	10.4
Hispanic or Latino	1,805	5.9
Poverty status[1]		
Poor	2,840	10.4
Near poor	3,236	7.4
Not poor	8,580	5.6
Health insurance status[2]		
Private coverage	8,195	5.3
Medicaid/CHIP[3]	2,289	12.1
Other coverage[4]	3,027	5.8
No coverage	2,896	8.1
Geographic region		
Northeast	2,610	6.3
Midwest	3,353	6.8
South	5,400	6.6
West	3,403	6.5
County type		
Large metro	7,649	6.4
Small metro	4,538	6.6
Nonmetro	2,579	7.0
Current employment		
Full-time	6,130	5.4
Part-time	2,306	7.3
Unemployed	1,427	9.7
Other[5]	4,902	7.5

See notes on 91.

Table 3 notes

*Estimates are considered unreliable because of low precision.

[1] Poverty status is based on respondent age, family income, family size, and composition using the U.S. Census Bureau's poverty thresholds. "Poor" persons are defined as living in households where the family income is less than 100 percent of the U.S. Census poverty threshold. "Near poor" persons have incomes of 100 percent to less than 200 percent of the poverty threshold. "Not poor" persons have incomes that are 200 percent of the poverty threshold or greater.

[2] Respondents could indicate multiple types of health insurance; thus, these response categories are not mutually exclusive.

[3] CHIP is the Children's Health Insurance Program (formerly State Children's Health Insurance Program [SCHIP]). Individuals aged 19 or younger are eligible for this plan.

[4] Other health insurance is defined as having Medicare, Civilian Health and Medical Program of the Uniformed Services (CHAMPUS), TRICARE, Civilian Health and Medical Program of the Department of Veterans Affairs (CHAMPVA), Veterans Administration (VA), military health care, or any other type of health insurance.

[5] The other employment category includes retired persons, disabled persons, homemakers, students, or other persons not in the labor force.

NOTES: The National Survey on Drug Use and Health is a nationally representative survey of the civilian, noninstitutionalized population of the United States aged 12 or older. The survey interviews approximately 67,500 persons each year.

Major depressive episode (MDE) is defined as a period of at least 2 weeks when a person experienced a depressed mood or loss of interest or pleasure in daily activities and had a majority of specified depression symptoms. According to the *Diagnostic and Statistical Manual of Mental Disorders, Fourth Edition* (DSM-IV) (APA, 1994), two or more MDEs are necessary to meet the criteria for recurrent major depressive disorder.

SOURCE: National Survey on Drug Use and Health, 2009, Substance Abuse and Mental Health Services Administration, Office of Applied Studies.

Table 4. Number and percentage of persons aged 18 or older with a past year major depressive episode (MDE), by age, sex, and Hispanic origin and race, United States, 2005–2009

[Data are based on a survey of a representative sample of the national population]

Characteristic	2005		2006		2007		2008		2009	
	Number (1,000s)	Percent	Number (1,000s)	Percent	Number (1,000s)	Percent	Number (1,000s)	Percent	Number (1,000s)	Percent
Total	**15,772**	**7.3**	**15,796**	**7.2**	**16,462**	**7.5**	**14,297**	**6.4**	**14,766**	**6.5**
Age										
18–25	3,135	9.7	2,920	9.0	2,891	8.9	2,862	8.7	2,656	8.0
26–49	8,358	8.4	8,482	8.5	8,417	8.5	7,302	7.4	7,514	7.6
50 or older	4,280	5.1	4,393	5.1	5,155	5.8	4,133	4.5	4,595	4.9
Sex										
Male	5,397	5.2	5,604	5.3	5,607	5.3	4,949	4.6	5,209	4.8
Female	10,375	9.3	10,191	9.0	10,855	9.5	9,348	8.1	9,557	8.2
Hispanic origin and race										
Not Hispanic or Latino	13,854	7.3	14,255	7.5	14,611	7.6	12,734	6.6	12,960	6.7
White	11,534	7.6	11,909	7.8	12,355	8.1	10,712	7.0	10,854	7.0
Black or African American	1,585	6.5	1,579	6.3	1,520	6.1	1,236	4.9	1,424	5.4
American Indian or Alaska Native	104	9.4	132	12.1	101	9.2	67	4.9	70	6.5
Native Hawaiian or Other Pacific Islander	*	*	48	5.8	*	*	*	*	*	*
Asian	324	3.6	273	3.0	275	2.9	345	3.6	320	3.2
Two or more races	221	10.1	315	14.3	278	12.1	294	12.7	251	10.4
Hispanic or Latino	1,918	7.0	1,541	5.4	1,851	6.3	1,564	5.2	1,805	5.9

*Estimates are considered unreliable because of low precision.

NOTES: The National Survey on Drug Use and Health is a nationally representative survey of the civilian, noninstitutionalized population of the United States aged 12 or older. The survey interviews approximately 67,500 persons each year.

Major depressive episode (MDE) is defined as a period of at least 2 weeks when a person experienced a depressed mood or loss of interest or pleasure in daily activities and had a majority of specified depression symptoms. According to the *Diagnostic and Statistical Manual of Mental Disorders, Fourth Edition* (DSM-IV) (APA, 1994), two or more MDEs are necessary to meet the criteria for recurrent major depressive disorder.

SOURCE: National Survey on Drug Use and Health, 2005–2009, Substance Abuse and Mental Health Services Administration, Office of Applied Studies.

Table 5. Number and percentage of persons aged 18 or older with past 30-day serious psychological distress (SPD), by selected characteristics, United States, 2009

[Data are based on household interviews of a representative sample of the national population]

Characteristic	Number (1,000s)	Percent
Total[1]	**7,357**	**3.2**
Age		
18–44	3,609	3.3
45–64	2,965	3.7
65 or older	783	2.1
Sex		
Male	3,038	2.8
Female	4,319	3.7
Hispanic origin and race		
White-alone, non-Hispanic	4,917	3.1
Black-alone, non-Hispanic	1,123	4.2
Hispanic[2]	997	3.2
Other, non-Hispanic and multiple races	319	2.5
Poverty status		
Poor	2,399	8.4
Near poor	1,971	4.7
Not poor	2,987	1.9
Health insurance status (persons younger than age 65)[3]		
Private coverage[4]	2,144	3.5
Public	2,265	1.7
Other coverage	30	11.1
Uninsured	2,082	5.2
Health insurance status (persons aged 65 or older)[3]		
Private coverage[4]	364	1.5
Public, besides Medicare	162	6.6
Medicare only	252	2.2
Other coverage	0	0.0
Uninsured	6	2.0
Geographic region		
Northeast	1,182	3.0
Midwest	1,928	3.5
South	2,921	3.6
West	1,326	2.6

[1] Estimates are total, not age-adjusted.

[2] Persons of Hispanic or Latino origin may be of any race or combination of races.

[3] Health insurance status is unknown for approximately 0.50 percent of the adult population younger than age 65 and approximately 0.15 percent of the adult population aged 65 or older.

[4] The private category includes people with both private and public insurance.

Table 5 notes *(continued)*

NOTES: The National Health Interview Survey provides national estimates for a broad range of health measures for the U.S. civilian noninstitutionalized population. The interviewed sample for 2009 consisted of 33,856 households, which yielded 88,446 persons in 34,640 families.

Six psychological distress questions are included in the National Health Interview Survey's Sample Adult Core component. These questions ask how often a respondent experienced certain symptoms of psychological distress during the past 30 days. The response codes (0 to 4) of the six items for each person are summed to yield a scale ranging from 0 to 24. A value of 13 or more for this scale is used here to define serious psychological distress.

SOURCE: National Health Interview Survey, 2009, Centers for Disease Control and Prevention, National Center for Health Statistics.

Table 6. Number and percentage of persons aged 18 or older with past 30-day serious psychological distress (SPD), by age, sex, and Hispanic origin and race, United States, 2004–2009

[Data are based on household interviews of a representative sample of the national population]

Characteristic	2004		2005		2006		2007		2008		2009	
	Number (1,000s)	Percent	Number (1,000s)	Percent	Number (1,000s)	Percent	Number (1,000s)	Percent	Number (1,000s)	Percent	Number (1,000s)	Percent
Total[1]	**6,578**	**3.1**	**6,469**	**3.0**	**6,575**	**3.0**	**6,047**	**2.7**	**7,061**	**3.1**	**7,357**	**3.2**
Age												
18–44	3,116	2.8	3,027	2.7	2,878	2.6	2,687	2.4	3,165	2.9	3,609	3.3
45–64	2,686	3.8	2,516	3.5	2,972	4.0	2,606	3.4	2,876	3.7	2,965	3.7
65 or older	776	2.2	927	2.7	724	2.0	755	2.1	1,020	2.7	783	2.1
Sex												
Male	2,434	2.4	2,361	2.3	2,569	2.4	2,084	1.9	2,807	2.6	3,038	2.8
Female	4,144	3.7	4,108	3.6	4,006	3.5	3,964	3.4	4,254	3.7	4,319	3.7
Hispanic origin and race[2]												
White-alone, non-Hispanic	4,669	3.0	4,388	2.8	4,493	2.9	4,090	2.6	5,013	3.2	4,917	3.1
Black-alone, non-Hispanic	836	3.4	910	3.7	959	3.7	794	3.0	926	3.5	1,123	4.2
Hispanic[3]	889	3.3	948	3.4	762	2.7	959	3.2	1,051	3.4	997	3.2

[1] Estimates are total, not age-adjusted.

[2] Estimates for other non-Hispanic and multiple races are not currently available.

[3] Persons of Hispanic or Latino origin may be of any race or combination of races.

NOTES: The National Health Interview Survey provides national estimates for a broad range of health measures for the U.S. civilian noninstitutionalized population. The interviewed sample for 2009 consisted of 33,856 households, which yielded 88,446 persons in 34,640 families.

Six psychological distress questions are included in the National Health Interview Survey's Sample Adult Core component. These questions ask how often a respondent experienced certain symptoms of psychological distress during the past 30 days. The response codes (0 to 4) of the six items for each person are summed to yield a scale ranging from 0 to 24. A value of 13 or more for this scale is used here to define serious psychological distress.

SOURCE: National Health Interview Survey, 2004–2009, Centers for Disease Control and Prevention, National Center for Health Statistics.

Table 7. Number and percentage of persons aged 18 or older with past 30-day serious psychological distress (SPD), by selected physical disorders, United States, 2009

[Data are based on household interviews of a representative sample of the national population]

Physical disorder	Number (1,000s)	Percent
Current asthma[1]	1,550	21.2
Lifetime diabetes[2]	1,220	17.2
Lifetime total heart disease[3]	1,825	24.9
Lifetime arthritic diagnosis[4]	3,218	43.8
History of any cancer[5]	924	12.6

[1] Respondents were asked in two separate questions if they had ever been told by a doctor or other health professional that they had asthma. Respondents who had been told they had asthma were asked if they still had asthma.

[2] Respondents were asked if they had ever been told by a doctor or other health professional that they had diabetes (or sugar diabetes; female respondents were instructed to exclude pregnancy-related diabetes). Responses from persons who said they had "borderline" diabetes were treated as unknown with respect to diabetes.

[3] Heart disease includes coronary heart disease, angina pectoris, heart attack, or any other heart condition or disease.

[4] Respondents were asked if they had ever been told by a doctor or other health professional that they had some form of arthritis, rheumatoid arthritis, gout, lupus, or fibromyalgia. Respondents who answered yes were classified as having an arthritis diagnosis.

[5] Respondents were asked if they had ever been told by a doctor or other health professional that they had a cancer or a malignancy of any kind. Respondents who answered yes were asked to name the kind of cancer they had.

NOTES: The National Health Interview Survey provides national estimates for a broad range of health measures for the U.S. civilian noninstitutionalized population. The interviewed sample for 2009 consisted of 33,856 households, which yielded 88,446 persons in 34,640 families.

Six psychological distress questions are included in the National Health Interview Survey's Sample Adult Core component. These questions ask how often a respondent experienced certain symptoms of psychological distress during the past 30 days. The response codes (0 to 4) of the six items for each person are summed to yield a scale ranging from 0 to 24. A value of 13 or more for this scale is used here to define serious psychological distress.

SOURCE: National Health Interview Survey, 2009, Centers for Disease Control and Prevention, National Center for Health Statistics.

7. TABLES

Table 8. Percentage of persons aged 4 to 17 with reported emotional and behavioral difficulties, by level of severity and selected characteristics, United States, 2009

[Data are based on household interviews of a sample of the civilian noninstitutionalized population]

Characteristic	Definite or severe difficulties (percent)	Minor difficulties (percent)	No difficulties (percent)
Age and sex			
Total ages 4–17	5.3	13.7	81.0
Ages 4–7	3.2	11.6	85.3
Ages 8–10	6.3	15.6	78.1
Ages 11–14	5.6	14.3	80.0
Ages 15–17	6.5	14.0	79.5
Males ages 4–17	6.6	16.3	77.1
Ages 4–7	4.1	13.8	82.2
Ages 8–10	8.2	19.5	72.4
Ages 11–14	7.1	17.0	75.9
Ages 15–17	7.7	15.9	76.4
Females ages 4–17	3.9	11.0	85.1
Ages 4–7	2.1	9.1	88.8
Ages 8–10	4.4	11.7	83.9
Ages 11–14	4.1	11.5	84.4
Ages 15–17	5.3	12.0	82.7
Hispanic origin and race			
White-alone, non-Hispanic	5.5	13.9	80.7
Black-alone, non-Hispanic	7.0	17.6	75.4
Hispanic[1]	4.1	12.0	83.9
Other, non-Hispanic and multiple races	2.5	8.4	89.0
Poverty status[2]			
Poor	8.2	18.1	73.7
Near poor	6.5	14.6	79.0
Not poor	3.8	11.9	84.4

[1] Persons of Hispanic or Latino origin may be of any race or combination of races.

[2] Poverty status is based on respondent age, family income, family size, and composition using the U.S. Census Bureau's poverty thresholds. "Poor" persons are defined as living in households where the family income is less than 100 percent of the U.S. Census poverty threshold. "Near poor" persons have incomes of 100 percent to less than 200 percent of the poverty threshold. "Not poor" persons have incomes that are 200 percent of the poverty threshold or greater.

NOTES: The National Health Interview Survey provides national estimates for a broad range of health measures for the U.S. civilian noninstitutionalized population. The interviewed sample for 2009 consisted of 33,856 households, which yielded 88,446 persons in 34,640 families. A total of 12,404 children aged 17 or younger were eligible for the Sample Child Questionnaire. Children with emotional and behavioral difficulties are defined as those whose parent responded "yes, definite" or "yes, severe" to the following question on the Strengths and Difficulties Questionnaire: "Overall, do you think that (child) has any difficulties in one or more of the following areas: emotions, concentration, behavior, or being able to get along with other people?" Response choices were (1) no; (2) yes, minor difficulties; (3) yes, definite difficulties; and (4) yes, severe difficulties.

SOURCES: National Health Interview Survey, 2009, Centers for Disease Control and Prevention, National Center for Health Statistics.

Goodman, R. (1999). The extended version of the Strengths and Difficulties Questionnaire as a guide to child psychiatric caseness and consequent burden. *Journal of Child Psychology and Psychiatry, 40*(5), 791–799.

. Percentage of persons aged 8 to 15 with a past year mental disorder with or without severe impairment, United 2001–2004

ased on evaluations of a sample of the civilian noninstitutionalized population]

M-IV–defined disorder	Disorder without severe impairment					Disorder with severe impairment[1]				
	Total (percent)	Male (percent)	Female (percent)	Aged 8 to 11 (percent)	Aged 12 to 15 (percent)	Total (percent)	Male (percent)	Female (percent)	Aged 8 to 11 (percent)	Age 12 to (perc
deficit hyperactivity disorder	8.6	11.6	5.4	9.9	7.4	7.8	10.8	4.7	9.1	6.
isorder	2.1	2.3	1.9	1.5	2.7	1.7	2.0	1.4	1.2	2.
isorder	0.7	0.4	0.9	0.4	0.8	0.4	0.4	0.4	0.3	0.
ed anxiety	0.3	0.3	0.4	0.1	0.7	0.2	0.3	0.1	0.0	0.
order	0.4	0.2	0.6	0.4	0.4	0.3	0.2	0.4	0.3	0.
order	0.1	0.1	0.2	0.1	0.2	0.0	0.0	0.1	0.0	0.1
order	3.7	2.5	4.9	2.5	4.8	2.9	1.7	4.1	1.8	3.
depression	2.7	1.8	3.7	1.6	3.8	2.4	1.6	3.2	1.4	3.
ymia	1.0	0.7	1.2	0.8	1.1	0.5	0.1	0.9	0.4	0.
ove	13.1	14.5	11.6	12.8	13.4	11.3	13.0	9.4	11.0	11.

er with severe impairment indicates two intermediate ratings or one severe rating on the six impairment questions regarding personal distress and social (at ho peers) or academic difficulties.

Table 9 notes *(continued)*

NOTES: The National Health and Nutrition Examination Survey is a nationally representative probability sample of noninstitutionalized U.S. civilians. The sample shown includes 3,024 children aged 8 to 15 who were evaluated in person at mobile examination survey centers.

Diagnostic categories are not mutually exclusive. Disorder without impairment is the total prevalence for the population (i.e., the 12-month prevalence rate of attention deficit hyperactivity disorder with or without impairment is 8.6 percent). The notes and source for this table have been reordered at the express wish of the copyright holding organization. Mental disorders were assessed using the National Institute of Mental Health Diagnostic Interview Schedule for Children (DISC), Version IV, a structured diagnostic interview administered by lay interviewers to assess *Diagnostic and Statistical Manual of Mental Disorders, Fourth Edition* (DSM-IV) (APA, 1994) diagnostic criteria for mental disorders in children and adolescents. Diagnostic modules within DISC include an assessment of both symptoms and functional impairment. Six impairment items assess personal distress and social (at home or with peers) or academic difficulties within each diagnostic module; these items are rated from "mild" to "severe." This study assessed only certain childhood mental disorders by parent or youth report. Modules for generalized anxiety disorder (GAD), panic disorder, eating disorders (anorexia nervosa and bulimia nervosa), and major depressive disorder (MDD)/dysthymic disorder (DD) were administered to youth; and modules for MDD/DD, eating disorders, attention deficit hyperactivity disorder (ADHD), and conduct disorder were administered to the primary caretakers. The diagnoses of GAD and panic disorder were based on youth reports alone, the diagnoses of ADHD and conduct disorder were based on parent reports alone, and the diagnoses of MDD/DD and eating disorders were based on either youth or parent report. The prevalence of mental disorders found in this study may be underestimated due to study methods. This study did not assess two common childhood anxiety disorders: separation anxiety and phobias. And, as described above, certain diagnoses were assessed by either youth or parent report, counter to methods used in previous research. See Merikangas et al. (2010) for additional details on the disorders presented.

At the request of the publisher, Table 9a is the original, published form of the table, and the source reference is listed directly below the table.

SOURCE: Merikangas, K. R., He, J.-P., Brody, D., Fisher, P. W., Bourdon, K., & Koretz, D. S. (2010). Prevalence and treatment of mental disorders among US children in the 2001–2004 NHANES. *Pediatrics, 125*(1), 75–81. *Reproduced with permission from Pediatrics, 125*(1), 75–81, Copyright © 2010 by the American Academy of Pediatrics.

a. Percentage of persons aged 8 to 15 with a 12-month mental disorder with or without severe impairment, Uni
2001–2004: Original exhibit

title: Prevalence of 12-month, DSM-IV-defined disorders according to gender and age in US children 8 to 15 years of a

-IV–Defined isorder	Prevalence, Estimate ± SE, %									
	Disorder Without Impairment					Disorder With Severe Impairment (Level D)[a]				
	Gender		Age		Total (*N* = 3,042)	Gender		Age		Total (*N* = 3,04
	Male (*N* = 1,492)	Female (*N* = 1,550)	8–11 y (*N* = 1,148)	12–15 y (*N* = 1,894)		Male (*N* = 1,492)	Female (*N* = 1,550)	8–11 y (*N* = 1,148)	12–15 y (*N* = 1,894)	
	11.6 ± 1.0	5.4 ± 0.6	9.9 ± 1.0	7.4 ± 1.0	8.6 ± 0.7	10.8 ± 0.9	4.7 ± 0.7	9.1 ± 1.0	6.7 ± 0.8	7.8 ± 0.
	$X_1^2 = 45.18$, $P < .001$		$X_1^2 = 3.23$, $P = .082$			$X_1^2 = 46.86$, $P < .001$		$X_1^2 = 4.29$, $P = .047$		
ion deficit	5.4 ± 0.9	3.1 ± 0.5	4.6 ± 0.8	4.0 ± 0.8	4.3 ± 0.6					
	$X_1^2 = 5.59$, $P = .025$		$X_1^2 = 0.43$, $P = .517$							
activity	2.8 ± 0.7	1.2 ± 0.3	2.8 ± 0.7	1.3 ± 0.3	2.0 ± 0.4					
	$X_1^2 = 4.56$, $P = .041$		$X_1^2 = 3.85$, $P = .059$							
ned	3.4 ± 0.4	1.1 ± 0.2	2.4 ± 0.5	2.1 ± 0.3	2.2 ± 0.2					
	$X_1^2 = 20.99$, $P =< .001$		$X_1^2 = 0.27$, $P = .610$							
isorder	2.3 ± 0.3	1.9 ± 0.5	1.5 ± 0.3	2.7 ± 0.5	2.1 ± 0.3	2.0 ± 0.3	1.4 ± 0.4	1.2 ± 0.2	2.2 ± 0.5	1.7 ± 0.
	$X_1^2 = 0.71$, $P = .406$		$X_1^2 = 5.76$, $P = .023$			$X_1^2 = 1.26$, $P = .271$		$X_1^2 = 3.90$, $P = .058$		
sorder	0.4 ± 0.2	0.9 ± 0.3	0.4 ± 0.2	0.8 ± 0.3	0.7 ± 0.2	0.4 ± 0.2	0.4 ± 0.2	0.3 ± 0.2	0.5 ± 0.2	0.4 ± 0.
	$X_1^2 = 1.74$, $P = .197$		$X_1^2 = 1.04$, $P = .317$			$X_1^2 = 0.004$, $P = .948$		$X_1^2 = 0.20$, $P = .656$		
ed anxiety	0.3 ± 0.2	0.4 ± 0.2	0.1 ± 0.1	0.7 ± 0.3	0.3 ± 0.1	0.3 ± 0.2	0.1 ± 0.1	0.0 ± 0.0	0.4 ± 0.2	0.2 ± 0.
	$X_1^2 = 0.33$, $P = .569$		$X_1^2 = 3.54$, $P = .070$			$X_1^2 = 0.33$, $P = .571$		$X_1^2 = 3.29$, $P = .081$		
rder	0.2 ± 0.1	0.6 ± 0.2	0.4 ± 0.2	0.4 ± 0.2	0.4 ± 0.1	0.2 ± 0.1	0.4 ± 0.2	0.3 ± 0.2	0.2 ± 0.1	0.3 ± 0.
	$X_1^2 = 2.51$, $P = .124$		$X_1^2 = 0.003$, $P = .955$			$X_1^2 = 0.71$, $P = .406$		$X_1^2 = 0.172$, $P = .681$		
order	0.1 ± 0.0	0.2 ± 0.1	0.1 ± 0.1	0.2 ± 0.1	0.1 ± 0.1	0.0 ± 0.0	0.1 ± 0.0	0.0 ± 0.0	0.1 ± 0.0	0.03 ± 0
	$X_1^2 = 2.01$, $P = .167$		$X_1^2 = 1.07$, $P = .309$			$X_1^2 = 2.86$, $P = .101$		$X_1^2 = 2.85$, $P = .102$		
order	2.5 ± 0.7	4.9 ± 0.9	2.5 ± 0.7	4.8 ± 0.9	3.7 ± 0.6	1.7 ± 0.5	4.1 ± 0.8	1.8 ± 0.5	3.9 ± 0.8	2.9 ± 0.
	$X_1^2 = 6.64$, $P = .015$		$X_1^2 = 7.08$, $P = .012$			$X_1^2 = 7.37$, $P = .011$		$X_1^2 = 7.26$, $P = .011$		
depression	1.8 ± 0.6	3.7 ± 0.8	1.6 ± 0.5	3.8 ± 0.8	2.7 ± 0.6	1.6 ± 0.5	3.2 ± 0.7	1.4 ± 0.4	3.2 ± 0.7	2.4 ± 0.
	$X_1^2 = 4.65$, $P = .039$		$X_1^2 = 10.00$, $P = .004$			$X_1^2 = 3.90$, $P = .058$		$X_1^2 = 7.65$, $P = .010$		
ymia	0.7 ± 0.3	1.2 ± 0.4	0.8 ± 0.4	1.1 ± 0.3	1.0 ± 0.3	0.1 ± 0.1	0.9 ± 0.4	0.4 ± 0.2	0.7 ± 0.3	0.5 ± 0.
	$X_1^2 = 1.53$, $P = .225$		$X_1^2 = 0.28$, $P = .601$			$X_1^2 = 4.73$, $P = .038$		$X_1^2 = 0.91$, $P = .348$		
ove	14. 5 ± 1.0	11.6 ± 1.1	12.8 ± 1.3	13.4 ± 1.2	13.1 ± 0.9	13.0 ± 0.9	9.4 ± 1.2	11.0 ± 1.1	11.5 ± 1.3	11.3 ± 0.
	$X_1^2 = 6.47$, $P = .016$		$X_1^2 = 0.12$, $P = .731$			$X_1^2 = 9.73$, $P = .004$		$X_1^2 = 0.10$, $P = .758$		

on page 102.

Table 9a notes

[a] Impairment level D indicates ≥2 intermediate or 1 severe rating on the 6 impairment questions regarding personal distress and social (at home or with peers) or academic difficulties.

SOURCE: Merikangas, K. R., He, J.-P., Brody, D., Fisher, P. W., Bourdon, K., & Koretz, D. S. (2010). Prevalence and treatment of mental disorders among US children in the 2001–2004 NHANES. *Pediatrics, 125*(1), 75–81.

NOTES: Reproduced with permission from *Pediatrics, 125*(1), 75–81, Copyright © 2010 by the American Academy of Pediatrics.

At the request of the publisher, Table 9a is the original, published form of the table.

Table 10. Number and percentage of persons aged 3 to 17 ever told of having attention deficit hyperactivity disorder, by selected characteristics, United States, 2009

[Data are based on household interviews of a sample of the national population]

Characteristic	Number (1,000s)	Age-adjusted percent[1]
Total[2]	**5,288**	**8.6**
Age[3]		
3–4	133	1.5
5–11	2,121	7.6
12–17	3,035	12.2
Sex		
Male	3,689	11.8
Female	1,599	5.3
Hispanic origin and race		
One race[4]	5,012	8.5
White	4,057	8.7
Black or African American	904	9.8
American Indian or Alaska Native	*	*
Asian	21	0.8
Native Hawaiian or Other Pacific Islander	*	*
Two or more races[5]	277	13.4
Black or African American and white	158	16.8
American Indian or Alaska Native and white	74	16.1
Hispanic or Latino origin and race[6]	—	—
Hispanic or Latino	659	5.1
Mexican or Mexican American	395	4.4
Not Hispanic or Latino	4,629	9.5
White, single race	3,460	9.9
Black or African American, single race	857	10.0
Poverty status[7]		
Poor	1,215	11.0
Near poor	1,372	10.7
Not poor	2,384	7.2
Health insurance status[8]		
Private coverage	2,497	7.1
Medicaid or other public	2,321	12.6
Other coverage	137	8.2
Uninsured	305	5.1
Geographic region		
Northeast	1,013	9.6
Midwest	1,432	9.7
South	2,089	9.8
West	754	5.1
Place of residence[9]		
Large MSA	2,381	7.4
Small MSA	1,811	9.6
Not in MSA	1,096	10.8

See notes on page 104.

Table 10 notes

— Data not available.

*Estimates are considered unreliable because of low precision.

[1] Estimates are age adjusted using the projected 2000 U.S. population as the standard population and using age groups 3 to 4 years, 5 to 11 years, and 12 to 17 years.

[2] Total includes other races not shown separately and children with unknown family structure, parent's education, family income, poverty status, health insurance, or current health status. Additionally, numbers within selected characteristics may not add to totals because of rounding.

[3] Estimates for age groups are not age adjusted.

[4] In accordance with the 1997 standards for Federal data on race and Hispanic or Latino origin, the category "one race" refers to persons who indicated only a single race group. Persons who indicated a single race other than the groups shown are included in the total for "one race" but are not shown separately due to small sample sizes. Therefore, the frequencies for the category "one race" will be greater than the sum of the frequencies for the specific groups shown separately.

[5] The category "two or more races" refers to all persons who indicated more than one race group. Only two combinations of multiple race groups are shown due to small sample sizes for other combinations. Therefore, the frequencies for the category "two or more races" will be greater than the sum of the frequencies for the specific combinations shown separately.

[6] Persons of Hispanic or Latino origin may be of any race or combination of races. Similarly, the category "Not Hispanic or Latino" refers to all persons who are not of Hispanic or Latino origin, regardless of race.

[7] Poverty status is based on respondent age, family income, family size, and composition using the U.S. Census Bureau's poverty thresholds. "Poor" persons are defined as living in households where the family income is less than 100 percent of the U.S. Census poverty threshold. "Near poor" persons have incomes of 100 percent to less than 200 percent of the poverty threshold. "Not poor" persons have incomes that are 200 percent of the poverty threshold or greater.

[8] Classification of health insurance coverage is based on a hierarchy of mutually exclusive categories. Persons with more than one type of health insurance were assigned to the first appropriate category in the hierarchy. The category "Uninsured" includes persons who had no coverage as well as persons who had only Indian Health Service coverage or had only a private plan that paid for one type of service, such as accidents or dental care.

[9] MSA is metropolitan statistical area. Large MSAs have a population size of 1 million or more, and small MSAs have a population size of less than 1 million. "Not in MSA" consists of persons not living in a metropolitan statistical area.

NOTES: The National Health Interview Survey provides national estimates for a broad range of health measures for the U.S. civilian noninstitutionalized population. The interviewed sample for 2009 consisted of 33,856 households, which yielded 88,446 persons in 34,640 families. A total of 12,404 children aged 17 or younger were eligible for the Sample Child Questionnaire, and data were collected for 11,156 sample children.

Attention deficit hyperactivity disorder is based on the question, "Has a doctor or health professional ever told you that your child had attention deficit hyperactivity disorder (ADHD) or attention deficit disorder (ADD)?"

SOURCE: Sondik, E. J., Madans, J. H., & Gentleman, J. F. (2010). Summary health statistics for U.S. children: National Health Interview Survey, 2009. *Vital and Health Statistics, 10*(247). Hyattsville, MD: National Center for Health Statistics.

Table 11. Number and percentage of persons aged 12 to 17 with a past year major depressive episode (MDE), by selected characteristics, United States, 2009

[Data are based on a survey of a representative sample of the national population]

Characteristic	Number (1,000s)	Percent
Total	**1,950**	**8.1**
Age		
12–13	331	4.6
14–15	739	8.8
16–17	881	10.4
Sex		
Male	574	4.7
Female	1,376	11.7
Hispanic origin and race		
Not Hispanic or Latino	1,589	8.2
White	1,174	8.3
Black or African American	286	7.9
American Indian or Alaska Native	9	7.5
Native Hawaiian or Other Pacific Islander	*	*
Asian	73	7.6
Two or more races	41	7.9
Hispanic or Latino	361	7.7
Poverty status[1]		
Poor	338	7.4
Near poor	462	8.6
Not poor	1,151	8.1
Health insurance status[2]		
Private coverage	1,193	7.8
Medicaid/CHIP[3]	562	8.1
Other coverage[4]	95	8.9
No coverage	179	9.8
Geographic region		
Northeast	293	7.0
Midwest	455	8.6
South	667	7.6
West	536	9.3
County type		
Large metro	1,017	8.0
Small metro	607	8.1
Nonmetro	326	8.5

See notes on page 106.

Table 11 notes

*Estimates are considered unreliable because of low precision.

[1] Poverty status is based on respondent age, family income, family size, and composition using the U.S. Census Bureau's poverty thresholds. "Poor" persons are defined as living in households where the family income is less than 100 percent of the U.S. Census poverty threshold. "Near poor" persons have incomes of 100 percent to less than 200 percent of the poverty threshold. "Not poor" persons have incomes that are 200 percent of the poverty threshold or greater.

[2] Respondents could indicate multiple types of health insurance; thus, these response categories are not mutually exclusive.

[3] CHIP is the Children's Health Insurance Program (formerly State Children's Health Insurance Program [SCHIP]). Individuals aged 19 or younger are eligible for this plan.

[4] Other health insurance is defined as having Medicare, Civilian Health and Medical Program of the Uniformed Services (CHAMPUS), TRICARE, Civilian Health and Medical Program of the Department of Veterans Affairs (CHAMPVA), Veterans Administration (VA), military health care, or any other type of health insurance.

NOTES: The National Survey on Drug Use and Health is a nationally representative survey of the civilian, noninstitutionalized population of the United States aged 12 or older. The survey interviews approximately 67,500 persons each year. In 2009, 22,626 youth aged 12 to 17 were interviewed.

Major depressive episode (MDE) is defined as a period of at least 2 weeks when a person experienced a depressed mood or loss of interest or pleasure in daily activities and had a majority of specified depression symptoms. According to the *Diagnostic and Statistical Manual of Mental Disorders, Fourth Edition* (DSM-IV) (APA, 1994), two or more MDEs are necessary to meet the criteria for recurrent major depressive disorder.

SOURCE: National Survey on Drug Use and Health, 2009, Substance Abuse and Mental Health Services Administration, Office of Applied Studies.

Table 12. Number and percentage of persons aged 12 to 17 with a past year major depressive episode (MDE), by selected characteristics, United States, 2004–2009

[Data are based on a survey of a representative sample of the national population]

Characteristic	2004		2005		2006		2007		2008		2009	
	Number (1,000s)	Percent	Number (1,000s)	Percent	Number (1,000s)	Percent	Number (1,000s)	Percent	Number (1,000s)	Percent	Number (1,000s)	Percent
Total	**2,225**	**9.0**	**2,191**	**8.8**	**1,969**	**7.9**	**2,016**	**8.2**	**2,014**	**8.3**	**1,950**	**8.1**
Age												
12–13	445	5.4	417	5.2	383	4.9	336	4.3	364	4.8	331	4.6
14–15	783	9.2	811	9.5	685	7.9	706	8.4	703	8.4	739	8.8
16–17	997	12.3	964	11.5	901	10.7	973	11.5	947	11.1	881	10.4
Sex												
Male	637	5.0	571	4.5	540	4.2	582	4.6	538	4.3	574	4.7
Female	1,588	13.1	1,620	13.3	1,429	11.8	1,433	11.9	1,476	12.4	1,376	11.7
Hispanic origin and race												
Not Hispanic or Latino	1,848	8.9	1,802	8.7	1,610	7.9	1,691	8.4	1,666	8.4	1,589	8.2
White	1,413	9.2	1,390	9.1	1,215	8.1	1,282	8.7	1,253	8.7	1,174	8.3
Black or African American	287	7.7	288	7.6	245	6.4	293	7.8	260	7.0	286	7.9
American Indian or Alaska Native	13	7.8	10	6.1	12	9.3	7	4.6	13	10.1	9	7.5
Native Hawaiian or Other Pacific Islander	*	*	*	*	*	*	*	*	*	*	*	*
Asian	82	8.3	63	6.0	77	7.6	67	6.8	72	7.6	73	7.6
Two or more races	51	11.7	41	10.5	53	13.0	41	10.0	59	12.0	41	7.9
Hispanic or Latino	377	9.1	389	9.1	359	8.0	324	7.1	348	7.5	361	7.7

*Estimates are considered unreliable because of low precision.

NOTES: The National Survey on Drug Use and Health is a nationally representative survey of the civilian, noninstitutionalized population of the United States aged 12 or older. The survey interviews approximately 67,500 persons each year. The youth aged 12 to 17 sample includes approximately 22,500 respondents each year.

Major depressive episode (MDE) is defined as a period of at least 2 weeks when a person experienced a depressed mood or loss of interest or pleasure in daily activities and had a majority of specified depression symptoms. According to the *Diagnostic and Statistical Manual of Mental Disorders, Fourth Edition* (DSM-IV) (APA, 1994), two or more MDEs are necessary to meet the criteria for recurrent major depressive disorder.

SOURCE: National Survey on Drug Use and Health, 2004–2009, Substance Abuse and Mental Health Services Administration, Office of Applied Studies.

7. TABLES

7.1 Mental Health of the Population

Table 13. Number and percentage of persons aged 18 or older with past year any mental illness (AMI), serious mental illness (SMI), or major depressive episode (MDE), by substance dependence or abuse status, United States, 2009

[Data are based on a survey of a representative sample of the national population]

Dependence or abuse status	No past year mental illness		Past year AMI		Past year SMI		Past year MDE	
	Number (1,000s)	Percent	Number (1,000s)	Percent	Number (1,000s)	Percent	Number (1,000s)	Percent
Dependence								
Both illicit drugs and alcohol	408	0.2	814	1.8	333	3.0	372	2.5
Illicit drugs and/or alcohol	5,406	3.0	6,098	13.5	2,064	18.8	2,415	16.4
Illicit drugs only	1,724	0.9	2,582	5.7	946	8.6	1,025	6.9
Alcohol only	4,091	2.2	4,330	9.6	1,451	13.2	1,761	11.9
Dependence or abuse								
Both illicit drugs and alcohol	1,070	0.6	1,705	3.8	682	6.2	664	4.5
Illicit drugs and/or alcohol	11,904	6.5	8,892	19.7	2,814	25.7	3,305	22.4
Illicit drugs only	2,581	1.4	3,462	7.7	1,265	11.6	1,264	8.6
Alcohol only	10,393	5.7	7,135	15.8	2,231	20.4	2,704	18.3

See notes on page 111.

Table 13 notes

NOTES: The National Survey on Drug Use and Health (NSDUH) is a nationally representative survey of the civilian, noninstitutionalized population of the United States aged 12 or older. The survey interviews approximately 67,500 persons each year.

Mental illness among persons aged 18 or older is defined according to two dimensions: (1) the presence of a diagnosable mental, behavioral, or emotional disorder in the past year (excluding developmental and substance use disorders) of sufficient duration to meet diagnostic criteria specified in the *Diagnostic and Statistical Manual of Mental Disorders, Fourth Edition* (DSM-IV) (APA, 1994); and (2) the level of interference with or limitation of one or more major life activities resulting from a disorder (functional impairment). Adult NSDUH respondents' mental illness was determined based on modeling their responses to questions on distress (K6 scale) and impairment (truncated version of the World Health Organization Disability Assessment Schedule). Serious mental illness (SMI) among adults is defined as persons aged 18 or older who currently or at any time in the past year had a diagnosable mental, behavioral, or emotional disorder as defined above and resulting in substantial impairment in carrying out major life activities, based on Global Assessment of Functioning (GAF) scores of 50 or less. AMI among adults is defined as persons aged 18 or older who currently or at any time in the past year had a diagnosable mental, behavioral, or emotional disorder as defined above, regardless of the level of impairment in carrying out major life activities. AMI includes persons with mental illness having serious, moderate, or mild functional impairment; SMI is a subset of the AMI group. No mental illness includes adults who did not meet the criteria for any mental illness in the past year. Major depressive episode (MDE) is defined as a period of at least 2 weeks when a person experienced a depressed mood or loss of interest or pleasure in daily activities and had a majority of specified depression symptoms. According to DSM-IV, two or more MDEs are necessary to meet the criteria for recurrent major depressive disorder. See Table 1 for number of persons with past year AMI and SMI and Table 3 for number of persons with past year MDE. Illicit drugs include marijuana/hashish, cocaine (including crack), heroin, hallucinogens, inhalants, or prescription-type psychotropic medications used nonmedically, based on data from original questions not including methamphetamine items added in 2005 and 2006. Dependence or abuse is based on definitions in DSM-IV. Substance abuse and dependence are broad categories associated with a pattern of substance use that leads to clinically significant impairment. Abuse may include symptoms such as failure to fulfill major role obligations, legal problems, use in situations that are physically hazardous, and continued use despite persistent social or interpersonal problems. Substance dependence symptoms may include drug taking in larger amounts than intended, inability to cut down on drug use, a great deal of time spent on activities necessary to obtain the drug, and continued use despite knowledge of health or social problems caused by the drug.

SOURCE: National Survey on Drug Use and Health, 2009, Substance Abuse and Mental Health Services Administration, Office of Applied Studies.

Table 14. Number and percentage of persons aged 12 to 17 with a past year major depressive episode (MDE), by substance dependence or abuse status, United States, 2009

[Data are based on a survey of a representative sample of the national population]

Dependence or abuse status	Number (1,000s)	Percent
Dependence		
Both illicit drugs and alcohol	53	2.7
Illicit drugs and/or alcohol	237	12.2
Illicit drugs only	164	8.4
Alcohol only	126	6.5
Dependence or abuse		
Both illicit drugs and alcohol	110	5.6
Illicit drugs and/or alcohol	368	18.9
Illicit drugs only	246	12.6
Alcohol only	231	11.9

NOTES: The National Survey on Drug Use and Health is a nationally representative survey of the civilian, noninstitutionalized population of the United States aged 12 or older. The survey interviews approximately 67,500 persons each year. In 2009, 22,626 youth aged 12 to 17 were interviewed.

Major depressive episode (MDE) is defined as a period of at least 2 weeks when a person experienced a depressed mood or loss of interest or pleasure in daily activities and had a majority of specified depression symptoms. According to the *Diagnostic and Statistical Manual of Mental Disorders, Fourth Edition* (DSM-IV) (APA, 1994), two or more MDEs are necessary to meet the criteria for recurrent major depressive disorder. See Table 12 for number of youth aged 12 to 17 with past year MDE. Illicit drugs include marijuana/hashish, cocaine (including crack), heroin, hallucinogens, inhalants, or prescription-type psychotropic medications used nonmedically, based on data from original questions not including methamphetamine items added in 2005 and 2006. Dependence or abuse is based on definitions in DSM-IV. Substance abuse and dependence are broad categories associated with a pattern of substance use that leads to clinically significant impairment. Abuse may include symptoms such as failure to fulfill major role obligations, legal problems, use in situations that are physically hazardous, and continued use despite persistent social or interpersonal problems. Substance dependence symptoms may include drug taking in larger amounts than intended, inability to cut down on drug use, a great deal of time spent on activities necessary to obtain the drug, and continued use despite knowledge of health or social problems caused by the drug.

SOURCE: National Survey on Drug Use and Health, 2009, Substance Abuse and Mental Health Services Administration, Office of Applied Studies.

7. TABLES

7.1 Mental Health of the Population

Table 15. Number and age-adjusted death rates for suicide, by Hispanic origin, race, and sex: United States, 2007

[Data are based on death certificates]

Characteristic	Total		Male		Female	
	Number	Age-adjusted death rate (per 100,000 population)	Number	Age-adjusted death rate (per 100,000 population)	Number	Age-adjusted death rate (per 100,000 population)
Total[1]	**34,598**	**11.3**	**27,269**	**18.4**	**7,329**	**4.7**
Race[1,2]						
White	31,348	12.5	24,725	20.2	6,623	5.2
Black	1,958	5.0	1,606	8.8	352	1.7
American Indian or Alaska Native	392	11.5	310	18.1	82	4.9
Asian or Pacific Islander	900	6.1	628	9.0	272	3.5
Hispanic origin and race[1,3]						
Hispanic	2,465	6.0	2,078	10.1	387	1.9
Non-Hispanic[4]	32,061	12.0	25,133	19.7	6,928	5.0
White non-Hispanic	28,897	13.5	22,660	21.9	6,237	5.7
Black non-Hispanic	1,916	5.1	1,571	9.0	345	1.8

[1] Estimates are age-adjusted to the year 2000 standard population using 11 age groups: younger than 1 year (3,794,901 persons), 1 to 4 years (15,191,619), 5 to 14 years (39,976,619), 15 to 24 years (38,076,743), 25 to 34 years (37,233,437), 35 to 44 years (44,659,185), 45 to 54 years (37,030,152), 55 to 64 years (23,961,506), 65 to 74 years (18,135,514), 75 to 84 years (12,314,793), and 85 years or older (4,259,173).

[2] Data for specified races other than white and black should be interpreted with caution because of inconsistencies between reporting race on death certificates and on censuses and surveys.

[3] Race and Hispanic origin are reported separately on the death certificate. Persons of Hispanic origin may be of any race or combination of races. Data for Hispanic persons are not tabulated separately by race; data for non-Hispanic persons are tabulated by race. Data for Hispanic origin should be interpreted with caution because of inconsistencies between reporting Hispanic origin on death certificates and on censuses and surveys.

[4] Includes races other than white and black.

NOTES: The National Vital Statistics Report presents detailed data on deaths and death rates according to a number of social, demographic, and medical characteristics. In 2007, 2,423,712 deaths were reported in the United States.

Race categories are consistent with the 1977 Office of Management and Budget (OMB) standards. Multiple-race data were reported by 27 States and the District of Columbia in 2007. The multiple-race data for these reporting areas were matched to the single-race categories of the 1977 OMB standards for comparability with other reporting areas.

Age-adjusted rates per 100,000 U.S. standard population. Populations used for computing death rates are postcensal estimates based on the 2000 census, estimated as of July 1, 2007.

SOURCES: National Vital Statistics System, Centers for Disease Control and Prevention, National Center for Health Statistics.

Tejada-Vera, B., & Sutton, P. D. (2010). Births, marriages, divorces, and deaths: Provisional data for 2009. *National Vital Statistics Report, 58*(25). Hyattsville, MD: National Center for Health Statistics.

Table 16. Death rates for suicide, by age and sex, United States, selected years 1985–2007

[Data are based on death certificates]

Characteristic	Death rate per 100,000 population					
	1985	1990	1995	2000	2005	2007
Total[1]	**12.5**	**12.5**	**11.8**	**10.4**	**10.9**	**11.3**
Age						
5–14	0.8	0.8	0.9	0.7	0.7	0.5
15–24	12.8	13.2	13.0	10.2	10.0	9.7
25–34	15.3	15.2	15.0	12.0	12.4	13.0
35–44	14.6	15.3	15.1	14.5	14.9	15.6
45–54	15.7	14.8	14.4	14.4	16.5	17.7
55–64	16.8	16.0	13.2	12.1	13.9	15.5
65–74	18.7	17.9	15.7	12.5	12.6	12.6
75–84	23.9	24.9	20.6	17.6	16.9	16.3
85 or older	19.4	22.2	21.3	19.6	16.9	15.6
Sex[1]						
Male	21.1	21.5	20.3	18.1	18.0	18.4
Female	5.3	4.9	4.3	4.0	4.4	4.7

[1] Estimates are age-adjusted to the year 2000 standard population using 11 age groups: younger than 1 year (3,794,901 persons), 1 to 4 years (15,191,619), 5 to 14 years (39,976,619), 15 to 24 years (38,076,743), 25 to 34 years (37,233,437), 35 to 44 years (44,659,185), 45 to 54 years (37,030,152), 55 to 64 years (23,961,506), 65 to 74 years (18,135,514), 75 to 84 years (12,314,793), and 85 years or older (4,259,173).

NOTES: The National Vital Statistics Report presents detailed data on deaths and death rates according to a number of social, demographic, and medical characteristics. In 2007, 2,423,712 deaths were reported in the United States.

Age-adjusted rates per 100,000 U.S. standard population. Populations used for computing death rates are postcensal estimates based on the 2000 census, estimated as of July 1, 2007.

SOURCES: 1985–1995 data with age-adjusted rates obtained from National Vital Statistics System, Centers for Disease Control and Prevention, National Center for Health Statistics.

Xu, J. Q., Kochanek, K. D., Murphy, S. L., & Tejada-Vera, B. (2010). Deaths: Final data for 2007. *National Vital Statistics Reports, 58*(19). Hyattsville, MD: National Center for Health Statistics.

7. TABLES

Table 17. Number and percentage of persons aged 65 or older with past year any mental illness (AMI), serious mental illness (SMI), or major depressive episode (MDE), by sex and Hispanic origin and race, United States, 2009

[Data are based on a survey of a representative sample of the national population]

Characteristic	Past year AMI		Past year SMI		Past year MDE	
	Number (1,000s)	Percent	Number (1,000s)	Percent	Number (1,000s)	Percent
Total	**4,083**	**10.8**	**516**	**1.4**	**892**	**2.4**
Sex						
Male	1,073	6.5	78	0.5	183	1.1
Female	3,010	14.0	439	2.0	709	3.3
Hispanic origin and race						
Not Hispanic or Latino	3,781	10.7	455	1.3	773	2.2
White	3,374	11.1	424	1.4	727	2.4
Black or African American	277	8.7	31	1.0	46	1.5
American Indian or Alaska Native	*	*	*	*	*	*
Native Hawaiian or Other Pacific Islander	*	*	*	*	*	*
Asian	*	*	*	*	*	*
Two or more races	*	*	*	*	*	*
Hispanic or Latino	303	11.2	*	*	119	4.4

*Estimates are considered unreliable because of low precision.

NOTES: The National Survey on Drug Use and Health (NSDUH) is a nationally representative survey of the civilian, noninstitutionalized population of the United States aged 12 or older. The survey interviews approximately 67,500 persons each year.

Mental illness among persons aged 18 or older is defined according to two dimensions: (1) the presence of a diagnosable mental, behavioral, or emotional disorder in the past year (excluding developmental and substance use disorders) of sufficient duration to meet diagnostic criteria specified in the *Diagnostic and Statistical Manual of Mental Disorders, Fourth Edition* (DSM-IV) (APA, 1994); and (2) the level of interference with or limitation of one or more major life activities resulting from a disorder (functional impairment). Adult NSDUH respondents' mental illness was determined based on modeling their responses to questions on distress (K6 scale) and impairment (truncated version of the World Health Organization Disability Assessment Schedule). Serious mental illness (SMI) among adults is defined as persons aged 18 or older who currently or at any time in the past year had a diagnosable mental, behavioral, or emotional disorder as defined above and resulting in substantial impairment in carrying out major life activities, based on Global Assessment of Functioning (GAF) scores of 50 or less. Any mental illness (AMI) among adults is defined as persons aged 18 or older who currently or at any time in the past year had a diagnosable mental, behavioral, or emotional disorder as defined above, regardless of the level of impairment in carrying out major life activities. AMI includes persons with mental illness having serious, moderate, or mild functional impairment; SMI is a subset of the AMI group. Major depressive episode (MDE) is defined as a period of at least 2 weeks when a person experienced a depressed mood or loss of interest or pleasure in daily activities and had a majority of specified depression symptoms. According to DSM-IV, two or more MDEs are necessary to meet the criteria for recurrent major depressive disorder.

SOURCE: National Survey on Drug Use and Health, 2009, Substance Abuse and Mental Health Services Administration, Office of Applied Studies.

Table 18. Number and percentage of nursing home residents with a diagnosis of mental illness, United States, 2004

[Data are based on a sample of nursing homes]

Characteristic of residents	Number	Percent
Total population of residents	**1,492,207**	**100.0**
Primary diagnosis of a mental illness	101,667	6.8
Any diagnosis of a mental illness	734,139	49.2
Total population of residents aged 64 or younger	**174,915**	**11.7**
Primary diagnosis of a mental illness	22,636	12.9
Any diagnosis of a mental illness	98,184	56.1
Total population of residents aged 65 or older	**1,317,292**	**88.3**
Primary diagnosis of a mental illness	79,031	6.0
Any diagnosis of a mental illness	635,955	48.3

NOTES: The National Nursing Home Survey is a nationally representative probability sample of 1,500 nursing homes, their residents, and their staff. The sample shown consists of 1,492,207 nursing home residents.

Mental illness is defined as having *International Classification of Diseases, Ninth Revision (ICD-9-CM)* (WHO, 1977) diagnosis codes 295–302 or 306–314. Alzheimer's and dementia are not included. Table originally published in Substance Abuse and Mental Health Services Administration (SAMHSA). (2010). *Mental Health, United States, 2008* (DHHS Publication No. SMA 10-4590). Rockville, MD: Center for Mental Health Services, SAMHSA.

SOURCES: National Nursing Home Survey, 2004, Centers for Disease Control and Prevention.

Table 19. Percentage of active duty military personnel with self-reported serious psychological distress (SPD); need for further posttraumatic stress disorder (PTSD) evaluation, anxiety evaluation, and depression evaluation; suicide ideation; and suicide attempts, by service, United States, 2008

[Data are based on self-administered questionnaires of military personnel]

Reported outcome	Department of Defense (DoD) service					Coast Guard (percent)	All services[2] (percent)
	Army (percent)	Navy (percent)	Marine Corps (percent)	Air Force (percent)	Total DoD services[1] (percent)		
SPD,[3] past 12 months	15.8	14.3	17.6	10.5	14.4	12.3	14.3
Need for further PTSD evaluation, past 30 days	13.4	9.1	15.0	5.6	10.7	6.8	10.6
Need for further anxiety evaluation, past 30 days	17.1	13.0	17.3	8.9	14.2	10.2	14.0
Need for further depression evaluation, past 7 days	23.7	21.9	25.9	13.8	21.2	18.3	21.1
Seriously considered suicide[3]							
Past year	4.9	5.1	5.5	3.1	4.6	2.8	4.6
Not within past year but since joining service	3.5	3.6	3.9	2.5	3.3	3.3	3.3
Not within past year but before joining service	4.4	3.8	4.0	2.8	3.8	3.2	3.8
Attempted suicide[3]							
Past year	2.0	2.8	2.3	1.6	2.2	1.7	2.1
Not within past year but since joining service	1.3	1.3	1.1	0.5	1.1	0.7	1.1
Not within past year but before joining service	3.3	2.2	3.0	1.3	2.5	1.4	2.5

[1] "Total DoD services" includes Army, Navy, Marine Corps, and Air Force.

[2] "All services" includes Army, Navy, Marine Corps, Air Force, and Coast Guard.

[3] Because of improvements in question wording for the 2008 survey, estimates of serious psychological distress and suicide measures in this table are not directly comparable with estimates from previous years of the survey.

Table 19 notes *(continued)*

NOTES: The 2008 Department of Defense Survey of Health Related Behaviors Among Active Duty Military Personnel provides representative estimates on substance use and abuse, mental well-being, stress and coping, combat exposure experience, deployment experience, and selected general health topics for all active duty personnel. The final sample consisted of 28,546 military personnel (5,927 Army; 6,637 Navy; 5,117 Marine Corps; 7,009 Air Force; and 3,856 Coast Guard) who completed self-administered questionnaires anonymously.

Table displays the percentage of military personnel by service who reported the mental illness/suicide response as indicated in the rows of this table. Estimates have not been adjusted for sociodemographic differences across services.

Serious psychological distress (SPD) was measured by the six-item K6 scale (Kessler et al., 2002; OAS, 2008). Need for PTSD evaluation was measured by the PTSD Checklist-Civilian Version (Weathers, Litz, Huska, & Keane, 1994), which consists of a set of 17 items that ask about experiences related to PTSD. To screen for generalized anxiety disorder (GAD) symptoms, a set of items adapted from the Patient Health Questionnaire (Spitzer, Kroenke, & Williams, 1999) was used. Need for depression evaluation was measured by a Burnam depression screen that included one item from the Center for Epidemiologic Studies–Depression Scale (Radloff, 1977) and two items from the Diagnostic Interview Schedule (Robins, Helzer, Croughan, & Ratcliff, 1981). Meeting screening criteria for PTSD, anxiety, and depression suggests a need for further evaluation and is not a clinical diagnosis. Estimates for suicide ideation and attempts are based on a series of questions asking if and when the respondent has ever seriously considered or attempted suicide.

SOURCE: Department of Defense Survey of Health Related Behaviors Among Active Duty Military Personnel, 2008. As taken from Bray, R. M., Pemberton, M. R., Hourani, L. L., Witt, M., Rae Olmsted, K. L., Brown, J. M., ... Bradshaw, M. R. (2009). *2008 Department of Defense survey of health related behaviors among active duty military personnel.* Report prepared for TRICARE Management Activity, Office of the Assistant Secretary of Defense (Health Affairs) and U.S. Coast Guard. Retrieved from http://www.tricare.mil/2008HealthBehaviors.pdf. The views, opinions, and findings contained in this report are those of the authors and should not be construed as an official Department of Defense position, policy, or decision, unless so designated by other official documentation.

Table 20. Percentage of active duty, National Guard, and Reserve military personnel with need for further posttraumatic stress disorder (PTSD) or depression evaluation and suicide ideation, by service, United States, 2006

[Data are based on self-administered questionnaires of military personnel]

Service	Need for further evaluation for PTSD—past 30 days		Need for further evaluation for depression—past 7 days		Suicide ideation—past 12 months	
	Unadjusted (percent)	Adjusted[1] (percent)	Unadjusted (percent)	Adjusted[1] (percent)	Unadjusted (percent)	Adjusted[1] (percent)
Army—total	**9.5**	**9.1**	**24.0**	**22.7**	**6.1**	**5.8**
Active duty	9.3	9.1	27.6	27.7	5.6	5.5
National Guard	10.5	9.8	21.7	20.9	6.9	6.5
Reserve	8.3	8.5	20.3	19.6	5.6	5.5
Navy—total	**5.7**	**5.1**	**19.9**	**17.9**	**5.0**	**5.0**
Active duty	6.2	6.0	21.6	21.7	5.3	5.2
Reserve	3.3	4.2	12.8	14.0	3.7	4.7
Marine Corps—total	**7.5**	**6.5**	**24.3**	**21.3**	**5.9**	**4.9**
Active duty	7.6	6.4	25.4	24.2	5.9	5.1
Reserve	7.3	6.7	19.6	18.4	5.9	4.7
Air Force—total	**3.6**	**4.0**	**15.1**	**15.2**	**3.4**	**3.7**
Active duty	3.7	4.1	15.6	16.3	3.5	3.8
National Guard	3.5	4.1	14.4	15.0	2.9	3.2
Reserve	3.1	3.7	13.7	14.3	3.4	4.1
Total DoD	**7.1**	**6.3**	**20.9**	**19.2**	**5.1**	**4.8**
Active duty	6.7	6.4	22.3	22.5	4.9	4.9
Total National Guard and Reserve	**7.7**	**6.2**	**18.8**	**17.0**	**5.5**	**4.8**

[1] Adjusted estimates have been adjusted to correct for differences in the demographic distributions between the Reserve components. The main effects of age group, sex, race/ethnicity, enlisted/officer indicator, marital status, and education were used in this standardization process. Comparisons across Reserve service components should be based on adjusted estimates.

NOTES: The 2006 Department of Defense Survey of Health Related Behaviors Among the Guard and Reserve Force provides representative estimates on substance use, stress and mental health, healthy behaviors and lifestyles, and other specific issues, such as injuries and injury prevention, sleep habits, and risk taking for all Reserve component personnel. The final sample consisted of 18,342 military personnel (2,796 Army National Guard; 1,665 Army Reserve; 3,215 Navy Reserve; 1,159 Marine Corps Reserve; 2,851 Air National Guard; and 6,656 Air Force Reserve) who completed self-administered questionnaires anonymously.

Reserve component estimates exclude full-time or activated Guard and Reserve. The PTSD Checklist-Civilian screen (Weathers, Litz, Huska, & Keane, 1994) was used to assess potential PTSD. Need for further depression screening was measured using a composite indicator made up of an eight-item set of symptoms that included six items from the Center for Epidemiologic Studies–Depression Scale (Radloff, 1977) and two items from the Diagnostic Interview Schedule (Robins, Helzer, Croughan, & Ratcliff, 1981). Two additional measures assessed past year suicidal ideation and suicide attempt.

SOURCE: Department of Defense Survey of Health Related Behaviors Among the Guard and Reserve Force, 2006. As taken from Hourani, L. L., Bray, R. M., Marsden, M. E., Witt, M. B., Vandermaas-Peeler, R., Scheffler, S., ... Strange, L. B. (2007, September). *2006 Department of Defense survey of health related behaviors among the Guard and Reserve force.* Report prepared for TRICARE Management Activity. Retrieved from http://www.tricare.mil/hpae/_docs/RC_2006 Reserve Component_FR_9-07.pdf. The views, opinions, and findings contained in this report are those of the authors and should not be construed as an official Department of Defense position, policy, or decision, unless so designated by other official documentation.

Table 21. Percentage of inmates in State and Federal correctional facilities (2004) and in local jails (2002) experiencing any mental health problem, by age, sex, and Hispanic origin and race, United States

[Data are based on a survey of inmates]

Characteristic	State prison inmates, 2004 (percent)	Federal prison inmates, 2004 (percent)	Local jail inmates, 2002 (percent)
All inmates	**56.2**	**44.8**	**64.2**
Age			
24 or younger	62.6	57.8	70.3
25–34	57.9	48.2	64.8
35–44	55.9	40.1	62.0
45–54	51.3	41.6	52.5
55 or older	39.6	36.1	52.4
Sex			
Male	55.0	43.6	62.8
Female	73.1	61.2	75.4
Hispanic origin and race[1]			
White[2]	62.2	49.6	71.2
Black[2]	54.7	45.9	63.4
Hispanic	46.3	36.8	50.7
Other[2,3]	61.9	50.3	69.5

[1] Hispanic origin and race was not reported by an estimated 1,400 jail inmates who had a mental health problem.

[2] Excludes persons of Hispanic origin.

[3] Includes American Indians, Alaska Natives, Asians, Native Hawaiians, Other Pacific Islanders, and inmates who specified more than one race.

NOTES: The Survey of Inmates in State and Federal Correctional Facilities, 2004, and the Survey of Inmates in Local Jails, 2002, included a modified structured clinical interview for the *Diagnostic and Statistical Manual of Mental Disorders, Fourth Edition* (DSM-IV). The interviewed sample included 681,600 State prison inmates, 56,600 Federal prison inmates, and 398,800 local jail inmates.

Any mental health problem was defined by two measures: a recent history of a mental health problem, either in the year before arrest or since admission; or symptoms of a mental health problem that occurred within the 12 months prior to the interview. A recent history of a mental health problem included inmates self-reporting that they were diagnosed with a mental health problem by a mental health professional or that they received treatment for a mental health problem by a mental health professional. Symptoms of a mental disorder were based on criteria specified in the *Diagnostic and Statistical Manual of Mental Disorders, Fourth Edition* (DSM-IV) (APA, 1994).

Percent refers to inmates with mental health problems as a proportion of the total number of prisoners in each demographic category. Table originally published in Substance Abuse and Mental Health Services Administration (SAMHSA). (2010). *Mental Health, United States, 2008* (DHHS Publication No. SMA 10-4590). Rockville, MD: Center for Mental Health Services, SAMHSA.

SOURCES: Survey of Inmates in State and Federal Correctional Facilities (2004) and Survey of Inmates in Local Jails (2002), Bureau of Justice Statistics (BJS), Washington, DC. Unpublished data delivered upon special request by Lauren E. Glaze, BJS Statistician, and verified by Tracy L. Snell, BJS Statistician, March 2, 2009.

James, D. J., & Glaze, L. E. (2006). *Mental health problems of prison and jail inmates* (NCJ-213600). Washington, DC: U.S. Department of Justice, Office of Justice Programs, Bureau of Justice Statistics. Retrieved from http://bjs.ojp.usdoj.gov/content/pub/pdf/mhppji.pdf

Table 22. Percentage of persons with behavior problems aged 18 months to 17 years involved with the child welfare system, by selected characteristics, United States, 2008

[Data are based on a national sample of children involved with the child welfare system]

Characteristic	Internalizing behavior problem[1] (percent)	Externalizing behavior problem[2] (percent)	Any behavior problem[3] (percent)
Total	**17.7**	**21.1**	**22.6**
Age			
18 months–2 years	6.2	9.0	9.6
3–5 years	15.4	12.2	15.6
6–10 years	20.2	25.8	25.6
11–17 years	21.0	27.6	29.5
Sex			
Male	20.2	22.9	24.1
Female	15.1	19.2	21.0
Hispanic origin and race			
White	17.2	22.3	24.0
Black	16.9	20.1	24.0
Hispanic	17.8	19.1	19.1
Other	22.6	25.6	25.4
Child's current living situation			
In home with biological parent	17.0	20.6	22.2
Kin care[4]	21.5	22.1	21.6
Foster care	24.5	28.6	30.7
Group home or residential program	32.7	40.3	36.0

[1] Internalizing behavior problems include symptoms consistent with anxiety or depression.

[2] Externalizing behavior problems include behaviors consistent with attention deficit hyperactivity disorder or conduct disorder.

[3] Any behavior problem indicates a clinically elevated score on the Child Behavior Checklist Total Problems scale.

[4] A kin caregiver may be a grandparent, aunt or uncle, sibling, or other relative who currently serves as the child's primary caregiver.

NOTES: The National Survey of Child and Adolescent Well-Being II (NSCAW II) includes a longitudinal, national probability sample of 5,873 children from birth to 17 years of age who became involved with the child welfare system in 2008 when reported for child maltreatment.

The measure used to assess behavior problems was the Child Behavior Checklist (Achenbach, 1991; Achenbach & Rescorla, 2001), a parent-report measure that assesses social competencies and problem behaviors of children 18 months to 17 years of age. This table reports elevation of the Internalizing, Externalizing, and Total Problems scale standardized scores. Behavior ratings were considered clinically significant if the scale T scores were at or above 64. All analyses were on weighted data.

SOURCE: Casanueva, C., Ringeisen, H., Wilson, E., Smith, K., & Dolan, M. (2011). *NSCAW II baseline report: Child well-being* (OPRE Report #2011-27b). Washington, DC: Office of Planning, Research and Evaluation, Administration for Children and Families, U.S. Department of Health and Human Services. Retrieved from http://www.acf.hhs.gov/programs/opre/abuse_neglect/nscaw/reports/nscaw2_child/nscaw2_child.pdf

7. TABLES

7.2 Providers and Settings for Mental Health Services

7.2.1 Adult Mental Health Services

Specialty Mental Health Services
Tables 23–31

Nonspecialty Mental Health Services

Mental Health Service Capacity

7.2.2 Child Mental Health Services

Mental Health Services

Mental Health Service Capacity

7.2.3 Special Populations

Table 23. Past year service use in mental health specialty sector or nonspecialty sector among persons aged 18 or older, United States, 2001–2002

[Data are based on a survey of a sample of the civilian noninstitutionalized population]

Treatment	Total population (percent)	Any mental disorder (percent)	No mental disorder (percent)
Any service use	**18.0**	**40.1**	**9.7**
Any health care (mental health or general medical)			
General medical professional	9.3	22.1	4.5
Family doctor	6.8	16.7	3.1
Other medical doctor	1.7	4.1	0.9
Other medical professional	0.4	1.1	0.1
Any mental health professional	8.8	21.0	4.2
Psychiatrist	4.6	11.7	1.8
Other mental health professional	6.3	15.6	2.8
Any non-health care			
Human services	3.4	7.9	1.8
Social worker in human services setting	0.4	0.8	0.2
Counselor in human services setting	0.5	1.2	0.3
Spiritual advisor	2.7	6.3	1.4
Complementary and alternative medicine (CAM)[1]—total	2.8	6.4	1.4
CAM (e.g., spiritual advisors)	0.8	1.8	0.4
Internet	0.6	1.7	0.2
Self-help group	1.6	3.5	1.0

[1] Complementary and alternative medicine (CAM) is defined as a broad class of services that are not traditionally provided as billable services in the treatment system, including services from several types of healers, participation in an Internet support group, or participation in a self-help group. The three most commonly used CAMs in the National Comorbidity Survey Replication (NCS-R) were spiritual advisors, relaxation techniques, and use of multivitamins and herbs (Wang et al., 2005).

NOTES: NCS-R is a nationally representative household survey of 9,282 English speakers aged 18 or older in the United States.

Table originally published in Substance Abuse and Mental Health Services Administration (SAMHSA). (2010). *Mental Health, United States, 2008* (DHHS Publication No. SMA 10-4590). Rockville, MD: Center for Mental Health Services, SAMHSA.

SOURCES: Produced using NCS-R data for Substance Abuse and Mental Health Services Administration (SAMHSA). (2010). *Mental Health, United States, 2008* (DHHS Publication No. SMA 10-4590). Rockville, MD: Center for Mental Health Services, SAMHSA.

Wang, P. S., Lane, M., Olfson, M., Pincus, H. A., Wells, K. B., & Kessler, R. C. (2005). Twelve month use of mental health services in the United States: Results from the National Comorbidity Survey Replication. *Archives of General Psychiatry, 62*(6), 629–640.

Table 24. Number and percentage of persons aged 18 or older who received mental health treatment in the past year, by disorder severity, United States, 2009

[Data are based on a survey of a representative sample of the national population]

Type and location of mental health treatment/counseling[1]	Total		Any mental illness		Serious mental illness		Moderate mental illness		Mild mental illness		No mental illness	
	Number (1,000s)	Percent	Number (1,000s)	Percent	Number (1,000s)	Percent	Number (1,000s)	Percent	Number (1,000s)	Percent	Number (1,000s)	Percent
Outpatient mental health[2]	14,332	6.3	9,522	21.2	4,145	38.0	1,870	20.8	3,507	14.0	4,810	2.6
Outpatient mental health clinic or center	3,064	1.4	2,356	5.2	1,156	10.6	614	6.8	586	2.3	708	0.4
Office of a private therapist, psychologist, psychiatrist, social worker, or counselor—not part of a clinic	7,648	3.4	5,104	11.4	2,172	19.9	918	10.2	2,015	8.0	2,544	1.4
Doctor's office—not part of a clinic	3,317	1.5	2,186	4.9	968	8.9	404	4.5	814	3.2	1,131	0.6
Outpatient medical clinic	1,229	0.5	903	2.0	456	4.2	196	2.2	250	1.0	326	0.2
Partial day hospital or day treatment program	354	0.2	266	0.6	183	1.7	39	0.4	45	0.2	87	0.0
School or university setting/ clinic/center[3]	83	0.0	68	0.2	25	0.2	23	0.3	21	0.1	15	0.0
Some other place[4]	274	0.1	177	0.4	87	0.8	16	0.2	74	0.3	97	0.1
Inpatient mental health[5]	1,894	0.8	1,377	3.1	747	6.8	239	2.6	391	1.6	517	0.3
Prescription medication for mental health	25,573	11.3	14,619	32.4	5,902	54.0	2,878	32.0	5,840	23.2	10,953	6.0
Did not receive mental health services	196,405	86.7	27,930	62.1	4,344	39.8	5,578	62.2	18,009	71.7	168,474	92.8

[1] Respondents could indicate multiple service sources; thus, these response categories are not mutually exclusive.

[2] Outpatient treatment includes any mental health treatment or counseling received at an outpatient mental health clinic or center; the office of a private therapist, psychologist, psychiatrist, social worker, or counselor that was not part of a clinic; a doctor's office that was not part of a clinic; an outpatient medical clinic; a partial day hospital or day treatment program; or some other place.

[3] Respondents were permitted to specify other locations for receiving outpatient mental health treatment/counseling. This location was the most commonly reported other location for receiving outpatient treatment/counseling.

[4] Respondents with unknown or invalid responses to the location "some other place received outpatient mental health treatment/counseling" were excluded.

[5] Inpatient treatment includes a stay of overnight or longer in a hospital or other facility for mental health problems.

Table 24 notes *(continued)*

NOTES: The National Survey on Drug Use and Health (NSDUH) is a nationally representative survey of the civilian, noninstitutionalized population of the United States aged 12 or older. The survey interviews approximately 67,500 persons each year.

Mental health treatment/counseling is defined as having received inpatient care or outpatient care or having used prescription medication for problems with emotions, nerves, or mental health. Respondents were not to include treatment for drug or alcohol use. Respondents with unknown treatment/counseling information were excluded. Estimates were based only on responses to items in the Adult Mental Health Service Utilization module. Mental illness among persons aged 18 or older is defined according to two dimensions: (1) the presence of a diagnosable mental, behavioral, or emotional disorder in the past year (excluding developmental and substance use disorders) of sufficient duration to meet diagnostic criteria specified in the *Diagnostic and Statistical Manual of Mental Disorders, Fourth Edition* (DSM-IV) (APA, 1994); and (2) the level of interference with or limitation of one or more major life activities resulting from a disorder (functional impairment). Adult NSDUH respondents' mental illness was determined based on modeling their responses to questions on distress (K6 scale) and impairment (truncated version of the World Health Organization Disability Assessment Schedule). Any mental illness (AMI) among adults is defined as persons aged 18 or older who currently or at any time in the past year had a diagnosable mental, behavioral, or emotional disorder as defined above, regardless of the level of impairment in carrying out major life activities. AMI includes persons with mental illness having serious, moderate, or mild functional impairment. Serious mental illness (SMI), moderate mental illness, and mild mental illness among adults are defined as persons aged 18 or older who currently or at any time in the past year had a diagnosable mental, behavioral, or emotional disorder as defined above and resulting in substantial, moderate, or mild impairment in carrying out major life activities, based on Global Assessment of Functioning (GAF) scores of 50 or less for SMI, GAF scores of 51 to 59 for moderate mental illness, and GAF scores of greater than 59 for mild mental illness.

SOURCE: National Survey on Drug Use and Health, 2009, Substance Abuse and Mental Health Services Administration, Office of Applied Studies.

Table 25. Percentage of persons aged 18 or older who received mental health treatment or counseling in the past year, by selected characteristics, United States, 2009

[Data are based on a survey of a representative sample of the national population]

Characteristic	Any treatment		Outpatient treatment[1]		Inpatient treatment[2]		Prescription medication	
	Number (1,000s)	Percent	Number (1,000s)	Percent	Number (1,000s)	Percent	Number (1,000s)	Percent
Total	**30,179**	**13.3**	**14,332**	**6.3**	**1,894**	**0.8**	**25,573**	**11.3**
Age								
18–25	3,705	11.1	2,019	6.0	356	1.1	2,826	8.4
26–49	14,415	14.6	7,338	7.4	972	1.0	12,139	12.2
50 or older	12,059	12.8	4,975	5.3	566	0.6	10,608	11.3
Sex								
Male	10,107	9.2	4,753	4.3	837	0.8	8,371	7.6
Female	20,072	17.1	9,579	8.2	1,056	0.9	17,202	14.7
Hispanic origin and race								
Not Hispanic or Latino	27,906	14.3	13,142	6.7	1,576	0.8	23,912	12.2
White	24,754	16.0	11,383	7.3	1,149	0.7	21,629	13.9
Black or African American	2,021	7.7	1,111	4.2	354	1.3	1,481	5.6
American Indian or Alaska Native	*	*	102	9.4	13	1.2	*	*
Native Hawaiian or Other Pacific Islander	*	*	*	*	3	0.4	41	5.6
Asian	353	3.5	234	2.3	23	0.2	186	1.8
Two or more races	463	19.1	233	9.6	35	1.4	376	15.5
Hispanic or Latino	2,274	7.3	1,190	3.8	317	1.0	1,661	5.3
Poverty status[3]								
Poor	4,318	15.8	2,429	8.8	626	2.3	3,629	13.2
Near poor	5,595	12.8	2,485	5.7	596	1.4	4,718	10.8
Not poor	20,113	13.0	9,317	6.0	664	0.4	17,129	11.1
Health insurance status[4]								
Private coverage	19,579	12.7	9,073	5.9	656	0.4	16,419	10.6
Medicaid/CHIP[5]	4,507	23.6	2,510	13.1	655	3.4	3,943	20.6
Other coverage[6]	7,383	14.0	3,275	6.2	654	1.2	6,555	12.5
No coverage	3,286	9.1	1,340	3.7	304	0.8	2,806	7.8

(continued)

Table 25. Percentage of persons aged 18 or older who received mental health treatment or counseling in the past year, by selected characteristics, United States, 2009 *(continued)*

Characteristic	Any treatment		Outpatient treatment[1]		Inpatient treatment[2]		Prescription medication	
	Number (1,000s)	Percent	Number (1,000s)	Percent	Number (1,000s)	Percent	Number (1,000s)	Percent
Geographic region								
Northeast	5,300	12.6	2,966	7.1	310	0.7	4,335	10.3
Midwest	7,187	14.5	3,266	6.6	447	0.9	6,306	12.7
South	11,148	13.5	4,738	5.7	731	0.9	9,717	11.7
West	6,544	12.5	3,362	6.4	407	0.8	5,215	10.0
County type								
Large metro	14,968	12.4	7,564	6.3	1,044	0.9	12,074	10.0
Small metro	9,930	14.4	4,652	6.8	618	0.9	8,605	12.5
Nonmetro	5,282	14.2	2,116	5.7	232	0.6	4,894	13.1
Current employment								
Full-time	12,791	11.2	5,909	5.2	381	0.3	10,614	9.3
Part-time	4,885	15.4	2,675	8.5	247	0.8	3,921	12.3
Unemployed	1,870	12.7	738	5.0	232	1.6	1,669	11.3
Other[7]	10,633	16.2	5,010	7.6	1,034	1.6	9,368	14.2

*Estimates are considered unreliable.

[1] Outpatient treatment includes any mental health treatment or counseling received at an outpatient mental health clinic or center; the office of a private therapist, psychologist, psychiatrist, social worker, or counselor that was not part of a clinic; a doctor's office that was not part of a clinic; an outpatient medical clinic; a partial day hospital or day treatment program; or some other place.

[2] Inpatient treatment includes a stay of overnight or longer in a hospital or other facility for mental health problems.

[3] Poverty status is based on respondent age, family income, family size, and composition using the U.S. Census Bureau's poverty thresholds. "Poor" persons are defined as living in households where the family income is less than 100 percent of the U.S. Census poverty threshold. "Near poor" persons have incomes of 100 percent to less than 200 percent of the poverty threshold. "Not poor" persons have incomes that are 200 percent of the poverty threshold or greater.

[4] Respondents could indicate multiple types of health insurance; thus, these response categories are not mutually exclusive.

[5] CHIP is the Children's Health Insurance Program (formerly State Children's Health Insurance Program [SCHIP]). Qualified individuals aged 19 or younger are eligible for this plan.

[6] Other health insurance is defined as having Medicare, Civilian Health and Medical Program of the Uniformed Services (CHAMPUS), TRICARE, Civilian Health and Medical Program of the Department of Veterans Affairs (CHAMPVA), Veterans Administration (VA), military health care, or any other type of health insurance.

[7] The other employment category includes retired persons, disabled persons, homemakers, students, or other persons not in the labor force.

Table 25 notes *(continued)*

NOTES: The National Survey on Drug Use and Health is a nationally representative survey of the civilian, noninstitutionalized population of the United States aged 12 or older. The survey interviews approximately 67,500 persons each year.

Mental health treatment/counseling is defined as having received inpatient care or outpatient care or having used prescription medication for problems with emotions, nerves, or mental health. Respondents were not to include treatment for drug or alcohol use. Respondents with unknown treatment/counseling information were excluded. Estimates were based only on responses to items in the Adult Mental Health Service Utilization module.

SOURCE: National Survey on Drug Use and Health, 2009, Substance Abuse and Mental Health Services Administration, Office of Applied Studies.

Table 26. Number and percentage of persons aged 18 or older who received mental health treatment in the past year, United States, 2005–2009

[Data are based on a survey of a representative sample of the national population]

Type and location of mental health treatment/counseling[1]	2005		2006		2007		2008		2009	
	Number (1,000s)	Percent	Number (1,000s)	Percent	Number (1,000s)	Percent	Number (1,000s)	Percent	Number (1,000s)	Percent
Outpatient[2]	14,856	6.8	14,673	6.7	15,344	6.9	15,241	6.8	14,332	6.3
Outpatient mental health clinic or center	3,612	1.7	3,326	1.5	3,128	1.4	3,352	1.5	3,064	1.4
Office of a private therapist, psychologist, psychiatrist, social worker, or counselor—not part of a clinic	8,038	3.7	7,775	3.5	8,380	3.8	8,744	3.9	7,648	3.4
Doctor's office—not part of a clinic	3,159	1.5	3,287	1.5	3,281	1.5	2,992	1.3	3,317	1.5
Outpatient medical clinic	1,126	0.5	1,157	0.5	1,370	0.6	1,345	0.6	1,229	0.5
Partial day hospital or day treatment program	311	0.1	189	0.1	348	0.2	234	0.1	354	0.2
School or university setting/clinic/center[3]	93	0.0	87	0.0	65	0.0	98	0.0	83	0.0
Some other place[4]	144	0.1	257	0.1	326	0.1	248	0.1	274	0.1
Inpatient[5]	2,129	1.0	1,591	0.7	2,126	1.0	1,963	0.9	1,894	0.8
Prescription medication	23,305	10.7	23,920	10.9	24,730	11.1	25,422	11.3	25,573	11.3
Did not receive mental health services	189,085	87.0	191,647	87.1	192,541	86.8	194,249	86.6	196,405	86.7

[1] Respondents could indicate multiple service sources; thus, these response categories are not mutually exclusive.

[2] Outpatient treatment includes any mental health treatment or counseling received at an outpatient mental health clinic or center; the office of a private therapist, psychologist, psychiatrist, social worker, or counselor that was not part of a clinic; a doctor's office that was not part of a clinic; an outpatient medical clinic; a partial day hospital or day treatment program; or some other place.

[3] Respondents were permitted to specify other locations for receiving outpatient mental health treatment/counseling. This location was the most commonly reported other location for receiving outpatient treatment/counseling.

[4] Respondents with unknown or invalid responses to the location "some other place received outpatient mental health treatment/counseling" were excluded.

[5] Inpatient treatment includes a stay of overnight or longer in a hospital or other facility for mental health problems.

NOTE: The National Survey on Drug Use and Health is a nationally representative survey of the civilian, noninstitutionalized population of the United States aged 12 or older. The survey interviews approximately 67,500 persons each year.

SOURCE: National Survey on Drug Use and Health, 2005–2009, Substance Abuse and Mental Health Services Administration, Office of Applied Studies.

Table 27. Number and percentage of persons aged 18 or older who received any mental health treatment, by disorder severity, United States, 2009

[Data are based on a survey of a representative sample of the national population]

Characteristic	Total		Any mental illness		Serious mental illness		Moderate mental illness		Mild mental illness		No mental illness	
	Number (1,000s)	Percent	Number (1,000s)	Percent	Number (1,000s)	Percent	Number (1,000s)	Percent	Number (1,000s)	Percent	Number (1,000s)	Percent
Total	**30,179**	**13.3**	**17,064**	**37.9**	**6,571**	**60.2**	**3,397**	**37.8**	**7,095**	**28.3**	**13,116**	**7.2**
Age												
18–25	3,705	11.1	2,599	25.9	1,091	44.6	576	26.6	932	17.2	1,106	4.7
26–49	14,415	14.6	8,831	40.0	3,655	62.5	1,622	37.8	3,555	29.8	5,584	7.3
50 or older	12,059	12.8	5,634	43.7	1,826	69.6	1,199	47.5	2,609	33.7	6,425	7.9
Sex												
Male	10,107	9.2	5,465	32.0	1,879	54.1	1,223	34.3	2,364	23.6	4,643	5.0
Female	20,072	17.1	11,599	41.5	4,692	63.0	2,175	40.2	4,732	31.4	8,473	9.5
Hispanic origin and race												
Not Hispanic or Latino	27,906	14.3	15,706	39.8	6,031	62.3	3,125	40.3	6,549	29.7	12,200	7.8
White	24,754	16.0	13,843	43.1	5,294	64.7	2,790	45.2	5,759	32.5	10,910	8.9
Black or African American	2,021	7.7	1,149	24.6	481	50.0	212	21.2	456	16.8	872	4.0
American Indian or Alaska Native	*	*	*	*	*	*	*	*	*	*	*	*
Native Hawaiian or Other Pacific Islander	*	*	*	*	*	*	*	*	*	*	*	*
Asian	353	3.5	236	15.2	*	*	*	*	125	13.0	117	1.4
Two or more races	463	19.1	358	45.1	*	*	*	*	*	*	105	6.4
Hispanic or Latino	2,274	7.3	1,358	24.6	540	43.8	272	22.4	546	17.7	916	3.6
Poverty status[1]												
Poor	4,318	15.8	2,991	36.3	1,486	59.0	600	34.1	905	22.9	1,326	6.9
Near poor	5,595	12.8	3,494	35.6	1,450	54.4	794	38.5	1,250	24.6	2,102	6.2
Not poor	20,113	13.0	10,457	39.4	3,582	63.5	1,975	39.0	4,900	31.0	9,656	7.6
Health insurance status[2]												
Private coverage	19,579	12.7	10,371	39.0	3,377	62.4	1,972	37.4	5,022	31.5	9,208	7.2
Medicaid/CHIP[3]	4,507	23.6	3,090	48.5	1,404	68.3	662	48.5	1,025	34.7	1,416	11.2
Other coverage[4]	7,383	14.0	3,683	43.5	1,444	69.3	855	49.7	1,385	29.7	3,699	8.4
No coverage	3,286	9.1	2,204	24.5	995	42.7	454	25.9	755	15.4	1,082	4.0

See notes on page 134.

Table 27 notes

*Estimates are considered unreliable because of low precision.

[1] Poverty status is based on respondent age, family income, family size, and composition using the U.S. Census Bureau's poverty thresholds. "Poor" persons are defined as living in households where the family income is less than 100 percent of the U.S. Census poverty threshold. "Near poor" persons have incomes of 100 percent to less than 200 percent of the poverty threshold. "Not poor" persons have incomes that are 200 percent of the poverty threshold or greater.

[2] Respondents could indicate multiple types of health insurance; thus, these response categories are not mutually exclusive.

[3] CHIP is the Children's Health Insurance Program (formerly State Children's Health Insurance Program [SCHIP]). Qualified individuals aged 19 or younger are eligible for this plan.

[4] Other health insurance is defined as having Medicare, Civilian Health and Medical Program of the Uniformed Services (CHAMPUS), TRICARE, Civilian Health and Medical Program of the Department of Veterans Affairs (CHAMPVA), Veterans Administration (VA), military health care, or any other type of health insurance.

NOTES: The National Survey on Drug Use and Health (NSDUH) is a nationally representative survey of the civilian, noninstitutionalized population of the United States aged 12 or older. The survey interviews approximately 67,500 persons each year.

Mental health treatment/counseling is defined as having received inpatient care or outpatient care or having used prescription medication for problems with emotions, nerves, or mental health. Respondents were not to include treatment for drug or alcohol use. Respondents with unknown treatment/counseling information were excluded. Estimates were based only on responses to items in the Adult Mental Health Service Utilization module. Mental illness among persons aged 18 or older is defined according to two dimensions: (1) the presence of a diagnosable mental, behavioral, or emotional disorder in the past year (excluding developmental and substance use disorders) of sufficient duration to meet diagnostic criteria specified in the *Diagnostic and Statistical Manual of Mental Disorders, Fourth Edition* (DSM-IV) (APA, 1994); and (2) the level of interference with or limitation of one or more major life activities resulting from a disorder (functional impairment). Adult NSDUH respondents' mental illness was determined based on modeling their responses to questions on distress (K6 scale) and impairment (truncated version of the World Health Organization Disability Assessment Schedule). Any mental illness (AMI) among adults is defined as persons aged 18 or older who currently or at any time in the past year had a diagnosable mental, behavioral, or emotional disorder as defined above, regardless of the level of impairment in carrying out major life activities. AMI includes persons with mental illness having serious, moderate, or mild functional impairment. Serious mental illness (SMI), moderate mental illness, and mild mental illness among adults are defined as persons aged 18 or older who currently or at any time in the past year had a diagnosable mental, behavioral, or emotional disorder as defined above and resulting in substantial, moderate, or mild impairment in carrying out major life activities, based on Global Assessment of Functioning (GAF) scores of 50 or less for SMI, GAF scores of 51 to 59 for moderate mental illness, and GAF scores of greater than 59 for mild mental illness.

SOURCE: National Survey on Drug Use and Health, 2009, Substance Abuse and Mental Health Services Administration, Office of Applied Studies.

Table 28. Number and percentage of persons aged 18 or older with a past year major depressive episode (MDE) who received mental health treatment, United States, 2009

[Data are based on a survey of a representative sample of the national population]

Characteristic	Saw or talked to medical doctor or other professional OR used prescription medication		Saw or talked to medical doctor or other professional AND used prescription medication		Saw or talked to medical doctor or other professional only		Used prescription medication only	
	Number (1,000s)	Percent	Number (1,000s)	Percent	Number (1,000s)	Percent	Number (1,000s)	Percent
Total	**9,491**	**64.4**	**6,581**	**44.6**	**2,111**	**14.3**	**798**	**5.4**
Sex								
Male	3,071	59.0	2,074	39.8	701	13.5	295	5.7
Female	6,420	67.4	4,507	47.2	1,410	14.8	504	5.3
Hispanic origin and race								
Not Hispanic or Latino	8,602	66.5	6,026	46.5	1,814	14.0	761	5.9
White	7,436	68.7	5,418	49.9	1,344	12.4	673	6.2
Black or African American	758	53.2	418	29.4	261	18.3	79	5.6
Other or two or more races	407	59.7	190	27.8	*	*	8	1.2
Hispanic or Latino	889	49.3	554	30.7	297	16.5	38	2.1
Poverty status[1]								
Poor	1,889	66.5	1,294	45.6	400	14.1	196	6.9
Near poor	1,855	57.4	1,287	39.8	404	12.5	163	5.0
Not poor	5,683	66.5	3,965	46.2	1,283	15.0	434	5.1
Health insurance status[2]								
Private coverage	5,321	65.1	3,678	44.9	1,276	15.6	366	4.5
Medicaid/CHIP[3]	1,799	78.6	1,301	56.9	329	14.4	169	7.4
Other coverage[4]	2,181	72.1	1,667	55.1	309	10.2	205	6.8
No coverage	1,383	47.8	838	29.0	349	12.0	196	6.8

See notes on page 136.

Table 28 notes

*Estimates are considered unreliable because of low precision.

[1] Poverty status is based on respondent age, family income, family size, and composition using the U.S. Census Bureau's poverty thresholds. "Poor" persons are defined as living in households where the family income is less than 100 percent of the U.S. Census poverty threshold. "Near poor" persons have incomes of 100 percent to less than 200 percent of the poverty threshold. "Not poor" persons have incomes that are 200 percent of the poverty threshold or greater.

[2] Respondents could indicate multiple types of health insurance; thus, these response categories are not mutually exclusive.

[3] CHIP is the Children's Health Insurance Program (formerly State Children's Health Insurance Program [SCHIP]). Qualified individuals aged 19 or younger are eligible for this plan.

[4] Other health insurance is defined as having Medicare, Civilian Health and Medical Program of the Uniformed Services (CHAMPUS), TRICARE, Civilian Health and Medical Program of the Department of Veterans Affairs (CHAMPVA), Veterans Administration (VA), military health care, or any other type of health insurance.

NOTES: The National Survey on Drug Use and Health is a nationally representative survey of the civilian, noninstitutionalized population of the United States aged 12 or older. The survey interviews approximately 67,500 persons each year.

Respondents with unknown past year treatment data were excluded.

Major depressive episode (MDE) is defined as a period of at least 2 weeks when a person experienced a depressed mood or loss of interest or pleasure in daily activities and had a majority of specified depression symptoms. According to the *Diagnostic and Statistical Manual of Mental Disorders, Fourth Edition* (DSM-IV) (APA, 1994), two or more MDEs are necessary to meet the criteria for recurrent major depressive disorder.

SOURCE: National Survey on Drug Use and Health, 2009, Substance Abuse and Mental Health Services Administration, Office of Applied Studies.

Table 29. Number of admissions to and year-end residents in State and county psychiatric hospitals, by selected characteristics, United States, 2002 and 2005

[Data are based on reporting by State and county psychiatric hospitals]

Characteristic	Admissions		Residents	
	2002	2005	2002	2005
Total	**155,740**	**188,649**	**49,443**	**49,947**
Age				
Younger than 18	15,416	19,574	2,865	2,476
18–24	24,079	28,853	4,552	4,134
25–44	76,212	88,230	21,602	21,210
45–64	35,144	46,854	16,569	18,755
65 or older	4,889	5,138	3,855	3,372
Sex				
Male	103,156	132,154	—	—
Female	52,584	56,495	—	—
Hispanic origin and race				
White	89,973	117,702	28,820	28,469
African American	46,639	51,261	15,689	15,752
Asian or Pacific Islander	6,310	2,184	836	927
Hispanic	10,534	14,433	3,693	4,320
American Indian	2,284	3,069	405	479
Diagnosis				
Affective disorders	40,882	47,547	6,482	6,583
Schizophrenia	46,163	56,856	25,524	26,298
Alcohol use related	9,502	8,075	1,388	847
Substance use related	13,356	15,717	2,017	2,146
Other psychotic	12,852	15,682	3,253	2,857
Other nonpsychotic	18,038	24,561	2,320	2,489
All other	14,947	20,211	8,459	8,727

— Data not available.

NOTE: Annual Census of Admission and Resident Patient Characteristics, State and County Mental Hospital 24-Hour Services, collects annual aggregate data from each State on age, sex, race, and ethnicity, by diagnosis, for annual admissions and year-end residents.

SOURCES: Annual Census of State and County Mental Health Hospitals, 2002 and 2005, Center for Mental Health Services, Substance Abuse and Mental Health Services Administration.

Manderscheid, R. W., Atay, J. E., & Crider, R. A. (2009). Changing trends in State psychiatric hospital use from 2002 to 2005. *Psychiatric Services, 60*(1), 29–34. Reprinted with permission from *Psychiatric Services* (Copyright © 2010). American Psychiatric Association.

Table 30. Number and percentage of prescription mental health/substance abuse (MH/SA) medication fills for all medical conditions among persons aged 18 or older, by selected medication class, United States, 1996–2008

[Data are based on a nationally representative survey of households, medical providers, and employers]

Medication class	1996	1997	1998	1999	2000	2001	2002	2003	2004	2005	2006	2007	2008
All MH and/or SA medications (percent of all prescription fills)	9.2	10.0	10.1	9.7	10.5	10.9	11.1	10.9	11.1	12.0	11.6	11.8	12.0
All MH and/or SA medications (millions)	155.8	173.0	184.1	185.1	211.1	253.9	278.3	284.0	305.8	337.4	336.3	341.3	358.8
Antianxiety, all classes[1] (millions)	58.3	62.1	60.7	55.8	62.6	73.7	79.8	76.5	79.7	92.6	85.5	90.1	98.1
Antidepressants, all classes (millions)	76.0	84.0	93.9	94.9	109.1	133.6	150.7	158.1	172.2	183.8	185.5	181.1	186.3
Antipsychotics, all classes (millions)	12.9	16.1	15.5	14.8	18.3	20.5	20.1	18.9	19.7	24.0	26.1	27.6	28.7
Antimanics, anticonvulsants (millions)	6.2	7.5	7.9	6.2	11.5	12.9	13.2	14.0	14.3	13.3	13.7	17.1	16.9

[1] Antianxiety medications include sedative and hypnotic medications.

NOTES: The Medical Expenditure Panel Survey (MEPS) is a set of large-scale surveys of families and individuals, their medical providers (e.g., doctors, hospitals, pharmacies), and employers across the United States. Since 1996, MEPS has collected data on the specific health services that Americans use, how frequently they use them, the cost of these services, and how they are paid for, as well as data on the cost, scope, and breadth of health insurance held by and available to U.S. workers.

All classes combined do not add to total because the table does not detail classes of medication with a relatively small number of fills.

See Appendix C for complete list of medications. Categorization of medications follows that of the National Institute of Mental Health (http://www.nimh.nih.gov/health/publications/mental-health-medications/alphabetical-list-of-medications.shtml).

SOURCES: Medical Expenditure Panel Survey, 1996–2008, Center for Financing, Access, and Cost Trends, Agency for Healthcare Research and Quality.

Zuvekas, S. H. (2005). Prescription drugs and the changing patterns of treatment for mental disorders, 1996–2001. *Health Affairs, 24*(1), 195–205.

Table 31. Number and percentage of prescription mental health/substance abuse (MH/SA) medication fills for MH/SA conditions among persons aged 18 or older, by selected medication class, United States, 1996–2008

[Data are based on a nationally representative survey of households, medical providers, and employers]

Medication class	1996	1997	1998	1999	2000	2001	2002	2003	2004	2005	2006	2007	2008
MH and/or SA medications (percent of all prescription fills)	6.2	6.8	7.0	6.9	7.5	7.5	8.0	7.9	8.0	8.5	8.3	8.6	8.8
MH and/or SA medications (millions)	105.4	116.9	127.2	131.3	150.3	175.0	200.4	206.1	221.5	239.9	242.6	248.8	263.0
Antianxiety, all classes[1] (millions)	32.6	31.8	30.6	29.5	33.0	39.4	44.4	40.8	41.5	48.7	46.1	48.2	54.3
Antidepressants, all classes (millions)	55.9	63.0	74.4	74.6	86.1	102.3	120.1	127.6	141.5	149.7	150.7	148.0	154.7
Antipsychotics, all classes (millions)	9.3	12.8	11.7	10.9	14.4	15.1	16.2	15.0	15.5	18.5	20.6	22.8	23.0
Antimanics, anticonvulsants (millions)	6.2	7.5	7.9	6.2	11.5	12.9	13.2	14.0	14.3	13.3	13.7	17.1	16.9

[1] Antianxiety medications include sedative and hypnotic medications.

NOTES: The Medical Expenditure Panel Survey (MEPS) is a set of large-scale surveys of families and individuals, their medical providers (e.g., doctors, hospitals, pharmacies), and employers across the United States. Since 1996, MEPS has collected data on the specific health services that Americans use, how frequently they use them, the cost of these services, and how they are paid for, as well as data on the cost, scope, and breadth of health insurance held by and available to U.S. workers.

All classes combined do not add to total because the table does not detail classes of medication with a relatively small number of fills.

See Appendix C for complete list of medications. Categorization of medications follows that of the National Institute of Mental Health (http://www.nimh.nih.gov/health/publications/mental-health-medications/alphabetical-list-of-medications.shtml).

SOURCES: Medical Expenditure Panel Survey, 1996–2008, Center for Financing, Access, and Cost Trends, Agency for Healthcare Research and Quality.

Zuvekas, S. H. (2005). Prescription drugs and the changing patterns of treatment for mental disorders, 1996–2001. *Health Affairs, 24*(1), 195–205.

7. TABLES

7.2 Providers and Settings for Mental Health Services

7.2.1 Adult Mental Health Services

Specialty Mental Health Services

Nonspecialty Mental Health Services
Tables 32–44

Mental Health Service Capacity

7.2.2 Child Mental Health Services

Mental Health Services

Mental Health Service Capacity

7.2.3 Special Populations

Table 32. Number and percentage of emergency department (ED) visits by persons aged 10 or older with a primary diagnosis of a mental disorder, by diagnosis, United States, 2008

[Data are based on reporting by a nationally representative sample of EDs]

Category of primary diagnosis	ED visits (number)	ED visits (percent)	ED visits with mental health diagnosis (percent)
All ED visits—all diagnoses	107,748,264	100.0	. . .
Any primary mental health diagnosis	4,686,580	4.3	100.0
Adjustment disorders	108,940	0.1	2.3
Anxiety disorders	811,743	0.8	17.3
Attention deficit, conduct, and disruptive behavior disorders	78,687	0.1	1.7
Delirium, dementia, and amnestic and other cognitive disorders	188,842	0.2	4.0
Developmental disorders	31,660	0.0	0.7
Disorders usually diagnosed in infancy, childhood, or adolescence	9,957	0.0	0.2
Impulse control disorders, not elsewhere classified	16,515	0.0	0.4
Mood disorders	1,216,680	1.1	26.0
Personality disorders	15,576	0.0	0.3
Schizophrenia and other psychotic disorders	537,634	0.5	11.5
Alcohol-related disorders	994,092	0.9	21.2
Substance-related disorders	487,803	0.5	10.4
Suicide and intentional self-inflicted injury	45,665	0.0	1.0
Miscellaneous mental disorders	142,785	0.1	3.0

... Category not applicable.

NOTES: The 2008 Nationwide Emergency Department Sample yields national estimates of ED visits.

Diagnostic categories follow the Healthcare Cost and Utilization Project Clinical Classifications Software, which categorizes diagnoses by *International Classification of Diseases, 9th Revision, Clinical Modification* (ICD-9-CM) (WHO, 1977) codes. See http://www.hcup-us.ahrq.gov/toolssoftware/ccs/CCSUsersGuide.pdf for more details on diagnosis categories. Omitted diagnoses include tobacco use disorders.

SOURCE: 2008 Nationwide Emergency Department Sample, Healthcare Cost and Utilization Project, Agency for Healthcare Research and Quality.

Table 33. Number and percentage of emergency department (ED) visits by persons aged 18 or older with a primary diagnosis of a mental disorder, by diagnosis and age group, United States, 2008

[Data are based on reporting by a nationally representative sample of EDs]

Category of primary diagnosis	Aged 18 to 44			Aged 45 to 64			Aged 65 or older		
	ED visits (number)	ED visits (percent)	ED visits with mental health diagnosis (percent)	ED visits (number)	ED visits (percent)	ED visits with mental health diagnosis (percent)	ED visits (number)	ED visits (percent)	ED visits with mental health diagnosis (percent)
All ED visits—all diagnoses	50,334,829	100.0	...	26,842,045	100.0	...	21,338,810	100.0	...
Any primary mental health diagnosis	2,492,675	5.0	100.0	1,342,897	5.0	100.0	436,818	2.0	100.0
Adjustment disorders	59,028	0.1	2.4	19,996	0.1	1.5	4,966	0.0	1.1
Anxiety disorders	484,066	1.0	19.4	193,682	0.7	14.4	72,264	0.3	16.5
Attention deficit, conduct, and disruptive behavior disorders	16,435	0.0	0.7	5,579	0.0	0.4	4,050	0.0	0.9
Delirium, dementia, and amnestic and other cognitive disorders	26,241	0.1	1.1	19,471	0.1	1.4	134,938	0.6	30.9
Developmental disorders	11,803	0.0	0.5	7,094	0.0	0.5	8,342	0.0	1.9
Disorders usually diagnosed in infancy, childhood, or adolescence	2,923	0.0	0.1	349	0.0	0.0	*	*	*
Impulse control disorders, not elsewhere classified	8,374	0.0	0.3	1,714	0.0	0.1	*	*	*
Mood disorders	676,316	1.3	27.1	329,766	1.2	24.6	67,172	0.3	15.4
Personality disorders	8,203	0.0	0.3	2,610	0.0	0.2	1,280	0.0	0.3
Schizophrenia and other psychotic disorders	271,630	0.5	10.9	190,345	0.7	14.2	62,927	0.3	14.4
Alcohol-related disorders	492,542	1.0	19.8	412,493	1.5	30.7	44,981	0.2	10.3
Substance-related disorders	315,360	0.6	12.7	122,252	0.5	9.1	25,972	0.1	5.9
Suicide and intentional self-inflicted injury	26,066	0.1	1.0	10,195	0.0	0.8	985	0.0	0.2
Miscellaneous mental disorders	93,689	0.2	3.8	27,353	0.1	2.0	8,522	0.0	2.0

See notes on page 144.

Table 33 notes

*Estimates are considered unreliable.

... Category not applicable.

NOTES: The 2008 Nationwide Emergency Department Sample yields national estimates of ED visits.

Diagnostic categories follow the Healthcare Cost and Utilization Project Clinical Classifications Software, which categorizes diagnoses by *International Classification of Diseases, 9th Revision, Clinical Modification* (ICD-9-CM) (WHO, 1977) codes. See http://www.hcup-us.ahrq.gov/toolssoftware/ccs/CCSUsersGuide.pdf for more details on diagnosis categories. Omitted diagnoses include tobacco use disorders.

SOURCE: 2008 Nationwide Emergency Department Sample, Healthcare Cost and Utilization Project, Agency for Healthcare Research and Quality.

Table 34. Number and percentage of emergency department (ED) visits by persons aged 10 to 17 with a primary diagnosis of a mental disorder, by diagnosis, United States, 2008

[Data are based on reporting by a nationally representative sample of EDs]

Category of primary diagnosis	ED visits (number)	ED visits (percent)	ED visits with mental health diagnosis (percent)
All ED visits—all diagnoses	9,232,580	100.0	...
Any primary mental health diagnosis	414,189	4.5	100.0
Adjustment disorders	24,950	0.3	6.0
Anxiety disorders	61,732	0.7	14.9
Attention deficit, conduct, and disruptive behavior disorders	52,622	0.6	12.7
Delirium, dementia, and amnestic and other cognitive disorders	8,193	0.1	2.0
Developmental disorders	4,421	0.0	1.1
Disorders usually diagnosed in infancy, childhood, or adolescence	6,547	0.1	1.6
Impulse control disorders, not elsewhere classified	6,146	0.1	1.5
Mood disorders	143,427	1.6	34.6
Personality disorders	3,483	0.0	0.8
Schizophrenia and other psychotic disorders	12,733	0.1	3.1
Alcohol-related disorders	44,076	0.5	10.6
Substance-related disorders	24,218	0.3	5.8
Suicide and intentional self-inflicted injury	8,419	0.1	2.0
Miscellaneous mental disorders	13,221	0.1	3.2

... Category not applicable.

NOTES: The 2008 Nationwide Emergency Department Sample yields national estimates of ED visits.

Diagnostic categories follow the Healthcare Cost and Utilization Project Clinical Classifications Software, which categorizes diagnoses by *International Classification of Diseases, 9th Revision, Clinical Modification* (ICD-9-CM) (WHO, 1977) codes. See http://www.hcup-us.ahrq.gov/toolssoftware/ccs/CCSUsersGuide.pdf for more details on diagnosis categories. Omitted diagnoses include tobacco use disorders.

SOURCE: 2008 Nationwide Emergency Department Sample, Healthcare Cost and Utilization Project, Agency for Healthcare Research and Quality.

Table 35. Number and percentage of emergency department (ED) visits by persons aged 10 or older with a primary and/or secondary diagnosis of mental disorder, by diagnosis, United States, 2008

[Data are based on reporting by a nationally representative sample of EDs]

Category of primary or secondary diagnosis	ED visits (number)	ED visits (percent)	ED visits with mental health diagnosis (percent)
All ED visits—all diagnoses	107,748,264	100.0	...
Any primary or secondary mental health diagnosis[1]	12,171,621	11.3	100.0
Adjustment disorders	223,487	0.2	1.8
Anxiety disorders	3,577,736	3.3	29.4
Attention deficit, conduct, and disruptive behavior disorders	447,070	0.4	3.7
Delirium, dementia, and amnestic and other cognitive disorders	2,496,495	2.3	20.5
Developmental disorders	384,900	0.4	3.2
Disorders usually diagnosed in infancy, childhood, or adolescence	75,138	0.1	0.6
Impulse control disorders, not elsewhere classified	40,511	0.0	0.3
Mood disorders	5,924,267	5.5	48.7
Personality disorders	234,148	0.2	1.9
Schizophrenia and other psychotic disorders	1,265,830	1.2	10.4
Alcohol-related disorders	3,001,281	2.8	24.7
Substance-related disorders	2,263,900	2.1	18.6
Suicide and intentional self-inflicted injury[1]	1,048,235	1.0	8.6
Miscellaneous mental disorders	345,628	0.3	2.8

... Category not applicable.

[1] Includes some cases with an external cause of injury code (E-code) indicating suicide and no other mental health diagnoses.

NOTES: The 2008 Nationwide Emergency Department Sample yields national estimates of ED visits.

Multiple diagnoses within a single diagnosis category are counted as one occurrence. Diagnoses can total to more than 100 percent because a discharge may have more than one mental health diagnosis.

Diagnostic categories follow the Healthcare Cost and Utilization Project Clinical Classifications Software, which categorizes diagnoses by *International Classification of Diseases, 9th Revision, Clinical Modification* (ICD-9-CM) (WHO, 1977) codes. See http://www.hcup-us.ahrq.gov/toolssoftware/ccs/CCSUsersGuide.pdf for more details on diagnosis categories. Omitted diagnoses include tobacco use disorders.

SOURCE: 2008 Nationwide Emergency Department Sample, Healthcare Cost and Utilization Project, Agency for Healthcare Research and Quality.

Table 36. Number and percentage of emergency department (ED) visits by persons aged 18 or older with a primary and/or secondary diagnosis of mental disorder, by diagnosis and age group, United States, 2008

[Data are based on reporting by a nationally representative sample of EDs]

Category of primary or secondary diagnosis	Aged 18 to 44			Aged 45 to 64			Aged 65 or older		
	ED visits (number)	ED visits (percent)	ED visits with mental health diagnosis (percent)	ED visits (number)	ED visits (percent)	ED visits with mental health diagnosis (percent)	ED visits (number)	ED visits (percent)	ED visits with mental health diagnosis (percent)
All ED visits—all diagnoses	50,334,829	100.0	...	26,842,045	100.0	...	21,338,810	100.0	...
Any primary or secondary mental health diagnosis[1]	4,429,896	8.8	100.0	3,225,767	12.0	100.0	3,794,637	17.8	100.0
Adjustment disorders	107,513	0.2	2.4	50,861	0.2	1.6	29,046	0.1	0.8
Anxiety disorders	1,627,043	3.2	36.7	1,075,157	4.0	33.3	726,838	3.4	19.2
Attention deficit, conduct, and disruptive behavior disorders	158,616	0.3	3.6	36,161	0.1	1.1	14,666	0.1	0.4
Delirium, dementia, and amnestic and other cognitive disorders	60,763	0.1	1.4	139,202	0.5	4.3	2,282,225	10.7	60.1
Developmental disorders	147,550	0.3	3.3	128,067	0.5	4.0	72,741	0.3	1.9
Disorders usually diagnosed in infancy, childhood, or adolescence	29,125	0.1	0.7	6,726	0.0	0.2	1,765	0.0	0.0
Impulse control disorders, not elsewhere classified	21,012	0.0	0.5	5,732	0.0	0.2	1,464	0.0	0.0
Mood disorders	2,357,836	4.7	53.2	1,967,268	7.3	61.0	1,313,946	6.2	34.6
Personality disorders	142,636	0.3	3.2	66,567	0.2	2.1	12,769	0.1	0.3
Schizophrenia and other psychotic disorders	498,381	1.0	11.3	470,041	1.8	14.6	274,038	1.3	7.2
Alcohol-related disorders	1,349,513	2.7	30.5	1,314,309	4.9	40.7	264,487	1.2	7.0
Substance-related disorders	1,354,419	2.7	30.6	710,567	2.6	22.0	114,540	0.5	3.0
Suicide and intentional self-inflicted injury[1]	621,430	1.2	14.0	265,735	1.0	8.2	34,787	0.2	0.9
Miscellaneous mental disorders	213,407	0.4	4.8	69,279	0.3	2.1	35,772	0.2	0.9

See notes on page 148.

Table 36 notes

... Category not applicable.

[1] Includes some cases with an external cause of injury code (E-code) indicating suicide and no other mental health diagnoses.

NOTES: The 2008 Nationwide Emergency Department Sample yields national estimates of ED visits.

Multiple diagnoses within a single diagnosis category are counted as one occurrence. Diagnoses can total to more than 100 percent because a discharge may have more than one mental health diagnosis.

Diagnostic categories follow the Healthcare Cost and Utilization Project Clinical Classifications Software, which categorizes diagnoses by *International Classification of Diseases, 9th Revision, Clinical Modification* (ICD-9-CM) (WHO, 1977) codes. See http://www.hcup-us.ahrq.gov/toolssoftware/ccs/CCSUsersGuide.pdf for more details on diagnosis categories. Omitted diagnoses include tobacco use disorders.

SOURCE: 2008 Nationwide Emergency Department Sample, Healthcare Cost and Utilization Project, Agency for Healthcare Research and Quality.

Table 37. Number and percentage of emergency department (ED) visits by persons aged 10 to 17 with a primary and/or secondary diagnosis of mental disorder, by diagnosis, United States, 2008

[Data are based on reporting by a nationally representative sample of EDs]

Category of primary or secondary diagnosis	ED visits (number)	ED visits (percent)	ED visits with mental health diagnosis (percent)
All ED visits—all diagnoses	9,232,580	100.0	. . .
Any primary or secondary mental health diagnosis[1]	721,321	7.8	100.0
Adjustment disorders	36,066	0.4	5.0
Anxiety disorders	148,699	1.6	20.6
Attention deficit, conduct, and disruptive behavior disorders	237,627	2.6	32.9
Delirium, dementia, and amnestic and other cognitive disorders	14,305	0.2	2.0
Developmental disorders	36,541	0.4	5.1
Disorders usually diagnosed in infancy, childhood, or adolescence	37,522	0.4	5.2
Impulse control disorders, not elsewhere classified	12,303	0.1	1.7
Mood disorders	285,218	3.1	39.5
Personality disorders	12,176	0.1	1.7
Schizophrenia and other psychotic disorders	23,369	0.3	3.2
Alcohol-related disorders	72,972	0.8	10.1
Substance-related disorders	84,374	0.9	11.7
Suicide and intentional self-inflicted injury[1]	126,283	1.4	17.5
Miscellaneous mental disorders	27,170	0.3	3.8

... Category not applicable.

[1] Includes some cases with an external cause of injury code (E-code) indicating suicide and no other mental health diagnoses.

NOTES: The 2008 Nationwide Emergency Department Sample yields national estimates of ED visits.

Multiple diagnoses within a single diagnosis category are counted as one occurrence. Diagnoses can total to more than 100 percent because a discharge may have more than one mental health diagnosis.

Diagnostic categories follow the Healthcare Cost and Utilization Project Clinical Classifications Software, which categorizes diagnoses by *International Classification of Diseases, 9th Revision, Clinical Modification* (ICD-9-CM) (WHO, 1977) codes. See http://www.hcup-us.ahrq.gov/toolssoftware/ccs/CCSUsersGuide.pdf for more details on diagnosis categories. Omitted diagnoses include tobacco use disorders.

SOURCE: 2008 Nationwide Emergency Department Sample, Healthcare Cost and Utilization Project, Agency for Healthcare Research and Quality.

Table 38. Number of visits to physicians' offices and percentage of visits for mental health disorders, by physician specialty, age group, and primary or any mental health diagnosis, United States, 2008

[Data are based on reporting by a nationally representative sample of office-based physicians]

Physician category	All ages[1]			Aged 1 to 21			Aged 22 to 64			Aged 65 or older		
	All diagnoses (1,000s)	Primary mental diagnosis (percent)	Any mental diagnosis (percent)	All diagnoses (1,000s)	Primary mental diagnosis (percent)	Any mental diagnosis (percent)	All diagnoses (1,000s)	Primary mental diagnosis (percent)	Any mental diagnosis (percent)	All diagnoses (1,000s)	Primary mental diagnosis (percent)	Any mental diagnosis (percent)
Total[1]	**955,969**	**3.9**	**6.2**	**169,344**	**4.9**	**6.4**	**501,119**	**5.0**	**7.8**	**256,135**	**1.7**	**3.8**
General and family practice	224,443	3.6	8.1	33,977	4.8	7.9	138,876	3.9	9.1	47,785	*	6.0
Internal medicine	152,909	3.0	7.5	3,641	*	*	88,697	3.6	8.0	60,481	*	6.9
Pediatrics	119,797	2.0	3.1	92,939	2.5	4.0	*	...	...	...	...	...
Psychiatry	22,990	92.3	95.3	4,234	93.6	94.3	16,896	91.7	95.4	1,833	93.9	96.1
All other specialties (combined)	435,830	0.3	1.0	34,553	*	1.1	254,645	*	1.3	145,689	*	0.6

*Estimates are considered unreliable.

... Category not applicable.

[1] "All ages" group includes people younger than 1 year.

NOTE: The National Ambulatory Medical Care Survey is a national probability sample survey of visits to office-based physicians.

SOURCE: National Ambulatory Medical Care Survey, 2008, Centers for Disease Control and Prevention, National Center for Health Statistics.

Table 39. Number and percentage of visits to physicians' offices for primary mental health diagnosis, by physician specialty and age group, United States, 2008

[Data are based on reporting by a nationally representative sample of office-based physicians]

Physician category	All ages[1]		Aged 1 to 21		Aged 22 to 64		Aged 65 or older	
	Number (1,000s)	Percent	Number (1,000s)	Percent	Number (1,000s)	Percent	Number (1,000s)	Percent
Total[1]	**37,686**	**100.0**	**8,312**	**100.0**	**24,964**	**100.0**	**4,382**	**100.0**
General and family practice	8,149	21.6	1,637	19.7	5,477	21.9	*	*
Internal medicine	4,661	12.4	*	*	3,166	12.7	*	*
Pediatrics	2,359	6.3	2,342	28.2	...	...	...	...
Psychiatry	21,214	56.3	3,965	47.7	15,501	62.1	1,721	39.3
All other specialties (combined)	1,303	3.5	*	*	*	*	*	*

*Estimates are considered unreliable.

... Category not applicable.

[1] "All ages" group includes people younger than 1 year.

NOTE: The National Ambulatory Medical Care Survey is a national probability sample survey of visits to office-based physicians.

SOURCE: National Ambulatory Medical Care Survey, 2008, Centers for Disease Control and Prevention, National Center for Health Statistics.

Table 40. Number and percentage of visits to physicians' offices for any mental health diagnosis, by physician specialty and age group, United States, 2008

[Data are based on reporting by a nationally representative sample of office-based physicians]

Physician category	All ages[1]		Aged 1 to 21		Aged 22 to 64		Aged 65 or older	
	Number (1,000s)	Percent	Number (1,000s)	Percent	Number (1,000s)	Percent	Number (1,000s)	Percent
Total[1]	**59,730**	**100.0**	**10,893**	**100.0**	**39,137**	**100.0**	**9,673**	**100.0**
General and family practice	18,149	30.4	2,680	24.6	12,590	32.2	2,878	29.8
Internal medicine	11,398	19.1	*	*	7,092	18.1	4,164	43.0
Pediatrics	3,710	6.2	3,693	33.9	...	...	...	...
Psychiatry	21,908	36.7	3,992	36.7	16,126	41.2	1,762	18.2
All other specialties (combined)	4,566	7.6	385	3.5	3,311	8.5	870	9.0

*Estimates are considered unreliable.

... Category not applicable.

[1] "All ages" group includes people younger than 1 year.

NOTE: The National Ambulatory Medical Care Survey is a national probability sample survey of visits to office-based physicians.

SOURCE: National Ambulatory Medical Care Survey, 2008, Centers for Disease Control and Prevention, National Center for Health Statistics.

Table 41. Percentage of nursing homes, home health care agencies, and hospice facilities providing mental health services, United States, selected years 1999–2007

[Data are based on a nationally representative sample of nursing homes, home health care agencies, and hospice facilities]

Type of facility	1999–2000[1] (percent)	2004[1] (percent)	2007[1] (percent)
Nursing homes	79.5	77.7	...
Regular basis only	...	25.1	...
On-call only	...	24.2	...
Both regular and on-call	...	28.4	...
Home health care only	16.5	...	17.5
Hospice care only	55.0	...	45.0
Home health and hospice care	45.5	...	38.3

... Category not applicable.

[1] The National Nursing Home Survey was conducted in 1999 and 2004. The National Home and Hospice Care Survey was conducted in 2000 and 2007.

NOTES: The National Nursing Home Survey is a nationally representative probability sample of 1,500 nursing homes, their residents, and their staff. The sample shown consists of 1,492,207 nursing home residents.

The 2007 National Home and Hospice Care Survey is one in a continuing series of nationally representative sample surveys of U.S. home health and hospice agencies. It is designed to provide descriptive information on home health and hospice agencies, their staff, their services, and their patients. In 2000, 1,425 agencies participated in the survey. In 2007, 1,036 agencies participated. Agencies were asked whether they provided "psychological services" in the 2000 survey and whether they provided "mental health services" in the 2007 survey.

SOURCES: National Nursing Home Survey, 1999, Centers for Disease Control and Prevention; National Home and Hospice Care Survey, 2007, Centers for Disease Control and Prevention.

Table 42. Number of members served in clubhouses, United States, 2010

[Data are from an annual survey of clubhouses]

Membership	ICCD certified ($N = 80$)		Non-ICCD certified ($N = 34$)	
	Number of clubhouses responding	Mean	Number of clubhouses responding	Mean
Average daily attendance	79	51.4	31	31.3
Evening or weekend	77	77.5	31	29.4
Active membership	78	167.7	31	92.9
Total membership	72	970.9	29	494.0

NOTES: The International Survey of Clubhouses was conducted by the International Center for Clubhouse Development (ICCD). The survey gathers information about clubhouse characteristics, governance and administration, membership, staffing and staff credentials, unit structure, employment, housing activities, services, and participation in clubhouse training. In 2010, there were 197 ICCD clubhouses in the United States; however, data were only available for 114 of them. The number of clubhouses responding varied across the survey items.

Fountain House in New York City has been excluded because its membership is considerably larger in number than other clubhouses.

SOURCE: International Survey of Clubhouses, 2010, ICCD.

Table 43. Demographic and diagnostic information for members of clubhouses, United States, 2010

[Data are from an annual survey of clubhouses]

Characteristic	ICCD certified ($N = 80$)		Non-ICCD certified ($N = 34$)	
	Number of clubhouses responding	Mean (percent)	Number of clubhouses responding	Mean (percent)
Age				
Younger than 20	67	1.7	22	1.3
20–25	77	5.4	25	5.5
26–30	76	7.8	26	8.3
31–40	77	19.1	26	15.8
41–50	77	29.4	26	28.5
51–60	76	24.2	26	23.8
61–70	76	7.4	25	9.2
Older than 70	57	1.4	19	1.8
Unknown	40	3.6	40	6.0
Sex				
Male	67	57.1	26	55.9
Female	67	43.0	26	44.1
Race/ethnicity				
White/Caucasian	78	61.7	27	49.2
Hispanic	**	4.8	27	8.8
Black/African American	74	20.2	27	29.3
American Indian/Alaska Native	52	1.7	28	1.4
Asian	61	4.3	26	1.9
Native Hawaiian or Other Pacific Islander	47	1.6	17	0.1
Unknown	55	5.6	18	9.2
Diagnoses				
Schizophrenia or schizophreniform disorders	52	43.6	17	47.8
Bipolar disorder	52	18.2	17	18.3
Depression	51	14.5	17	14.2
Other	43	5.0	16	7.6
Unknown	38	18.6	6	12.2

**Original estimate omitted.

NOTE: The International Survey of Clubhouses was conducted by the International Center for Clubhouse Development (ICCD). The survey gathers information about clubhouse characteristics, governance and administration, membership, staffing and staff credentials, unit structure, employment, housing activities, services, and participation in clubhouse training. In 2010, there were 197 ICCD clubhouses in the United States; however, data were only available for 114 of them. The number of clubhouses responding varied across the survey items. Sex and age were available for clubhouses with active membership.

SOURCE: International Survey of Clubhouses, 2010, ICCD.

Table 44. Percentage of clubhouses, by funding source and management structure, United States, 2010

[Data are from an annual survey of clubhouses]

Funding source and management structure	ICCD certified ($N = 75$) (percent)	Non-ICCD certified ($N = 30$) (percent)
Funding source[1]		
State mental health agency	46.2	31.8
Social services	0.3	1.8
Vocational rehabilitation agency	2.9	1.6
Labor department	0.0	0.0
County/borough government	8.6	18.0
Local/municipal government	4.5	0.5
National grants	0.3	0.1
Public insurance programs (e.g., Medicaid)	23.3	27.3
Other government funding	2.5	7.1
Private insurance programs	0.1	1.0
Foundations/grants	3.7	2.3
Donations and other private sources	1.4	0.8
Income generating activities (e.g., thrift shop, food sales, rents)	2.5	3.8
Other private funding	1.8	1.1
Unknown	1.8	0.7
Management structure		
Clubhouse is funded all or in part by Medicaid	42.0	44.0[2]
Clubhouse has its own Board of Directors	38.0[3]	9.0[2]
Clubhouse has an Advisory Board	62.0[3]	66.0[2]

[1] Funding is averaged across all clubhouses.

[2] $N = 32$

[3] $N = 79$

NOTE: The International Survey of Clubhouses was conducted by the International Center for Clubhouse Development (ICCD). The survey gathers information about clubhouse characteristics, governance and administration, membership, staffing and staff credentials, unit structure, employment, housing activities, services, and participation in clubhouse training. In 2010, there were 197 ICCD clubhouses in the United States; however, data were only available for 114 of them.

SOURCE: International Survey of Clubhouses, 2010, ICCD.

7. TABLES

7.2 Providers and Settings for Mental Health Services

7.2.1 Adult Mental Health Services

Specialty Mental Health Services

Nonspecialty Mental Health Services

Mental Health Service Capacity
Tables 45–55

7.2.2 Child Mental Health Services

Mental Health Services

Mental Health Service Capacity

7.2.3 Special Populations

Table 45. Number and percentage of clinically trained mental health personnel, by discipline and distribution, by sex, age, and Hispanic origin and race, United States, selected years

[Data are based on association membership and certification data]

Characteristic	Psychiatry[1]: 2006	Psychology[2]: 2006	Advanced practice psychiatric nursing[3]: 2006	Counseling[4]: 2008	Marriage and family therapy[5]: 2006	Social work[6]: 2004
Total (N)	**24,758**	**92,227**	**9,742**	**128,886**	**48,666**	**244,900**
Male (N)	17,047	42,425	659	45,110	—	44,082
Age						
Younger than 35	0.7	3.5	4.6	11.4	1.7	8.1
35–44	11.8	12.7	14.6	20.8	7.9	17.3
45–54	21.8	22.8	29.8	21.1	20.5	32.2
55–64	26.3	36.9	20.6	32.8	41.6	32.6
65–69	39.2	24.0	1.4	13.2	22.0	9.8
Unknown	0.2	0.0	29.1	—	6.2	0.0
Hispanic origin and race						
American Indian/ Alaska Native	0.1	0.3	0.9	0.5	1.0	0.2
Asian/Pacific Islander	10.7	1.3	2.0	1.2	1.0	1.2
Hispanic	4.3	2.0	—	2.7	4.8	5.4
Black (not Hispanic)	2.3	1.5	2.7	5.9	1.0	5.6
White (not Hispanic)	73.5	79.4	82.2	78.8	97.1	84.5
Multiracial	1.1	...	...	...	...	...
Other	0.6	...	...	...	...	...
Not specified	7.4	—	12.1	10.8	0.0	3.1
Female (N)	7,661	49,802	9,083	83,776	—	200,818
Age						
Younger than 35	2.3	11.0	3.6	21.1	3.6	16.3
35–44	23.2	24.7	7.6	23.0	10.0	22.2
45–54	33.7	26.2	25.8	20.3	21.5	32.0
55–64	25.5	27.2	28.9	25.7	38.8	23.0
65 or older	14.9	10.9	6.5	9.4	19.7	6.3
Unknown	0.4	0.0	27.6	—	6.3	0.2
Hispanic origin and race						
American Indian/ Alaska Native	0.1	0.3	0.6	0.5	1.1	0.6
Asian/Pacific Islander	15.5	1.9	2.0	1.2	1.1	1.7
Hispanic	4.4	2.5	—	2.6	3.4	4.2
Black (not Hispanic)	4.8	2.4	3.0	6.6	2.8	6.2
White (not Hispanic)	69.8	68.1	85.0	80.7	96.0	85.2
Multiracial	0.9	...	...	...	...	...
Other	0.7	...	...	...	...	...
Not specified	3.8	24.9	9.3	8.4	0.0	2.1

See notes on page 159.

Table 45 notes

— Data not available.

... Category not applicable.

[1] 2006 American Psychiatric Association membership residing in the United States, excluding medical students; psychiatric residents; international members and fellows; inactive members, associates, and fellows; and honorary fellows. Sex was not reported for 50 psychiatrists.

[2] American Psychological Association Member Directory 2006, compiled by American Psychological Association Center for Workforce Studies. For men, "not specified" includes 15.3 percent not specified and 0.2 percent multiethnic; for women, "not specified" includes 24.4 percent not specified and 0.5 percent multiethnic.

[3] The data source is the American Nurses Credentialing Center (ANCC) of all Advanced Practice Psychiatric Nurses who are certified in 2006.

[4] 2008 National Board for Certified Counselors certification directory and national job analysis, American Counseling Association membership directory, and licensure data provided by individual States.

[5] Data on age were obtained from the American Association for Marriage and Family Therapy (AAMFT) Membership Database of clinical members of AAMFT as of the end of 2006. Data on race were obtained from the 2004 AAMFT Practice Research Network project funded by the Center for Substance Abuse Treatment. Data were collected from a random sample of AAMFT clinical members. The "Hispanic" category was treated as a separate question; accordingly, percentages do not sum up to 100 percent.

[6] For social work, the Association for Social Work Boards estimates the number of licensed social workers to be 310,000. This number excludes bachelor level, doctorate level, and nondegreed licensed social workers. An estimated 79 percent of this number, or 244,900, have MSWs and are thus eligible to hold clinical licenses. The proportion of these MSWs that actually do hold clinical licenses is unknown. Hence, for purposes of this table, the total number of clinically trained social workers is considered to be 244,900.

NOTES: Originally published in Substance Abuse and Mental Health Services Administration (SAMHSA). (2010). *Mental Health, United States, 2008* (DHHS Publication No. SMA 10-4590). Rockville, MD: Center for Mental Health Services, SAMHSA.

Counts of mental health personnel are for clinically active and clinically trained personnel.

SOURCE: Data are drawn from multiple sources and are delineated in the footnotes.

Table 46. Number of mental health organizations with 24-hour hospital/residential treatment settings and number of beds, by type of organization, United States, selected years 1986–2004

[Data are based on reporting by a sample of mental health organizations and general hospitals with separate psychiatric services]

Type of organization	1986	1990	1992	1994	1998	2000	2002	2004
Total mental health organizations								
All organizations[1]	3,039	3,430	3,415	3,827	3,729	3,199	3,032	2,891
Department of Veterans Affairs Medical Centers[2]	124	130	133	135	123	133	131	—
State and county mental hospitals	285	273	273	256	229	223	222	237
Private psychiatric hospitals	314	462	475	430	348	269	253	264
Non-Federal general hospitals with separate psychiatric services	1,287	1,571	1,517	1,531	1,593	1,325	1,232	1,230
All other mental health organizations[3]	592	493	520	1,016	975	774	686	702
Beds per 100,000 civilian population[3]								
All organizations[1]	111.7	111.6	107.5	112.1	99.5	75.4	73.3	71.2
Department of Veterans Affairs Medical Centers[2]	11.2	8.9	8.9	8.2	6.3	3.3	3.4	—
State and county mental hospitals	49.7	40.5	36.9	31.6	25.6	21.5	19.9	19.1
Private psychiatric hospitals	12.6	18.4	17.3	16.4	12.4	9.4	8.7	9.5
Non-Federal general hospitals with separate psychiatric services	19.1	21.9	20.7	20.4	20.2	14.1	14	13.9
All other mental health organizations[3]	8.8	9.7	11.7	23.2	23.1	15.3	13.9	17.3

— Data not available.

[1] This table excludes residential treatment centers for children with emotional disturbance, so the sum of the organizations does not add up to the total of "all organizations." Data on residential treatment centers for children with emotional disturbance are presented in Tables 64 and 65.

[2] Department of Veterans Affairs Medical Centers were not included in the 2004 survey.

[3] Includes freestanding psychiatric outpatient clinics, partial care organizations, and multiservice mental health organizations.

[4] Civilian population estimates for 2000 and beyond are based on the 2000 census as of July 1; population estimates for 1992–1998 are 1990 postcensal estimates.

NOTES: The Survey of Mental Health Organizations was a biennial survey with two phases. In the first phase, limited data were collected from all mental health organizations. In the second phase, more detailed data were collected from a sample of specialty mental health organizations.

Changes to the design of the survey do not permit updates to be made to the Survey of Mental Health Organizations. Updates may be possible in the future.

SOURCE: Survey of Mental Health Organizations, 1986–2004, Substance Abuse and Mental Health Services Administration.

Table 47. Number of mental health organizations with 24-hour hospital/residential treatment settings and number of beds, by type of organization, United States, 2008

[Data are based on reporting by a sample of mental health facilities]

Type of organization	Number
Total mental health organizations	
All organizations[1]	3,130
Department of Veterans Affairs Medical Centers	130
State and county mental hospitals[2]	241
Private psychiatric hospitals	256
Non-Federal general hospitals with separate psychiatric services	1,292
All other mental health organizations[3]	673
Beds per 100,000 civilian population	
All organizations[1]	78.6
Department of Veterans Affairs Medical Centers	3.9
State and county mental hospitals[2]	12.3
Private psychiatric hospitals	8.4
Non-Federal general hospitals with separate psychiatric services	17.9
All other mental health organizations[3]	19.6

[1] This table excludes residential treatment centers for children with emotional disturbance, so the sum of the organizations does not add up to the total of "all organizations." Data on residential treatment centers for children with emotional disturbance are presented in Tables 64 and 65.

[2] Includes hospitals owned by district/regional authority.

[3] Includes freestanding psychiatric outpatient clinics, partial care organizations, and multiservice mental health organizations.

NOTE: The 2008 National Survey of Mental Health Treatment Facilities includes approximately 15,000 point-of-contact facilities nationwide representing approximately 4,400 mental health organizations nationwide.

SOURCE: 2008 National Survey of Mental Health Treatment Facilities, Substance Abuse and Mental Health Services Administration.

Table 48. Number and percentage of State correctional facilities offering various mental health services, by type of facility, United States, 2000

[Data are based on reporting by a sample of State and Federal adult correctional facilities]

Mental health service	All facilities		Confinement facilities[1]		Community-based facilities[2]	
	Number	Percent	Number	Percent	Number	Percent
Total	**1,558**	**100.0**	**1,109**	**100.0**	**449**	**100.0**
Any screening/treatment	1,394	91.8	1,047	95.4	347	82.2
Screen inmates at intake	1,055	69.5	855	77.9	200	47.4
Conduct psychiatric assessments	990	65.2	864	78.8	126	29.9
Provide 24-hour mental health care	776	51.1	693	63.2	83	19.7
Provide therapy/counseling	1,073	70.6	926	84.4	147	34.8
Distribute psychotropic medications	1,115	73.4	910	83.0	205	48.6
Help released inmates obtain services	1,006	66.2	790	72.0	216	51.2
No screening/treatment	125	8.2	50	4.6	75	17.8
Not reported	39	2.5	12	1.1	27	6.0

[1] Correctional facilities were classified as confinement facilities if fewer than 50 percent of the inmates were regularly permitted to leave unaccompanied.

[2] Facilities were classified as community-based if 50 percent or more of their inmates were regularly permitted to leave unaccompanied or if their primary function was community corrections. Such facilities include halfway houses and restitution, prerelease, work release, and study release centers.

NOTES: *Mental Health Treatment in State Prisons, 2000*, reports on facility policies related to screening inmates at intake, conducting psychiatric or psychological evaluations, and providing treatment (including 24-hour mental health care, therapy/counseling, and use of psychotropic medications) in State prisons. This report is based on the 2000 Census of State and Federal Adult Correctional Facilities, which gathered data from 1,668 separate institutions. *Mental Health Treatment in State Prisons* excludes 84 Federal facilities and 26 privately operated facilities in which at least half of the inmates were under Federal authority.

Table originally published in Substance Abuse and Mental Health Services Administration (SAMHSA). (2010). *Mental Health, United States, 2008* (DHHS Publication No. SMA 10-4590). Rockville, MD: Center for Mental Health Services, SAMHSA.

SOURCE: Beck, A. J., & Maruschak, L. M. (2001). *Mental health treatment in State prisons, 2000* (NCJ 188215). Washington, DC: U.S. Department of Justice, Office of Justice Programs, Bureau of Justice Statistics. Retrieved from http://bjs.ojp.usdoj.gov/content/pub/pdf/mhtsp00.pdf

Table 49. Percentage of inmates with a mental health problem in State and Federal correctional facilities (2004) and in local jails (2002) receiving mental health treatment, United States

[Data are based on a survey of inmates]

Type of mental health treatment	2004		2002
	State prison inmates (percent)	Federal prison inmates (percent)	Local jail inmates (percent)
Ever received mental health treatment	49.3	35.3	42.7
Had overnight hospital stay	20.0	9.5	18.0
Used prescribed medications	39.5	28.0	32.7
Had professional mental health therapy	35.4	25.6	31.1
Received treatment during year before arrest	22.3	14.9	22.6
Had overnight hospital stay	5.8	3.2	6.6
Used prescribed medications	15.8	10.1	16.9
On prescribed medication at time of arrest	11.3	7.3	12.3
Had professional mental health therapy	11.5	8.0	12.3
Received treatment after admission	33.8	24.0	17.5
Had overnight hospital stay	5.4	2.7	2.2
Used prescribed medications	26.8	19.5	14.8
Had professional mental health therapy	22.6	15.1	7.3

NOTES: The Survey of Inmates in State and Federal Correctional Facilities, 2004, and the Survey of Inmates in Local Jails, 2002, included a modified structured clinical interview for the *Diagnostic and Statistical Manual of Mental Disorders, Fourth Edition* (DSM-IV) (APA, 1994). The interviewed sample included 681,600 State prison inmates; 56,600 Federal prison inmates; and 398,800 local jail inmates.

Any mental health problem was defined by two measures: (1) a recent history of a mental health problem, either in the year before arrest or since admission; or (2) symptoms of a mental health problem that occurred within the 12 months prior to the interview. A recent history of a mental health problem included inmates self-reporting that they were diagnosed with a mental health problem by a mental health professional or that they received treatment for a mental health problem by a mental health professional. Symptoms of a mental disorder were based on criteria specified in the DSM-IV.

Percent refers to inmates receiving treatment as a proportion of inmates with mental health problems.

SOURCE: James, D. J., & Glaze, L. E. (2006). *Mental health problems of prison and jail inmates* (NCJ-213600). Washington, DC: U.S. Department of Justice, Office of Justice Programs, Bureau of Justice Statistics. Retrieved from http://bjs.ojp.usdoj.gov/content/pub/pdf/mhppji.pdf

Table 50. Selected characteristics of mental health and substance abuse services provided by community health centers (CHCs), United States, 2007

[Data are based on reporting from federally funded CHCs]

Mental health/substance abuse services	Service provided by CHC		Service referred elsewhere and funded by CHC		Service referred elsewhere and not funded by CHC		Service through either type of referral/funding source	
	Number	Percent	Number	Percent	Number	Percent	Number	Percent
All community health centers (CHCs)	1,067	...	1,067	...	1,067	...	1,067	...
Mental health treatment/counseling	822	77.0	129	12.1	816	76.5	1,058	99.2
Developmental screening	765	71.7	54	5.1	685	64.2	1,044	97.8
24-hour crisis intervention/counseling	211	19.8	39	3.7	947	88.8	1,030	96.5
Other mental health services	513	48.1	77	7.2	833	78.1	1,022	95.8
Substance abuse treatment/ counseling	543	50.9	93	8.7	907	85.0	1,047	98.1
Other substance abuse services	367	34.4	69	6.5	905	84.8	1,019	95.5
Comprehensive mental health/ substance abuse screening	450	42.2	57	5.3	815	76.4	1,003	94.0

... Category not applicable.

NOTES: The Uniform Data System is a set of electronic files compiled by the Health Resources and Services Administration (HRSA) from reports submitted annually by all U.S. federally funded CHCs on administration, patient population, demographic characteristics, utilization, and finances.

Community health centers (CHCs) are community-based and patient-directed organizations that serve populations with limited access to health care. These centers are public and private nonprofit health care organizations that meet certain criteria under the Medicare and Medicaid programs and serve a variety of underserved populations and areas. (See U.S. Department of Health and Human Services, HRSA. What is a health center? Available at: http://bphc.hrsa.gov/about/.) The centers included in the table received grants from HRSA to deliver services. A CHC may be counted in more than one service type. Table originally published in Substance Abuse and Mental Health Services Administration (SAMHSA). (2010). *Mental Health, United States, 2008* (DHHS Publication No. SMA 10-4590). Rockville, MD: Center for Mental Health Services, SAMHSA.

SOURCE: Grantees Uniform Data System National Rollup Report, 2007, HRSA.

Table 51. Number and percentage of community health centers (CHCs) with on-site behavioral health services, United States, 1998–2007

[Data are based on reporting from federally funded CHCs]

Year	CHCs (number)	CHCs with specialty mental health on site[1] (percent)	CHCs with crisis services on site (percent)	CHCs with substance abuse treatment on site (percent)
1998	694	53	17	43
1999	690	54	16	43
2000	730	58	18	44
2001	748	62	17	46
2002	843	67	19	48
2003	890	70	20	50
2004	914	72	19	48
2005	952	74	20	50
2006	1,002	76	20	51
2007	1,067	77	20	51

[1] Specialty mental health services were defined in the Uniform Data System documentation as "mental health therapy, counseling, or other treatment provided by a mental health professional."

NOTES: The Uniform Data System is a set of electronic files compiled by the Health Resources and Services Administration (HRSA) from reports submitted annually by all U.S. federally funded CHCs on administration, patient population, demographic characteristics, utilization, and finances.

Community health centers (CHCs) are community-based and patient-directed organizations that serve populations with limited access to health care. These centers are public and private nonprofit health care organizations that meet certain criteria under the Medicare and Medicaid programs and serve a variety of underserved populations and areas. (See U.S. Department of Health and Human Services, HRSA. What is a health center? Available at: http://bphc.hrsa.gov/about/.) "Grantees" refers to receipt of a grant from HRSA to deliver services.

A CHC may be counted in more than one service type.

SOURCES: Grantees Uniform Data System National Rollup Report, 2007, HRSA.

Wells, R., Morrissey, J. P., Lee, I.- H., & Radford, A. (2010). Trends in behavioral health care service provision by community health centers, 1998–2007. *Psychiatric Services, 61*(8), 759–764. Reprinted with permission from *Psychiatric Services* (Copyright © 2010). American Psychiatric Association.

Table 52. Number and percentage of encounters and patients receiving mental health services in community health centers (CHCs), United States, 2007

[Data are based on reporting from federally funded CHCs]

Diagnostic category	Encounters			Patients			Encounters per patient (percent)
	Number	Percent	Mental health encounters (percent)	Number	Percent	Mental health patients (percent)	
All diagnoses	**47,037,267**	**100.0**	...	**13,962,680**	**100.0**	...	**3.4**
Total mental health or substance-related diagnoses	4,450,166	9.5	100.0	1,357,188	9.7	100.0	3.3
Alcohol-related disorders	338,382	0.7	7.6	69,076	0.5	5.1	4.9
Other substance-related disorders (excluding tobacco use disorders)	579,997	1.2	13.0	79,664	0.6	5.9	7.3
Depression and other mood disorders	1,557,220	3.3	35.0	506,442	3.6	37.3	3.1
Anxiety disorders, including posttraumatic stress disorder	595,093	1.3	13.4	257,997	1.8	19.0	2.3
Attention deficit and disruptive behavior disorders	414,651	0.9	9.3	129,460	0.9	9.5	3.2
Other mental disorders, excluding drug or alcohol dependence (includes mental retardation)	964,823	2.1	21.7	314,549	2.3	23.2	3.1

... Category not applicable.

NOTES: The Uniform Data System is a set of electronic files compiled by the Health Resources and Services Administration (HRSA) from reports submitted annually by all U.S. federally funded CHCs on administration, patient population, demographic characteristics, utilization, and finances.

Community health centers (CHCs) are community-based and patient-directed organizations that serve populations with limited access to health care. These centers are public and private nonprofit health care organizations that meet certain criteria under the Medicare and Medicaid programs and serve a variety of underserved populations and areas. (See U.S. Department of Health and Human Services, HRSA. What is a health center? Available at: http://bphc.hrsa.gov/about/.) Table originally published in Substance Abuse and Mental Health Services Administration (SAMHSA). (2010). *Mental Health, United States, 2008* (DHHS Publication No. SMA 10-4590). Rockville, MD: Center for Mental Health Services, SAMHSA.

SOURCE: Grantees Uniform Data System National Rollup Report, 2007, HRSA.

Table 53. Number of specialty mental health and substance abuse encounters in community health centers (CHCs), United States, 1998–2007

[Data are based on reporting from federally funded CHCs]

Year	Specialty mental health encounters[1]	Substance abuse treatment encounters[2]
1998	913,828	571,496
1999	936,309	667,311
2000	1,083,855	682,925
2001	1,223,408	745,855
2002	1,418,752	927,866
2003	1,708,571	1,046,867
2004	1,798,197	934,374
2005	1,976,503	907,227
2006	2,317,997	916,613
2007	2,738,408	972,857

[1] Specialty mental health services were defined in the Uniform Data System documentation as "mental health therapy, counseling, or other treatment provided by a mental health professional."

[2] Substance abuse treatment was defined in the Uniform Data System documentation as "counseling and other medical and/or psychosocial treatment services provided to individuals with substance abuse (i.e., alcohol and/or other drug) problems."

NOTE: The Uniform Data System is a set of electronic files compiled by the Health Resources and Services Administration (HRSA) from reports submitted annually by all U.S. federally funded CHCs on administration, patient population, demographic characteristics, utilization, and finances.

SOURCES: Grantees Uniform Data System National Rollup Report, 2007, HRSA.

Wells, R., Morrissey, J. P., Lee, I.- H., & Radford, A. (2010). Trends in behavioral health care service provision by community health centers, 1998–2007. *Psychiatric Services, 61*(8), 759–764. Reprinted with permission from *Psychiatric Services* (Copyright © 2010). American Psychiatric Association.

Table 54. Percentage of clubhouses providing specific services, United States, 2010

[Data are from an annual survey of clubhouses]

Service/activity	ICCD certified ($N = 80$) (percent)	Non-ICCD certified ($N = 34$) (percent)
Transitional employment[1]	97	88
Independent employment	95	88
Supported employment	94	82
Low priced meals	91	79
Help with obtaining entitlements (e.g., disability insurance)	90	59
Reach out, home or hospital visits	90	76
Education	89	71
Social activities: recreational, sports, and/or cultural	86	68
Help finding housing	85	71
Wellness, nutrition, or health promotion activities	84	68
Links to physical health care/dental care	79	76
Linkage to colleges and universities	78	59
Money management	75	50
Transportation to clubhouse and/or appointments	71	56
Volunteer work to benefit the clubhouse	66	65
Political advocacy, board positions, legislative testimony	62	41
Arbitration of members' disputes (e.g., landlords, employers, family members)	60	44
Mobile outreach	59	44
Psychiatric medication linkage, advocacy, and/or planning	59	50
Substance use/abuse intervention or education	50	32
Nonreimbursed case management	49	32
Financial assistance with buying food or clothing	47	29
Volunteer work to benefit other persons or programs	44	47
Peer support groups	40	44
Adolescent or young adult services	36	21
24-hour crisis coverage	26	9
Reimbursed case management	25	18
Programs/supports for family members	23	24

[1] Two clubhouses lost their transitional employment placements after being certified by the International Center for Clubhouse Development (ICCD).

NOTE: The International Survey of Clubhouses was conducted by ICCD. The survey gathers information about clubhouse characteristics, governance and administration, membership, staffing and staff credentials, unit structure, employment, housing activities, services, and participation in clubhouse training. In 2010, there were 197 ICCD clubhouses in the United States; however, data were only available for 114 of them.

SOURCE: International Survey of Clubhouses, 2010, ICCD.

Table 55. Characteristics of psychiatric discharges from community hospital scatter beds and psychiatric units, United States, 2003

[Data are based on community hospital psychiatric discharges]

Characteristic	Total scatter bed discharges[1]		Scatter bed in hospital with psychiatric unit[2]		Scatter bed in hospital without psychiatric unit[3]		Psychiatric unit[4]	
	Number	Percent	Number	Percent	Number	Percent	Number	Percent
Total discharges = 397,953	**26,969**	**6.8**	**14,130**	**3.6**	**12,839**	**3.2**	**370,984**	**93.2**
Age								
0–17	3,755	13.9	2,878	20.4	877	6.8	38,579	10.4
18–34	4,807	17.8	2,515	17.8	2,292	17.9	110,521	29.8
35–44	4,409	16.3	2,303	16.3	2,106	16.4	90,461	24.4
45–54	4,220	15.6	2,119	15.0	2,101	16.4	67,389	18.2
55–64	2,986	11.1	1,418	10.0	1,568	12.2	29,972	8.1
65 or older	6,791	25.2	2,896	20.5	3,895	30.3	34,052	9.2
Sex								
Male	10,519	39.0	5,743	40.6	4,776	37.2	170,794	46.0
Female	16,449	61.0	8,386	59.3	8,063	62.8	200,180	54.0
Primary expected payer								
Medicare	9,198	34.1	4,007	28.4	5,191	40.4	101,651	27.4
Medicaid	5,872	21.8	3,679	26.0	2,193	17.1	123,820	33.4
Private insurance	8,158	30.2	4,578	32.4	3,580	27.9	99,627	26.9
Uninsured	2,442	9.1	1,188	8.4	1,254	9.8	31,503	8.5
Other	1,227	4.5	637	4.5	590	4.6	12,774	3.4
Admission source								
Emergency department	17,254	64.0	8,505	60.2	8,749	68.1	200,768	54.1
Another hospital	933	3.5	602	4.3	331	2.6	23,998	6.5
Other health facility, including long-term care	386	1.4	189	1.3	197	1.5	12,072	3.3
Court or law enforcement	158	0.1	109	0.1	49	0.4	6,856	1.8
Routine	7,881	29.2	4,389	31.1	3,492	27.2	124,829	33.6

(continued)

Table 55. Characteristics of psychiatric discharges from community hospital scatter beds and psychiatric units, United States, 2003 *(continued)*

Characteristic	Total scatter bed discharges[1]		Scatter bed in hospital with psychiatric unit[2]		Scatter bed in hospital without psychiatric unit[3]		Psychiatric unit[4]	
	Number	Percent	Number	Percent	Number	Percent	Number	Percent
Discharge disposition								
Routine	19,258	71.4	10,358	73.3	8,900	69.3	310,668	83.7
Short-term hospital	869	3.2	407	2.9	462	3.6	8,404	2.3
Other facility	5,187	19.2	2,536	17.9	2,651	20.6	37,455	10.1
Home health care	910	3.4	436	3.1	474	3.7	4,042	1.1
Against medical advice	568	2.1	313	2.2	255	2.0	8,663	2.3
Died	53	0.2	25	0.2	28	0.2	322	0.1

... Category not applicable.

[1] For total scatter bed discharges, mean total charge is $9,790, and mean length of stay is 5 days.

[2] For scatter bed in hospital with psychiatric unit, mean total charge is $10,206, and mean length of stay is 6 days.

[3] For scatter bed in hospital without psychiatric unit, mean total charge is $9,330, and mean length of stay is 4 days.

[4] For psychiatric unit, mean total charge is $15,456, and mean length of stay is 10 days.

NOTES: The State Inpatient Databases consist of data from 43 States on the number of community hospitals and discharges from those hospitals, which account for approximately 90 percent of all community hospital discharges.

Percent is the percentage of the total discharges.

Discharges were identified as psychiatric based on patient discharge diagnoses as well as revenue codes indicating discharge from a psychiatric unit. Community hospitals are defined by the American Hospital Association as all non-Federal, short-term general, and other specialty hospitals and include academic medical centers or other teaching hospitals if they are non-Federal short-term hospitals. Excluded are hospitals not accessible by the general public, such as prison hospitals or college infirmaries. Scatter beds refer to inpatient psychiatric care provided outside of psychiatric units through general medical beds.

SOURCES: Mark, T. L., Vandivort-Warren, R., Owens, P. L., Buck, J. A., Levit, K. R., Coffey, R. M., & Stocks, C. (2010). Psychiatric discharges in community hospitals with and without psychiatric units: How many and for whom? *Psychiatric Services, 61*(6), 562–568. Reprinted with permission from *Psychiatric Services* (Copyright © 2010). American Psychiatric Association.

State Inpatient Databases, Healthcare Cost and Utilization Project, 2003, Agency for Healthcare Research and Quality.

7. TABLES

7.2 Providers and Settings for Mental Health Services

7.2.1 Adult Mental Health Services

Specialty Mental Health Services

Nonspecialty Mental Health Services

Mental Health Service Capacity

7.2.2 Child Mental Health Services

Mental Health Services
Tables 56–63

Mental Health Service Capacity

7.2.3 Special Populations

Table 56. Number and percentage of persons aged 12 to 17 who received mental health treatment in the past year, by type of treatment, United States, 2009

[Data are based on a survey of a representative sample of the national population]

Source of mental health service[1]	Number (1,000s)	Percent
Specialty mental health	**2,920**	**12.0**
Outpatient[2]		
Total	2,635	10.8
Private therapist, psychologist, psychiatrist, social worker, or counselor	2,281	9.3
Mental health clinic or center	533	2.2
Partial day hospital or day treatment program	339	1.4
In-home therapist, counselor, or family preservation worker	651	2.7
Inpatient or residential (overnight or longer stay)		
Total	565	2.3
Hospital	435	1.8
Residential treatment center	211	0.9
Foster care or therapeutic foster care home	92	0.4
Education[3,4]		
Total	2,919	12.1
School social worker, school psychologist, or school counselor	2,276	9.4
Special school or program within a regular school for students with emotional or behavioral problems	970	4.0
Medical		
Pediatrician or other family doctor	603	2.5
Specialty mental health and education or medical[4,5]	1,190	4.9
Juvenile justice[6]		
Juvenile detention center, prison, or jail[7]	109	0.4

[1] Respondents could indicate multiple service sources; thus, these response categories are not mutually exclusive.

[2] Outpatient treatment includes treatment/counseling from a (1) private therapist, psychologist, psychiatrist, social worker, or counselor; (2) mental health clinic or center; (3) partial day hospital or day treatment program; or (4) in-home therapist, counselor, or family preservation worker.

[3] Respondents who did not report their school enrollment status, who reported not being enrolled in school in the past 12 months, or who reported being home-schooled were not asked about receipt of mental health treatment/counseling from this source; however, respondents who reported not being enrolled in school in the past 12 months were classified as not having received treatment/counseling from this source.

[4] Because of revisions to the "source of youth mental health education services" questions in 2009, these estimates are not comparable with the education services estimates presented before the 2009 National Survey on Drug Use and Health (NSDUH).

[5] Includes receipt of any specialty mental health services and receipt of services from either education or medical sources.

[6] A question on receiving juvenile justice youth mental health services was added to NSDUH in 2009, so data are not available for 2008.

[7] These services were often provided by psychiatrists, psychologists, social workers, or counselors who work for the court system.

NOTE: The National Survey on Drug Use and Health is a nationally representative survey of the civilian, noninstitutionalized population of the United States aged 12 or older. The survey interviews approximately 67,500 persons each year. In 2009, 22,626 youth aged 12 to 17 were interviewed.

SOURCE: National Survey on Drug Use and Health, 2009, Substance Abuse and Mental Health Services Administration, Office of Applied Studies.

Table 57. Percentage of persons aged 8 to 15 who used mental health services in the past year, United States, 2001–2004

[Data are based on evaluations of a sample of the civilian noninstitutionalized population]

12-month disorder	All cases (percent)	Cases with severe impairment[1] (percent)
Any disorder	50.6	52.8
Attention deficit hyperactivity disorder	47.7	48.5
Conduct disorder	46.4	44.2
Anxiety disorders[2]	32.2	33.9
Mood disorders	43.8	50.7

[1] Impairment was assessed using six items. Cases with severe impairment received either a severe rating on any question or an intermediate rating on two questions or more.

[2] Anxiety disorders include generalized anxiety disorder (GAD) and panic disorders.

NOTES: The National Health and Nutrition Examination Survey (NHANES) is a nationally representative probability sample of noninstitutionalized U.S. civilians and in the sample shown includes 3,024 children aged 8 to 15 who were evaluated in person at the mobile examination centers of the 2001–2004 NHANES.

Not all mental health diagnoses are included under "any disorder."

The notes and source for this table have been reordered at the express wish of the copyright holding organization. Service use indicated that the respondent saw someone at a hospital, clinic, or office because of a specific disorder in the previous 12 months.

Mental disorders were assessed using the National Institute of Mental Health Diagnostic Interview Schedule for Children (DISC) Version IV, 1997, a structured diagnostic interview administered by lay interviewers to assess *Diagnostic and Statistical Manual of Mental Disorders, Fourth Edition* (DSM-IV) (APA, 1994) diagnostic criteria for mental disorders in children and adolescents. Diagnostic modules within DISC include an assessment of both symptoms and functional impairment. Six impairment items assess personal distress and social (at home or with peers) or academic difficulties within each diagnostic module; these items are rated from "mild" to "severe." Disorder with severe impairment indicates two "intermediate" or one "severe" rating on the six impairment questions within that diagnostic module. This study assessed only certain childhood mental disorders by parent or youth report. Modules for GAD, panic disorder, eating disorders (anorexia nervosa and bulimia nervosa), and major depressive disorder (MDD)/dysthymic disorder (DD) were administered to youth; and modules for MDD/DD, eating disorders, attention deficit hyperactivity disorder (ADHD), and conduct disorder were administered to the primary caretakers. The diagnoses of GAD and panic disorder were based on youth reports alone, those of ADHD and conduct disorder were based on parent reports alone, and those of MDD/DD and eating disorders were based on either youth or parent reports. The prevalence of mental disorders found in this study may be underestimated due to study methods. This study did not assess two common childhood anxiety disorders: separation anxiety and phobias. And, as described above, certain diagnoses were assessed by either youth or parent report, counter to methods used in previous research. See Merikangas et al. (2010) for additional details on the disorders presented.

At the request of the publisher, Table 57a is the original, published form of the table, and the source reference is listed directly below the table.

SOURCE: Merikangas, K. R., He, J.-P., Brody, D., Fisher, P. W., Bourdon, K., & Koretz, D. S. (2010). Prevalence and treatment of mental disorders among US children in the 2001–2004 NHANES. *Pediatrics, 125*(1), 75–81. *Reproduced with permission from Pediatrics, 125*(1), 75–81, Copyright © 2010 by the American Academy of Pediatrics.

Table 57a. Percentage of persons aged 8 to 15 who used mental health services in the past year, United States, 2001–2004: Original exhibit

Original title: Past-year mental health service use among children 8 to 15 years of age with 12-month, DSM-IV–defined disorder

12-mo Disorder	All Cases		Cases With Severe Impairment[a]	
	n	Proportion, Estimate ± SE, %	*n*	Proportion, Estimate ± SE, %
Any disorder	366	50.6 ± 3.4	305	52.8 ± 3.7
ADHD	218	47.7 ± 4.4	195	48.5 ± 4.5
Conduct disorder	68	46.4 ± 8.0	63	44.2 ± 8.4
Anxiety disorders (GAD or panic disorder)	21	32.2 ± 14.3	12	33.9 ± 19.0
Mood disorders	128	43.8 ± 6.0	95	50.7 ± 6.0

Service use indicated the respondent saw someone at a hospital, clinic, or office because of [specific disorder] in the previous 12 months.

[a] Impairment level D.

SOURCE: Merikangas, K. R., He, J.-P., Brody, D., Fisher, P. W., Bourdon, K., & Koretz, D. S. (2010). Prevalence and treatment of mental disorders among US children in the 2001–2004 NHANES. *Pediatrics, 125*(1), 75–81.

NOTES: Reproduced with permission from *Pediatrics, 125*(1), 75–81, Copyright © 2010 by the American Academy of Pediatrics.

At the request of the publisher, Table 57a is the original, published form of the table.

Table 58. Number and percentage of persons aged 2 to 17 using prescription medication for attention deficit hyperactivity disorder (ADHD), by selected characteristics, United States, 2007

[Data are based on a nationally representative survey of children]

Characteristic	Taking medication		Not taking medication	
	Number (1,000s)[1]	Percent[2]	Number (1,000s)[1]	Percent[2]
Total	**2,744**	**4.2**	**1,413**	**2.2**
Age				
2–5	51	0.3	98	0.6
6–11	1,263	5.3	518	2.2
12–17	1,430	5.7	797	3.2
Sex				
Male	2,036	6.1	991	3.0
Female	702	2.2	422	1.3
Hispanic origin and race[3]				
Hispanic	270	2.1	207	1.6
White, non-Hispanic	1,802	5.0	780	2.2
Black, non-Hispanic	433	4.7	247	2.7
Multiracial, non-Hispanic	159	6.0	88	3.3
Other, non-Hispanic	46	1.5	37	1.2
Poverty[4,5]				
0–99 percent of Federal poverty level	647	5.5	299	2.6
100–199 percent of Federal poverty level	563	4.1	369	2.7
200–399 percent of Federal poverty level	805	4.0	398	2.0
400 percent of Federal poverty level or higher	729	3.8	347	1.8
Any health care coverage				
Public insurance, such as Medicaid/CHIP[6]	1,181	6.5	539	3.0
Private health insurance	1,459	3.6	729	1.8
Currently uninsured	93	1.5	106	1.7

[1] Estimated number of children in population after applying sampling weights. In some cases, this number may be underestimated because unknown values are not included in its calculation. Unknown values are less than 1 percent for most questions. Among the exceptions is household income, with nearly 10 percent unknown values.

[2] Estimated percentage of specified child population after applying sampling weights.

[3] Hispanic includes all children reporting Hispanic/Latino origin; non-Hispanic children reporting a single race category of either white or black are grouped respectively; non-Hispanic children reporting more than one race category are grouped as "multiracial"; and non-Hispanic children reporting only one race category of Asian, American Indian, Alaska Native, Native Hawaiian, or Pacific Islander are grouped as "other" because of small sample sizes. Race data were missing for approximately 2 percent of respondents.

[4] The Federal poverty level (FPL) numbers are based on the Federal poverty guidelines issued annually by the U.S. Department of Health and Human Services. FPL is used as a measure of eligibility for a wide variety of State and Federal programs. For more information, visit http://aspe.hhs.gov/poverty.

[5] Household poverty level for the 9.3 percent of households in the sample with unknown values for income, household size, or both was calculated using single imputation methods. The poverty level estimates and confidence intervals based on single imputed poverty level may differ slightly from those obtained using multiple imputation methods.

[6] CHIP is the Children's Health Insurance Program (formerly State Children's Health Insurance Program [SCHIP]).

NOTE: The National Survey of Children's Health is a nationally representative survey of 91,642 noninstitutionalized children aged 0 to 17 and provides a range of children's health and well-being information.

SOURCE: National Survey of Children's Health, 2007, Child and Adolescent Health Measurement Initiative, Oregon Health and Science University. Computed from data retrieved December 28, 2010, from http://www.nschdata.org

Table 59. Number and percentage of persons aged 12 to 17 who received mental health treatment in the past year, by selected characteristics, United States, 2009

[Data are based on a survey of a representative sample of the national population]

Characteristic	Specialty mental health service—total		Specialty mental health service—outpatient[1]		Specialty mental health service—inpatient or residential[2]		Education[3,4]		Medical[5]		Juvenile justice[4,6]	
	Number (1,000s)	Percent	Number (1,000s)	Percent	Number (1,000s)	Percent	Number (1,000s)	Percent	Number (1,000s)	Percent	Number (1,000s)	Percent
Total	**2,920**	**12.0**	**2,635**	**10.8**	**565**	**2.3**	**2,919**	**12.1**	**603**	**2.5**	**109**	**0.4**
Age												
12–13	851	11.6	778	10.6	137	1.8	965	13.3	165	2.2	21	0.3
14–15	1,043	12.3	925	10.9	223	2.6	1,107	13.1	199	2.3	32	0.4
16–17	1,026	12.1	932	11.0	205	2.4	846	10.0	239	2.8	56	0.7
Sex												
Male	1,249	10.1	1,066	8.6	300	2.4	1,306	10.6	252	2.0	65	0.5
Female	1,671	14.0	1,569	13.1	265	2.2	1,613	13.6	350	2.9	44	0.4
Hispanic origin and race												
Not Hispanic or Latino	2,439	12.4	2,205	11.3	452	2.3	2,331	11.9	492	2.5	72	0.4
White	1,819	12.8	1,684	11.8	288	2.0	1,549	10.9	366	2.6	40	0.3
Black or African American	444	12.2	362	9.9	122	3.3	594	16.4	94	2.6	24	0.7
American Indian or Alaska Native	19	14.9	18	14.5	5	3.9	14	10.8	1	1.1	1	0.6
Native Hawaiian or Other Pacific Islander	*	*	*	*	*	*	*	*	*	*	*	*
Asian	64	6.6	55	5.7	15	1.5	99	10.3	11	1.1	0	0.0
Two or more races	86	16.4	78	14.9	22	4.1	70	13.5	20	3.8	6	1.1
Hispanic or Latino	481	10.2	430	9.1	113	2.4	587	12.6	110	2.3	37	0.8
Poverty status[7]												
Poor	562	12.3	450	9.9	176	3.8	660	14.6	136	3.0	40	0.9
Near poor	693	12.8	615	11.4	171	3.1	735	13.7	150	2.8	39	0.7
Not poor	1,666	11.6	1,570	10.9	218	1.5	1,523	10.6	316	2.2	30	0.2
Geographic region												
Northeast	551	13.0	510	12.0	91	2.1	549	13.0	102	2.4	16	0.4
Midwest	689	12.9	615	11.5	131	2.4	681	12.8	136	2.5	28	0.5
South	987	11.1	857	9.6	234	2.6	1,023	11.5	242	2.7	36	0.4
West	693	11.9	652	11.2	110	1.9	666	11.5	123	2.1	29	0.5

(continued)

Table 59. Number and percentage of persons aged 12 to 17 who received mental health treatment in the past year, by selected characteristics, United States, 2009 *(continued)*

Characteristic	Specialty mental health service—total		Specialty mental health service—outpatient[1]		Specialty mental health service—inpatient or residential[2]		Education[3,4]		Medical[5]		Juvenile justice[4,6]	
	Number (1,000s)	Percent	Number (1,000s)	Percent	Number (1,000s)	Percent	Number (1,000s)	Percent	Number (1,000s)	Percent	Number (1,000s)	Percent
County type												
Large metro	1,567	12.2	1,417	11.0	281	2.2	1,583	12.4	273	2.1	53	0.4
Small metro	916	12.1	834	11.0	169	2.2	907	12.0	209	2.7	38	0.5
Nonmetro	437	11.3	384	9.9	115	2.9	429	11.1	122	3.1	18	0.5

*Estimates are considered unreliable.

[1] Includes treatment/counseling from a (1) private therapist, psychologist, psychiatrist, social worker, or counselor; (2) mental health clinic or center; (3) partial day hospital or day treatment program; or (4) in-home therapist, counselor, or family preservation worker.

[2] Includes treatment/counseling from an overnight or longer stay in a (1) hospital, (2) residential treatment center, or (3) foster care or therapeutic foster care home.

[3] Includes treatment/counseling from (1) a school social worker, school psychologist, or school counselor; or (2) a special school or program within a regular school for students with emotional or behavioral problems. Respondents who did not report their school enrollment status, who reported not being enrolled in school in the past 12 months, or who reported being home-schooled were not asked about receipt of mental health treatment/counseling from this source; however, respondents who reported not being enrolled in school in the past 12 months were classified as not having received treatment/counseling from this source.

[4] Because of revisions to the "source of youth mental health education services" questions in 2009, these estimates are not comparable with the education services estimates presented before the 2009 National Survey on Drug Use and Health (NSDUH).

[5] Includes treatment/counseling from a pediatrician or other family doctor.

[6] Includes treatment/counseling received in juvenile detention centers, prisons, or jails, and often provided by psychiatrists, psychologists, social workers, or counselors who work for the court system. A question on receiving juvenile justice youth mental health services was added to NSDUH in 2009, so data are not available for 2008.

[7] Poverty status is based on respondent age, family income, family size, and composition using the U.S. Census Bureau's poverty thresholds. "Poor" persons are defined as living in households where the family income is less than 100 percent of the U.S. Census poverty threshold. "Near poor" persons have incomes of 100 percent to less than 200 percent of the poverty threshold. "Not poor" persons have incomes that are 200 percent of the poverty threshold or greater.

NOTES: The National Survey on Drug Use and Health (NSDUH) is a nationally representative survey of the civilian, noninstitutionalized population of the United States aged 12 or older. The survey interviews approximately 67,500 persons each year. In 2009, 22,626 youth aged 12 to 17 were interviewed.

Receipt of mental health services for persons aged 12 to 17 is defined as having received treatment/counseling for emotional or behavioral problems not caused by drug or alcohol use. Respondents with unknown receipt of mental health service information were excluded. Respondents could indicate multiple service sources; thus, the response categories are not mutually exclusive.

SOURCE: National Survey on Drug Use and Health, 2009, Substance Abuse and Mental Health Services Administration, Office of Applied Studies.

Table 60. Number and percentage of persons aged 12 to 17 with a past year major depressive episode (MDE) who received particular types of care, by selected characteristics, United States, 2009

[Data are based on a survey of a representative sample of the national population]

Characteristic	Saw or talked to medical doctor or other professional OR used prescription medication		Saw or talked to medical doctor or other professional AND used prescription medication		Saw or talked to medical doctor or other professional only		Used prescription medication only	
	Number (1,000s)	Percent	Number (1,000s)	Percent	Number (1,000s)	Percent	Number (1,000s)	Percent
Total	**674**	**34.7**	**234**	**12.0**	**394**	**20.3**	**45**	**2.3**
Sex								
Male	167	29.3	52	9.1	107	18.8	8	1.4
Female	507	37.0	182	13.2	287	20.9	38	2.7
Hispanic origin and race								
Not Hispanic or Latino	556	35.1	200	12.6	324	20.5	30	1.9
White	440	37.6	178	15.2	237	20.2	26	2.2
Black or African American	72	25.4	*	*	55	19.4	4	1.2
Other or two or more races	*	*	9	6.9	*	*	1	0.6
Hispanic or Latino	118	33.1	33	9.3	70	19.5	15	4.3
Poverty status[1]								
Poor	110	32.9	35	10.5	66	19.7	9	2.6
Near poor	147	32.1	45	9.8	83	18.3	18	3.9
Not poor	417	36.3	153	13.3	244	21.3	18	1.6
Health insurance status[2]								
Private coverage	418	35.1	156	13.1	246	20.7	14	1.2
Medicaid/CHIP[3]	200	36.0	67	11.9	116	20.8	18	3.1
Other coverage[4]	*	*	*	*	*	*	*	*
No coverage	45	25.6	11	6.3	22	12.5	*	*

See notes on page 179.

Table 60 notes

*Estimates are considered unreliable.

[1] Poverty status is based on respondent age, family income, family size, and composition using the U.S. Census Bureau's poverty thresholds. "Poor" persons are defined as living in households where the family income is less than 100 percent of the U.S. Census poverty threshold. "Near poor" persons have incomes of 100 percent to less than 200 percent of the poverty threshold. "Not poor" persons have incomes that are 200 percent of the poverty threshold or greater.

[2] Respondents could indicate multiple types of health insurance; thus, these response categories are not mutually exclusive.

[3] CHIP is the Children's Health Insurance Program (formerly State Children's Health Insurance Program [SCHIP]). Qualified individuals aged 19 or younger are eligible for this plan.

[4] Other health insurance is defined as having Medicare, Civilian Health and Medical Program of the Uniformed Services (CHAMPUS), TRICARE, Civilian Health and Medical Program of the Department of Veterans Affairs (CHAMPVA), Veterans Administration (VA), military health care, or any other type of health insurance.

NOTES: The National Survey on Drug Use and Health is a nationally representative survey of the civilian, noninstitutionalized population of the United States aged 12 or older. The survey interviews approximately 67,500 persons each year. In 2008, 22,546 youth aged 12 to 17 were interviewed. In 2009, 22,626 youth aged 12 to 17 were interviewed.

Respondents with unknown past year treatment data were excluded.

Major depressive episode (MDE) is defined as a period of at least 2 weeks when a person experienced a depressed mood or loss of interest or pleasure in daily activities and had a majority of specified depression symptoms. According to the *Diagnostic and Statistical Manual of Mental Disorders, Fourth Edition* (DSM-IV) (APA, 1994), two or more MDEs are necessary to meet the criteria for recurrent major depressive disorder.

SOURCE: National Survey on Drug Use and Health, 2009, Substance Abuse and Mental Health Services Administration, Office of Applied Studies.

Table 61. Use of residential treatment centers by children with emotional disturbance, by type of facility, United States, selected years 1986–2004

[Data are based on reporting by a sample of mental health organizations and general hospitals with separate psychiatric services]

Year	24-hour hospital and residential treatment		Less than 24-hour care[3]	
	Admissions[1]	Admission rate per 100,000 civilian population[2]	Admissions[1]	Admission rate per 100,000 civilian population[2]
1986	24,511	10.2	67,344	28.1
1990	41,588	17.0	99,503	40.8
1992	36,388	14.4	121,131	48.0
1994	46,704	18.0	167,344	64.6
1998	44,930	16.7	128,271	47.4
2000	45,841	16.2	199,201	70.6
2002	59,633	20.7	207,722	72.1
2004	60,620	20.3	194,294	65.2

[1] Admissions sometimes are referred to as additions, because they can be duplicated counts across a year.

[2] Civilian population estimates for 2000 and beyond are based on the 2000 census as of July 1; population estimates for 1992–1998 are 1990 postcensal estimates.

[3] Includes freestanding psychiatric outpatient clinics, partial care organizations, and multiservice mental health organizations.

NOTES: The Survey of Mental Health Organizations was a biennial survey with two phases. In the first phase, limited data were collected from all mental health organizations. In the second phase, more detailed data were collected from a sample of specialty mental health organizations.

Changes to the design of the survey do not permit updates to be made to the Survey of Mental Health Organizations at this time. Updates may be possible in the future.

SOURCE: Survey of Mental Health Organizations, 1986–2004, Substance Abuse and Mental Health Services Administration, Center for Mental Health Services.

Table 62. Number and percentage of prescription mental health/substance abuse (MH/SA) medication fills for all medical conditions among persons aged 17 or younger, by selected medication class, United States, 1996–2008

[Data are based on a nationally representative survey of households, medical providers, and employers]

Medication class	1996	1997	1998	1999	2000	2001	2002	2003	2004	2005	2006	2007	2008
All MH and/or SA medications													
(percent of all prescription fills)	10.9	13.1	14.3	13.9	15.2	15.5	15.4	17.1	18.6	18.3	17.9	17.2	18.7
All MH and/or SA medications (millions)	**18.2**	**19.8**	**21.4**	**21.3**	**23.3**	**26.1**	**27.3**	**32.6**	**32.5**	**33.7**	**34.3**	**29.8**	**31.6**
Antianxiety, all classes (millions)	2.1	1.5	1.8	2.3	1.6	2.2	2.2	2.0	1.7	1.4	1.8	1.8	0.9
Antidepressants, all classes (millions)	3.1	4.3	4.1	4.0	6.1	5.8	7.2	8.5	6.9	7.2	6.4	4.8	5.3
Antipsychotics, all classes (millions)	*	*	*	*	1.4	1.8	2.0	2.2	2.9	4.1	3.8	2.6	3.9
Stimulants (millions)	11.5	12.3	13.8	13.9	13.2	15.1	14.2	17.8	18.9	18.9	20.3	19.1	20.6

*Estimates are considered unreliable.

[1] Antianxiety medications include sedative and hypnotic medications.

NOTES: The Medical Expenditure Panel Survey (MEPS) is a set of large-scale surveys of families and individuals, their medical providers (e.g., doctors, hospitals, pharmacies), and employers across the United States. Since 1996, MEPS has collected data on the specific health services that Americans use, how frequently they use them, the cost of these services, and how they are paid for, as well as data on the cost, scope, and breadth of health insurance held by and available to U.S. workers.

All classes combined do not add to total because the table does not detail classes of medication with a relatively small number of fills.

See Appendix C for complete list of medications. Categorization of medications follows that of the National Institute of Mental Health (http://www.nimh.nih.gov/health/publications/mental-health-medications/alphabetical-list-of-medications.shtml).

SOURCES: Medical Expenditure Panel Survey, 1996–2008, Center for Financing, Access, and Cost Trends, Agency for Healthcare Research and Quality.

Zuvekas, S. H. (2005). Prescription drugs and the changing patterns of treatment for mental disorders, 1996–2001. *Health Affairs, 24*(1), 195–205.

Table 63. Number and percentage of prescription mental health/substance abuse (MH/SA) medication fills for an MH/SA condition among persons aged 17 or younger, by selected medication class, United States, 1996–2008

[Data are based on a nationally representative survey of households, medical providers, and employers]

Medication class	1996	1997	1998	1999	2000	2001	2002	2003	2004	2005	2006	2007	2008
MH and/or SA medications													
(percent of all prescription fills)	9.3	11.5	12.5	12.2	13.2	13.3	13.7	15.3	16.9	17.1	16.8	16.0	17.9
MH and/or SA medications (millions)	**15.6**	**17.5**	**18.7**	**18.6**	**20.2**	**22.4**	**24.2**	**29.0**	**29.5**	**31.4**	**32.2**	**27.6**	**30.2**
Antianxiety, all classes (millions)	*	*	*	*	*	*	*	*	*	*	*	*	*
Antidepressants, all classes (millions)	2.6	3.9	3.5	3.5	5.5	5.2	6.5	7.3	6.1	6.5	5.8	4.2	4.9
Antipsychotics, all classes (millions)	*	*	*	*	*	1.4	1.5	2.0	2.6	4.0	3.7	2.5	3.8
Stimulants (millions)	11.1	11.9	13.2	13.8	12.2	14.2	13.4	17.1	18.5	18.7	19.9	18.8	20.6

*Estimates are considered unreliable.

[1] Antianxiety medications include sedative and hypnotic medications.

NOTES: The Medical Expenditure Panel Survey (MEPS) is a set of large-scale surveys of families and individuals, their medical providers (e.g., doctors, hospitals, pharmacies), and employers across the United States. Since 1996, MEPS has collected data on the specific health services that Americans use, how frequently they use them, the cost of these services, and how they are paid for, as well as data on the cost, scope, and breadth of health insurance held by and available to U.S. workers.

All classes combined do not add to total because the table does not detail classes of medication with a relatively small number of fills.

See Appendix C for complete list of medications. Categorization of medications follows that of the National Institute of Mental Health (http://www.nimh.nih.gov/health/publications/mental-health-medications/alphabetical-list-of-medications.shtml).

SOURCES: Medical Expenditure Panel Survey, 1996–2008, Center for Financing, Access, and Cost Trends, Agency for Healthcare Research and Quality.

Zuvekas, S. H. (2005). Prescription drugs and the changing patterns of treatment for mental disorders, 1996–2001. *Health Affairs, 24*(1), 195–205.

7. TABLES

7.2 Providers and Settings for Mental Health Services

7.2.1 Adult Mental Health Services

Specialty Mental Health Services

Nonspecialty Mental Health Services

Mental Health Service Capacity

7.2.2 Child Mental Health Services

Mental Health Services

Mental Health Service Capacity
Tables 64–66

7.2.3 Special Populations

Table 64. Number of residential treatment centers for children with emotional disturbance and number of beds among persons aged 17 or younger, United States, selected years 1986–2004

[Data are based on reporting by a sample of mental health organizations and general hospitals with separate psychiatric services]

Year	Number of treatment centers	Number of filled residential treatment beds	Filled beds per 100,000 civilian population[1]
1986	437	24,547	10.3
1990	501	35,170	13.9
1992	497	34,952	13.7
1994	472	32,691	12.4
1998	462	32,040	11.2
2000	476	33,508	11.7
2002	510	39,407	13.5
2004	458	33,835	11.4

[1] Civilian population estimates for 2000 and beyond are based on the 2000 census as of July 1; population estimates for 1992–1998 are 1990 postcensal estimates.

NOTES: The Survey of Mental Health Organizations was a biennial survey with two phases. In the first phase, limited data were collected from all mental health organizations. In the second phase, more detailed data were collected from a sample of specialty mental health organizations.

Changes to the design of the survey do not permit updates to be made to the Survey of Mental Health Organizations at this time. Updates may be possible in the future.

SOURCE: Survey of Mental Health Organizations, 1986–2004, Substance Abuse and Mental Health Services Administration, Center for Mental Health Services.

Table 65. Number of residential treatment centers for children with emotional disturbance and number of beds among persons aged 17 or younger, United States, 2008

[Data are based on reporting by a sample of mental health facilities]

Type of facility	Number of beds
Total number of treatment centers	551
Number of treatment centers with 24-hour hospital or residential treatment service	538
Number of treatment centers with less than 24-hour care	219
Number of 24-hour hospital and residential treatment beds	50,063
Inpatient beds	1,717
Residential care beds	48,346
Number of 24-hour hospital and residential treatment beds per 100,000 civilian population	16.5
Inpatient beds per 100,000 civilian population	0.6
Residential care beds per 100,000 civilian population	15.9
Number of inpatient or residential care residents	44,900
Number of inpatient or residential care residents per 100,000 civilian population	14.8

NOTE: The 2008 National Survey of Mental Health Treatment Facilities includes approximately 15,000 point-of-contact facilities nationwide representing approximately 4,400 mental health organizations nationwide.

SOURCE: National Survey of Mental Health Treatment Facilities, 2008, Substance Abuse and Mental Health Services Administration.

Table 66. Percentage of schools that provided mental health or social services and methods of service delivery, United States, 2006

[Data are based on a survey of schools]

Type of service	Percent
Mental health or social service[1]	
Alcohol or other drug use treatment[2]	53.8
Counseling after a natural disaster or other emergency or crisis situation	94.2
Counseling for emotional or behavioral disorders (e.g., anxiety, depression, ADHD)	86.2
Crisis intervention for personal problems	95.4
Eating disorders treatment[2]	46.2
Identification of emotional or behavioral disorders (e.g., anxiety, depression, ADHD)	81.7
Identification of or referral for physical, sexual, or emotional abuse	93.8
Identification of or referral for students with family problems	94.0
Services for gay, lesbian, or bisexual students[2]	59.0
Stress management	83.6
Method of service delivery[1]	
Case management for students with chronic health conditions (e.g., asthma, diabetes)	40.3
Case management for students with emotional or behavioral problems (e.g., anxiety, depression, ADHD)	83.7
Comprehensive assessment or intake evaluation	65.1
Family counseling	49.7
Group counseling	78.6
Individual counseling	92.9
Peer counseling or mediation	67.9
Self-help or support groups	64.4

[1] Services provided by mental health and social services staff, such as counselors, psychologists, and social workers. Did not include activities by teachers in the classroom or activities by nurses or physicians.

[2] Only asked in middle schools and high schools.

NOTES: The School Health Policies and Programs Study is a nationally representative survey of State education agency personnel in all 50 States plus the District of Columbia; school districts (*n* = 538); elementary, middle, and high schools (*n* = 1,103); teachers of classes covering required health instruction in elementary schools and required health education courses in middle and high schools (*n* = 912); and teachers of required physical education classes and courses (*n* = 1,194).

ADHD, attention deficit hyperactivity disorder.

SOURCE: Brener, N. D., Weist, M., Adelman, H., Taylor, L., & Vernon-Smiley, M. (2007). Mental health and social services: Results from the School Health Policies and Programs Study 2006. *Journal of School Health, 77*(8), 486–499. This material is reproduced with permission of John Wiley & Sons, Inc.

7 TABLES

7.2 Providers and Settings for Mental Health Services

Table 67. Percentage of active duty military who received mental health treatment in the past year, United States, 2008

[Data are based on a national survey of active duty service members]

Mental health measure	Army (percent)	Navy (percent)	Marine Corps (percent)	Air Force (percent)	DoD services[1] (percent)	Coast Guard (percent)	All services[2] (percent)
Receipt of prescribed medication for depression, anxiety, or sleeping problems	10.7	6.2	7.9	8.1	8.6	6.3	8.5
Receipt of mental health counseling							
Any mental health counseling	24.2	17.4	19.9	16.0	20.0	17.1	19.9
From a military mental health professional	13.0	7.7	9.8	8.6	10.2	6.4	10.1
From a general physician at a military facility	9.3	6.3	8.0	5.0	7.3	5.3	7.3
From a military chaplain	8.0	5.2	7.1	3.4	6.1	2.6	6.0
From a civilian mental health professional	6.2	3.8	5.1	3.0	4.7	6.3	4.7
From a general physician at a civilian facility	3.8	2.0	3.4	1.4	2.7	2.5	2.7
From a civilian pastoral counselor	3.3	2.7	3.7	1.7	2.8	1.9	2.8
From a self-help group (e.g., Alcoholics Anonymous, Narcotics Anonymous)	2.7	2.5	3.5	1.2	2.4	1.9	2.4
Concerns sought help for							
Depression	9.9	6.8	8.1	5.5	7.8	6.1	7.8
Anxiety	7.8	4.9	5.6	4.0	5.9	4.7	5.9
Family problems	9.0	6.0	7.6	6.5	7.5	6.4	7.4
Substance use problems	1.7	1.5	2.8	0.9	1.6	1.1	1.6
Anger or stress management	9.6	5.9	7.9	5.1	7.4	5.0	7.3
Other	6.4	3.8	4.8	3.4	4.9	3.5	4.8

[1] "DoD services" includes Army, Navy, Marine Corps, and Air Force.

[2] "All services" includes Army, Navy, Marine Corps, Air Force, and Coast Guard.

Table 67 notes *(continued)*

NOTES: The 2008 Department of Defense Survey of Health Related Behaviors Among Active Duty Military Personnel provides representative estimates on substance use and abuse, mental well-being, stress and coping, combat exposure experience, deployment experience, and selected general health topics for all active duty personnel. The final sample consisted of 28,546 military personnel (5,927 Army; 6,637 Navy; 5,117 Marine Corps; 7,009 Air Force; and 3,856 Coast Guard) who completed self-administered questionnaires anonymously.

Table displays the percentage of military personnel by service who reported the mental illness/suicide response as indicated in the rows of this table. Estimates have not been adjusted for sociodemographic differences across services.

SOURCE: Department of Defense Survey of Health Related Behaviors Among Active Duty Military Personnel, 2008. As taken from Bray, R. M., Pemberton, M. R., Hourani, L. L., Witt, M., Rae Olmsted, K. L., Brown, J. M., ... Bradshaw, M. R. (2009). *2008 Department of Defense survey of health related behaviors among active duty military personnel*. Report prepared for TRICARE Management Activity, Office of the Assistant Secretary of Defense (Health Affairs) and U.S. Coast Guard. Retrieved from http://www.tricare.mil/2008HealthBehaviors.pdf. The views, opinions, and findings contained in this report are those of the authors and should not be construed as an official Department of Defense position, policy, or decision, unless so designated by other official documentation.

Table 68. Percentage of active duty, National Guard, and Reserve personnel receiving mental health counseling, United States, 2006

[Data are based on self-administered questionnaires of military personnel]

Service	Unadjusted (percent)	Adjusted[1] (percent)
Army—total	15.5	15.1
Active duty	16.4	16.9
National Guard	14.8	14.5
Reserve	14.7	14.0
Navy—total	14.0	13.1
Active duty	14.8	15.1
Reserve	10.8	11.0
Marine Corps—total	12.5	12.2
Active duty	12.7	13.2
Reserve	*	*
Air Force—total	12.5	11.2
Active duty	13.3	13.2
National Guard	11.4	11.0
Reserve	9.7	9.5
Total DoD	14.1	13.0
Active duty	14.6	14.6
Total National Guard and Reserve	13.3	11.9

*Estimates are considered unreliable because of low precision.

[1] Adjusted estimates have been corrected for differences in the demographic distributions between the Reserve components. The main effects of sex, age group, enlisted/officer indicator, marital status, education, and race/ethnicity were used in this standardization process. Comparisons across Reserve service components should be based upon adjusted estimates.

NOTES: The 2006 Department of Defense Survey of Health Related Behaviors Among the Guard and Reserve Force provides representative estimates on substance use, stress and mental health, healthy behaviors and lifestyles, and other specific issues, such as injuries and injury prevention, sleep habits, and risk taking, for all Guard and Reserve component personnel. The final sample consisted of 18,342 military personnel (2,796 Army National Guard; 1,665 Army Reserve; 3,215 Navy Reserve; 1,159 Marine Corps Reserve; 2,851 Air National Guard; and 6,656 Air Force Reserve) who completed self-administered questionnaires anonymously.

Reserve component estimates exclude full-time or activated Guard and Reserve.

Mental health counseling refers to receiving services from a psychologist, psychiatrist, clinical social worker, other mental health counselor, or a general medical doctor at a military or civilian facility. Services could also be received from a military chaplain, civilian pastor, rabbi, other pastoral counselor, or a self-help group, such as Alcoholics Anonymous or Narcotics Anonymous.

SOURCES: Department of Defense Survey of Health Related Behaviors Among the Guard and Reserve Force, 2006. As taken from Hourani, L. L., Bray, R. M., Marsden, M. E., Witt, M. B., Vandermaas-Peeler, R., Scheffler, S., ... Strange, L. B. (2007, September). *2006 Department of Defense survey of health related behaviors among the Guard and Reserve force.* Report prepared for TRICARE Management Activity. Retrieved from http://www.tricare.mil/hpae/_docs/RC_2006 Reserve Component_FR_9-07.pdf. The views, opinions, and findings contained in this report are those of the authors and should not be construed as an official Department of Defense position, policy, or decision, unless so designated by other official documentation.

Table 69. Percentage of persons aged 10 to 20 in the juvenile justice system receiving mental health counseling, by selected characteristics, United States, 2003

[Data are based on a nationally representative survey of youth in residential placement]

Characteristic	Any counseling (percent)	Individual counseling (percent)	Group counseling (percent)	Family counseling (percent)
Total	**52.7**	**70.0**	**47.4**	**17.6**
Age				
10–12	56.9	72.3	32.0	26.6
13–15	53.3	69.3	41.2	22.7
16–17	51.7	70.5	49.8	16.3
18–20	54.2	69.7	54.2	10.3
Sex				
Male	51.9	67.1	49.0	16.4
Female	57.2	84.5	39.7	23.6
Hispanic origin and race				
Not Hispanic				
White	55.7	72.0	50.8	20.5
Black or African American	51.8	66.5	44.3	12.2
American Indian or Alaska Native	53.0	72.1	43.6	16.0
Asian	58.7	76.3	54.8	18.3
Native Hawaiian or Other Pacific Islander	58.4	92.7	*	*
Other two or more race groups (non-Hispanic)	57.6	79.4	44.1	21.0
Hispanic	47.6	66.9	48.6	20.0

*Estimates are considered unreliable.

NOTE: The Survey of Youth in Residential Placement is a nationally representative survey of offender youth aged 10 to 20 in State and local facilities. The final sample consisted of 7,073 youth who were interviewed using an audio computer-assisted self-interview system.

SOURCE: Survey of Youth in Residential Placement, 2003, Office of Juvenile Justice and Delinquency Prevention.

7. TABLES

7.3 Payers and Payment Mechanisms

Table 70. Mental health expenditures, by type of provider, United States, selected years 1986–2005

[Data are based on national expenditures for mental health services]

Type of provider	1986 (millions of dollars)	1993 (millions of dollars)	2000 (millions of dollars)	2003 (millions of dollars)	2005 (millions of dollars)
Total expenditures	$31,764	$54,249	$79,295	$100,302	$112,787
Total all service providers and products	30,222	51,138	74,225	92,872	104,403
Total all service providers	27,860	46,531	57,528	67,045	74,429
All hospitals	13,596	21,054	23,443	27,409	30,166
General hospitals	5,345	9,211	12,444	14,960	16,750
General hospital, specialty units[1]	3,026	6,474	9,131	10,831	11,540
General hospital, nonspecialty care	2,320	2,737	3,313	4,129	5,210
Specialty hospitals	8,251	11,843	10,999	12,449	13,416
All physicians	3,814	7,440	11,193	13,736	16,266
Psychiatrists	2,755	5,239	8,100	9,332	11,403
Nonpsychiatric physicians	1,058	2,201	3,093	4,405	4,864
Other professionals[2]	1,519	3,480	4,765	5,364	5,812
Freestanding nursing homes	4,903	5,593	5,313	6,266	6,855
Freestanding home health	112	376	609	832	1,070
All other personal and public health	3,916	8,588	12,205	13,438	14,259
Specialty facilities, nonhospital[3]	3,916	8,588	12,205	13,438	14,259
Retail prescription medication[4]	2,362	4,607	16,697	25,826	29,974
Insurance administration[5]	1,542	3,111	5,071	7,430	8,384
All specialty providers[6]	19,467	35,624	45,200	51,414	56,430
All nonspecialty providers[7]	8,393	10,907	12,328	15,632	17,999

[1] General hospital specialty units include all spending for mental health care in Veterans Affairs hospitals.

[2] Other professionals include paid specialty providers who are not physicians, such as counselors, psychologists, and social workers.

[3] Specialty facilities, nonhospital include organizations providing outpatient and/or residential services or a combination of services to individuals with mental illness or substance use diagnoses.

[4] Retail prescription medication includes psychotropic medications sold through retail outlets and mail order pharmacies; excluded are sales through hospitals, exclusive-to-patient health maintenance organizations, and nursing home pharmacies.

[5] Insurance administration includes spending for the cost of running various government health care insurance programs, as well as the administrative costs and profit of private health insurance.

[6] All specialty providers include community hospital specialty units, specialty hospitals, psychiatrists, other professionals, and specialty mental health centers.

[7] All nonspecialty providers include community hospital nonspecialty care, nonpsychiatric physicians, freestanding nursing homes, and freestanding home health.

Table 70 notes *(continued)*

NOTES: National Expenditures for Mental Health Services and Substance Abuse Treatment (Spending Estimates Project [SEP]) presents a broad overview of spending on mental health services and substance abuse treatment. SEP uses data from 15 national sources to produce these estimates.

These data include revisions and may differ from previously published data. These data are not adjusted for inflation.

SOURCE: Substance Abuse and Mental Health Services Administration (SAMHSA). (2010). *National expenditures for mental health services and substance abuse treatment, 1986–2005* (DHHS Publication No. SMA 10-4612). Rockville, MD: Center for Mental Health Services and Center for Substance Abuse Treatment, SAMHSA.

Table 71. Mental health expenditures and all health expenditures, by type of provider, United States, 1986 and 2005

[Data are based on national expenditures for mental health services]

Type of provider	1986			2005		
	Mental health (millions of dollars)	All health[1] (millions of dollars)	Mental health share (percent)	Mental health (millions of dollars)	All health[1] (millions of dollars)	Mental health share (percent)
Total expenditures	$31,764	$439,394	7.2	$112,787	$1,850,363	6.1
Total all service providers and products	30,222	416,515	7.3	104,403	1,711,708	6.1
Total all service providers	27,860	367,511	7.6	74,429	1,454,255	5.1
All hospitals	13,596	176,548	7.7	30,166	607,495	5.0
General hospitals	5,345	164,295	3.3	16,750	588,752	2.8
General hospital, specialty units[2]	3,026	—	—	11,540	—	—
General hospital, nonspecialty care	2,320	—	—	5,210	—	—
Specialty hospitals	8,251	12,253	67.3	13,416	18,743	71.6
All physicians	3,814	99,558	3.8	16,266	422,240	3.9
Psychiatrists	2,755	—	—	11,403	—	—
Nonpsychiatric physicians	1,058	—	—	4,864	—	—
Other professionals[3]	1,519	9,736	15.6	5,812	56,015	10.4
Freestanding nursing homes	4,903	33,945	14.4	6,855	120,597	5.7
Freestanding home health	112	6,388	1.8	1,070	48,085	2.2
All other personal and public health	3,916	18,226	21.5	14,259	113,434	12.6
Specialty facilities, nonhospital[4]	3,916	—	—	14,259	—	—
Retail prescription medication[5]	2,362	24,289	9.7	29,974	199,699	15.0
Insurance administration[6]	1,542	22,879	6.7	8,384	138,656	6.0
All specialty providers[7]	19,467	—	—	56,430	—	—
All nonspecialty providers[8]	8,393	—	—	17,999	—	—

—Data not available.

[1] For all health, the total includes spending not shown separately for dentists, other nondurable medical products, and durable medical products.

[2] General hospital specialty units include all spending for mental health care in Veterans Affairs hospitals.

[3] Other professionals include paid specialty providers who are not physicians, such as counselors, psychologists, and social workers.

[4] Specialty facilities, nonhospital include organizations providing outpatient and/or residential services or a combination of services to individuals with mental illness or substance use diagnoses.

[5] Retail prescription medication includes psychotropic medications sold through retail outlets and mail order pharmacies; excluded are sales through hospitals, exclusive-to-patient health maintenance organizations, and nursing home pharmacies.

[6] Insurance administration includes spending for the cost of running various government health care insurance programs, as well as the administrative costs and profit of private health insurance.

[7] All specialty providers include community hospital specialty units, specialty hospitals, psychiatrists, other professionals, and specialty mental health centers.

[8] All nonspecialty providers include community hospital nonspecialty care, nonpsychiatric physicians, freestanding nursing homes, and freestanding home health.

Table 71 notes *(continued)*

NOTES: National Expenditures for Mental Health Services and Substance Abuse Treatment (Spending Estimates Project [SEP]) presents a broad overview of spending on mental health services and substance abuse treatment. SEP uses data from 15 national sources to produce these estimates.

These data include revisions and may differ from previously published data. These data are not adjusted for inflation.

SOURCE: Substance Abuse and Mental Health Services Administration (SAMHSA). (2010). *National expenditures for mental health services and substance abuse treatment, 1986–2005* (DHHS Publication No. SMA 10-4612). Rockville, MD: Center for Mental Health Services and Center for Substance Abuse Treatment, SAMHSA.

Table 72. Percentage distribution of mental health expenditures and all health expenditures, by type of provider, United States, selected years 1986–2005

[Data are based on national expenditures for mental health services]

Type of provider	1986 (percent)	1993 (percent)	2000 (percent)	2003 (percent)	2005 (percent)
Mental health					
Total expenditures	100.0	100.0	100.0	100.0	100.0
Total all service providers and products	95.1	94.3	93.6	92.6	92.6
Total all service providers	87.7	85.8	72.5	66.8	66.0
All hospitals	42.8	38.8	29.6	27.3	26.7
General hospitals	16.8	17.0	15.7	14.9	14.9
General hospital, specialty units[1]	9.5	11.9	11.5	10.8	10.2
General hospital, nonspecialty care	7.3	5.0	4.2	4.1	4.6
Specialty hospitals	26.0	21.8	13.9	12.4	11.9
All physicians	12.0	13.7	14.1	13.7	14.4
Psychiatrists	8.7	9.7	10.2	9.3	10.1
Nonpsychiatric physicians	3.3	4.1	3.9	4.4	4.3
Other professionals[2]	4.8	6.4	6.0	5.3	5.2
Freestanding nursing homes	15.4	10.3	6.7	6.2	6.1
Freestanding home health	0.4	0.7	0.8	0.8	0.9
All other personal and public health	12.3	15.8	15.4	13.4	12.6
Specialty facilities, nonhospital[3]	12.3	15.8	15.4	13.4	12.6
Retail prescription medication[4]	7.4	8.5	21.1	25.7	26.6
Insurance administration[5]	4.9	5.7	6.4	7.4	7.4
All specialty providers[6]	61.3	65.7	57.0	51.3	50.0
All nonspecialty providers[7]	26.4	20.1	15.5	15.6	16.0
All health					
Total expenditures[8]	100.0	100.0	100.0	100.0	100.0
Total all service providers and products	94.8	93.8	93.5	92.5	92.5
Total all service providers	83.6	83.5	80.1	78.4	78.6
All hospitals	40.2	37.2	33.0	32.5	32.8
General hospitals	37.4	35.3	31.7	31.4	31.8
Specialty hospitals	2.8	1.9	1.2	1.1	1.0
All physicians	22.7	23.6	22.8	22.6	22.8
Other professionals[2]	2.2	2.9	3.1	3.0	3.0
Freestanding nursing homes	7.7	7.7	7.5	6.8	6.5
Freestanding home health	1.5	2.6	2.4	2.3	2.6
All other personal and public health	4.1	5.0	6.4	6.4	6.1
Retail prescription medication[4]	5.5	6.0	9.5	10.7	10.8
Insurance administration[5]	5.2	6.2	6.5	7.5	7.5

See notes on page 199.

Table 72 notes

[1] General hospital specialty units include all spending for mental health care in Veterans Affairs hospitals.

[2] Other professionals include paid specialty providers who are not physicians, such as counselors, psychologists, and social workers.

[3] Specialty facilities, nonhospital include organizations providing outpatient and/or residential services or a combination of services to individuals with mental illness or substance use diagnoses.

[4] Retail prescription medication includes psychotropic medications sold through retail outlets and mail order pharmacies; excluded are sales through hospitals, exclusive-to-patient health maintenance organizations, and nursing home pharmacies.

[5] Insurance administration includes spending for the cost of running various government health care insurance programs, as well as the administrative costs and profit of private health insurance.

[6] All specialty providers include community hospital specialty units, specialty hospitals, psychiatrists, other professionals, and specialty mental health centers.

[7] All nonspecialty providers include community hospital nonspecialty care, nonpsychiatric physicians, freestanding nursing homes, and freestanding home health.

[8] For all health, the total includes spending not shown separately for dentists, other nondurable medical products, and durable medical products.

NOTES: National Expenditures for Mental Health Services and Substance Abuse Treatment (Spending Estimates Project [SEP]) presents a broad overview of spending on mental health services and substance abuse treatment. SEP uses data from 15 national sources to produce these estimates.

These data include revisions and may differ from previously published data. These data are not adjusted for inflation.

SOURCE: Substance Abuse and Mental Health Services Administration (SAMHSA). (2010). *National expenditures for mental health services and substance abuse treatment, 1986–2005* (DHHS Publication No. SMA 10-4612). Rockville, MD: Center for Mental Health Services and Center for Substance Abuse Treatment, SAMHSA.

Table 73. Mental health expenditures, by payer, United States, selected years 1986–2005

[Data are based on national expenditures for mental health services]

Type of payer	1986 (millions of dollars)	1993 (millions of dollars)	2000 (millions of dollars)	2003 (millions of dollars)	2005 (millions of dollars)
Total expenditures	$31,764	$54,249	$79,295	$100,302	$112,787
Private—total	13,471	20,482	31,477	41,046	47,108
Out-of-pocket[1]	5,569	6,916	10,232	12,612	13,802
Private insurance[2]	6,308	11,160	19,106	25,964	30,417
Other private[3]	1,594	2,406	2,139	2,470	2,890
Public—total	18,293	33,767	47,818	59,255	65,678
Medicare[4]	2,099	4,812	6,629	7,641	8,630
Medicaid[5]	5,503	11,535	20,193	27,574	31,115
Other Federal[6]	1,993	2,752	3,777	5,066	5,673
Other State and local[6,7]	8,698	14,670	17,219	18,973	20,261
All Federal[8]	7,171	14,846	22,156	29,068	32,078
All State[9]	11,122	18,923	25,662	30,186	33,601

[1] Out-of-pocket expenditures account for direct spending by consumers for health care goods and services, including coinsurance, deductibles, and any amounts not covered by public or private insurance.

[2] Private insurance accounts for benefits paid by private health insurers, including behavioral health plans, to providers of service or for prescription medication, and for the administrative costs and profits of health plans.

[3] Other private includes spending from philanthropic and other nonpatient revenue sources.

[4] Medicare is the Federal government program that provides health insurance coverage to eligible aged and disabled persons.

[5] Medicaid is a program jointly funded by Federal and State governments that provides health care coverage to certain classes of people with limited income and resources.

[6] Children's Health Insurance Program (CHIP) is distributed across Medicaid, other Federal, and other State and local categories, depending on whether CHIP was run through Medicaid or as a separate State program.

[7] Other State and local accounts for programs funded primarily through State and local mental health and substance abuse agencies. Substance Abuse and Mental Health Services Administration (SAMHSA) block grant expenditures are included in other Federal expenditures. However, these funds are distributed from the Federal government to State and local governments that then distribute them to providers.

[8] All Federal category includes Federal share of Medicaid.

[9] All State category includes State and local share of Medicaid.

NOTES: National Expenditures for Mental Health Services and Substance Abuse Treatment (Spending Estimates Project [SEP]) presents a broad overview of spending on mental health services and substance abuse treatment. SEP uses data from 15 national sources to produce these estimates.

These data include revisions and may differ from previously published data. These data are not adjusted for inflation.

SOURCE: Substance Abuse and Mental Health Services Administration (SAMHSA). (2010). *National expenditures for mental health services and substance abuse treatment, 1986–2005* (DHHS Publication No. SMA 10-4612). Rockville, MD: Center for Mental Health Services and Center for Substance Abuse Treatment, SAMHSA.

Table 74. Mental health expenditures and all health expenditures, by payer, United States, 1986 and 2005

[Data are based on national expenditures for mental health services]

Type of payer	1986			2005		
	Mental health (millions of dollars)	All health[1] (millions of dollars)	Mental health share (percent)	Mental health (millions of dollars)	All health[1] (millions of dollars)	Mental health share (percent)
Total expenditures	$31,764	$439,394	7.2	$112,787	$1,850,363	6.1
Private—total	13,471	260,862	5.2	47,108	1,007,380	4.7
Out-of-pocket[2]	5,569	103,248	5.4	13,802	246,971	5.6
Private insurance[2]	6,308	135,865	4.6	30,417	689,997	4.4
Other private[4]	1,594	21,749	7.3	2,890	70,412	4.1
Public—total	18,293	178,532	10.2	65,678	842,983	7.8
Medicare[5]	2,099	76,395	2.7	8,630	339,357	2.5
Medicaid[6]	5,503	45,383	12.1	31,115	311,488	10.0
Other Federal[7]	1,993	20,809	9.6	5,673	83,593	6.8
Other State and local[7,8]	8,698	35,945	24.2	20,261	108,545	18.7
All Federal[9]	7,171	122,606	5.8	32,078	600,765	5.3
All State[10]	11,122	55,926	19.9	33,601	242,218	13.9

[1] For all health, the total includes spending not shown separately for dentists, other nondurable medical products, and durable medical products.

[2] Out-of-pocket expenditures account for direct spending by consumers for health care goods and services, including coinsurance, deductibles, and any amounts not covered by public or private insurance.

[3] Private insurance accounts for benefits paid by private health insurers, including behavioral health plans, to providers of service or for prescription medication, and for the administrative costs and profits of health plans.

[4] Other private includes spending from philanthropic and other nonpatient revenue sources.

[5] Medicare is the Federal government program that provides health insurance coverage to eligible aged and disabled persons.

[6] Medicaid is a program jointly funded by Federal and State governments that provides health care coverage to certain classes of people with limited income and resources.

[7] Children's Health Insurance Program (CHIP) is distributed across Medicaid, other Federal, and other State and local categories, depending on whether CHIP was run through Medicaid or as a separate State program.

[8] Other State and local accounts for programs funded primarily through State and local mental health and substance abuse agencies. Substance Abuse and Mental Health Services Administration (SAMHSA) block grant expenditures are included in other Federal expenditures. However, these funds are distributed from the Federal government to State and local governments that then distribute them to providers.

[9] All Federal category includes Federal share of Medicaid.

[10] All State category includes State and local share of Medicaid.

NOTES: National Expenditures for Mental Health Services and Substance Abuse Treatment (Spending Estimates Project [SEP]) presents a broad overview of spending on mental health services and substance abuse treatment. SEP uses data from 15 national sources to produce these estimates.

These data include revisions and may differ from previously published data. These data are not adjusted for inflation.

SOURCE: Substance Abuse and Mental Health Services Administration (SAMHSA). (2010). *National expenditures for mental health services and substance abuse treatment, 1986–2005* (DHHS Publication No. SMA 10-4612). Rockville, MD: Center for Mental Health Services and Center for Substance Abuse Treatment, SAMHSA.

Table 75. Percentage distribution of mental health expenditures and all health expenditures, by payer, United States, selected years 1986–2005

[Data are based on national expenditures for mental health services]

Type of payer	1986 (percent)	1993 (percent)	2000 (percent)	2003 (percent)	2005 (percent)
Mental health					
Total expenditures	100.0	100.0	100.0	100.0	100.0
Private—total	42.4	37.8	39.7	40.9	41.8
Out-of-pocket[1]	17.5	12.7	12.9	12.6	12.2
Private insurance[2]	19.9	20.6	24.1	25.9	27.0
Other private[3]	5.0	4.4	2.7	2.5	2.6
Public—total	57.6	62.2	60.3	59.1	58.2
Medicare[4]	6.6	8.9	8.4	7.6	7.7
Medicaid[5]	17.3	21.3	25.5	27.5	27.6
Other Federal[6]	6.3	5.1	4.8	5.1	5.0
Other State and local[6,7]	27.4	27.0	21.7	18.9	18.0
All Federal[8]	22.6	27.4	27.9	29.0	28.4
All State[9]	35.0	34.9	32.4	30.1	29.8
All health					
Total expenditures[10]	100.0	100.0	100.0	100.0	100.0
Private—total	59.4	56.2	55.8	55.0	54.4
Out-of-pocket[1]	23.5	17.0	15.2	13.8	13.3
Private insurance[2]	30.9	34.6	36.0	37.2	37.3
Other private[3]	4.9	4.6	4.6	4.0	3.8
Public—total	40.6	43.8	44.2	45.0	45.6
Medicare[4]	17.4	17.6	17.7	17.4	18.3
Medicaid[5]	10.3	14.3	15.9	16.7	16.8
Other Federal[6]	4.7	4.1	4.0	4.6	4.5
Other State and local[6,7]	8.2	7.7	6.6	6.3	5.9
All Federal[8]	27.9	30.7	31.0	31.9	32.5
All State[9]	12.7	13.1	13.2	13.1	13.1

See notes on page 203.

Table 75 notes

[1] Out-of-pocket expenditures account for direct spending by consumers for health care goods and services, including coinsurance, deductibles, and any amounts not covered by public or private insurance.

[2] Private insurance accounts for benefits paid by private health insurers, including behavioral health plans, to providers of service or for prescription medication, and for the administrative costs and profits of health plans.

[3] Other private includes spending from philanthropic and other nonpatient revenue sources.

[4] Medicare is the Federal government program that provides health insurance coverage to eligible aged and disabled persons.

[5] Medicaid is a program jointly funded by Federal and State governments that provides health care coverage to certain classes of people with limited income and resources.

[6] Children's Health Insurance Program (CHIP) is distributed across Medicaid, other Federal, and other State and local categories, depending on whether CHIP was run through Medicaid or as a separate State program.

[7] Other State and local accounts for programs funded primarily through State and local mental health and substance abuse agencies. Substance Abuse and Mental Health Services Administration (SAMHSA) block grant expenditures are included in other Federal expenditures. However, these funds are distributed from the Federal government to State and local governments that then distribute them to providers.

[8] All Federal category includes Federal share of Medicaid.

[9] All State category includes State and local share of Medicaid.

[10] For all health, the total includes spending not shown separately for dentists, other nondurable medical products, and durable medical products.

NOTES: National Expenditures for Mental Health Services and Substance Abuse Treatment (Spending Estimates Project [SEP]) presents a broad overview of spending on mental health services and substance abuse treatment. SEP uses data from 15 national sources to produce these estimates.

These data include revisions and may differ from previously published data. These data are not adjusted for inflation.

SOURCE: Substance Abuse and Mental Health Services Administration (SAMHSA). (2010). *National expenditures for mental health services and substance abuse treatment, 1986–2005* (DHHS Publication No. SMA 10-4612). Rockville, MD: Center for Mental Health Services and Center for Substance Abuse Treatment, SAMHSA.

Table 76. Mental health treatment expenditures, by site of service, United States, selected years 1986–2005

[Data are based on national expenditures for mental health services]

Site of service	1986 (millions of dollars)	1993 (millions of dollars)	2000 (millions of dollars)	2003 (millions of dollars)	2005 (millions of dollars)
All service providers	**$27,860**	**$46,531**	**$57,528**	**$67,045**	**$74,429**
Inpatient	13,314	18,998	18,915	20,887	21,653
Outpatient	7,559	17,042	26,271	31,865	37,195
Residential	6,988	10,492	12,341	14,294	15,581

NOTES: National Expenditures for Mental Health Services and Substance Abuse Treatment (Spending Estimates Project [SEP]) presents a broad overview of spending on mental health services and substance abuse treatment. SEP uses data from 15 national sources to produce these estimates.

These data are not adjusted for inflation.

SOURCE: Substance Abuse and Mental Health Services Administration (SAMHSA). (2010). *National expenditures for mental health services and substance abuse treatment, 1986–2005* (DHHS Publication No. SMA 10-4612). Rockville, MD: Center for Mental Health Services and Center for Substance Abuse Treatment, SAMHSA.

Table 77. Percentage distribution of mental health treatment expenditures, by site of service, United States, selected years 1986–2005

[Data are based on national expenditures for mental health services]

Site of service	1986 (percent)	1993 (percent)	2000 (percent)	2003 (percent)	2005 (percent)
All service providers	**100.0**	**100.0**	**100.0**	**100.0**	**100.0**
Inpatient	47.8	40.8	32.9	31.2	29.1
Outpatient	27.1	36.6	45.7	47.5	50.0
Residential	25.1	22.5	21.5	21.3	20.9

NOTES: National Expenditures for Mental Health Services and Substance Abuse Treatment (Spending Estimates Project [SEP]) presents a broad overview of spending on mental health services and substance abuse treatment. SEP uses data from 15 national sources to produce these estimates.

These data are not adjusted for inflation.

SOURCE: Substance Abuse and Mental Health Services Administration (SAMHSA). (2010). *National expenditures for mental health services and substance abuse treatment, 1986–2005* (DHHS Publication No. SMA 10-4612). Rockville, MD: Center for Mental Health Services and Center for Substance Abuse Treatment, SAMHSA.

7. TABLES

7.3 Payers and Payment Mechanisms: Tables

7.3.1 Mental Health Expenditures: Overview

7.3.2 Revenues and Expenditures by Public Funding Source

Medicaid
Tables 78–81

Medicare

Veterans Mental Health

State Mental Health Agencies

7.3.3 Private Employer-Sponsored Mental Health Benefits

7.3.4 Mental Health Prescription Medication Use

Table 78. Medicaid fee-for-service (FFS) mental health (MH) and substance abuse (SA) beneficiaries and expenditures, by selected characteristics, 13 States, 2003

[Data are based on Medicaid claims from 13 States]

Characteristic	FFS MH beneficiaries[1]				FFS SA beneficiaries[1]				FFS expenditures (millions of dollars)[3]	
	Number	Percentage of all FFS bene-ficiaries	Average number of months[2] in FFS	Average number of months receiving an MH service	Number	Percentage of all FFS bene-ficiaries	Average number of months[2] in FFS	Average number of months receiving an SA service	MH bene-ficiaries	SA bene-ficiaries
All	**1,292,854**	**11**	**10.5**	**4.3**	**87,336**	**1**	**9.8**	**3.0**	**$13,720**	**$812**
Age										
0–5	80,673	3	10.1	3.0	1,223	0	8.4	1.9	534	19
6–12	294,139	13	10.6	4.3	539	0	10.8	2.8	1,389	4
13–18	226,422	15	10.5	4.5	15,444	1	9.8	3.0	1,830	97
19–21	41,270	8	9.7	3.2	5,110	1	8.7	2.5	388	27
22–44	329,204	15	10.2	4.1	42,424	2	9.5	3.0	3,599	343
45–64	206,563	21	11.0	5.2	18,891	2	10.6	3.1	3,485	262
65 or older	114,582	8	11.0	4.4	3,705	0	11.0	3.2	2,496	60
Unknown	*	*	*	*	*	*	*	*	*	*
Sex										
Female	708,103	10	10.5	4.1	44,856	1	9.7	2.9	7,497	384
Male	584,625	12	10.6	4.6	42,475	1	9.9	3.0	6,223	429
Unknown	126	6	8.3	3.3	*	*	*	*	1	*
Race/ethnicity										
White	783,057	15	10.5	4.5	48,268	1	9.6	3.2	8,825	440
Black	310,275	9	10.7	4.2	28,202	1	10.2	2.8	3,144	284
Hispanic	129,516	6	10.3	3.7	6,328	0	9.5	2.3	984	46
American Indian/ Alaska Native	11,192	12	10.7	4.3	1,795	2	9.9	2.7	113	15
Asian/Hawaiian/ Pacific Islander	7,512	5	10.6	4.5	212	0	9.6	2.6	82	2
Other/unknown	51,302	12	10.9	4.6	2,531	1	10.0	2.9	573	26

(continued)

Table 78. Medicaid fee-for-service (FFS) mental health (MH) and substance abuse (SA) beneficiaries and expenditures, by selected characteristics, 13 States, 2003 *(continued)*

Characteristic	FFS MH beneficiaries[1]				FFS SA beneficiaries[1]				FFS expenditures (millions of dollars)[3]	
	Number	Percentage of all FFS bene-ficiaries	Average number of months[2] in FFS	Average number of months receiving an MH service	Number	Percentage of all FFS bene-ficiaries	Average number of months[2] in FFS	Average number of months receiving an SA service	MH bene-ficiaries	SA bene-ficiaries
Medicaid and Medicare dual eligibility status										
Aged duals with full Medicaid	103,073	9	11.0	4.5	3,215	0	11.0	3.4	$2,324	$54
Disabled duals with full Medicaid	153,553	29	11.3	5.9	9,101	2	11.1	3.4	2,716	86
Duals with limited Medicaid	24,440	6	10.9	3.7	1,321	0	10.7	2.0	124	6
Other duals	4,914	28	9.9	4.5	385	2	9.6	3.7	42	3
Disabled nonduals	290,115	29	11.1	5.4	20,860	2	10.8	3.1	4,833	340
All other nonduals	716,759	8	10.1	3.5	52,454	1	9.1	2.8	3,681	324
Eligibility group[4]										
Aged	101,319	7	11.0	4.3	3,120	0	10.9	3.2	2,206	51
Disabled	473,203	27	11.2	5.5	31,527	2	10.9	3.2	7,878	437
Adults (nondisabled)	193,563	9	9.3	2.5	34,804	2	8.9	2.8	956	208
Children (nondisabled)	524,769	8	10.4	3.9	17,885	0	9.5	2.9	2,681	116
Unknown	*	*	*	*	*	*	*	*	*	*

See notes on page 208.

Table 78 notes

*Estimates are considered unreliable.

[1] Fee-for-service (FFS) beneficiaries include beneficiaries enrolled in Medicaid, but not in comprehensive managed care or a behavioral health managed care plan, for at least 1 month during the year. FFS mental health (MH) beneficiaries include FFS beneficiaries who, during the year, (1) had at least one claim on which an MH disorder was the primary diagnosis or (2) received a clearly identifiable MH service. FFS substance abuse (SA) beneficiaries include FFS beneficiaries who, during the year, had at least one claim on which a substance use disorder was the primary diagnosis. If beneficiaries had at least one claim on which an MH disorder was the primary diagnosis and at least one claim on which a substance use disorder was the primary diagnosis, they are included in the category that represents the diagnosis most frequently listed during the year.

[2] Months receiving an MH service are those in which the beneficiary had at least one nonprescription medication claim on which the primary diagnosis was an MH disorder or in which the beneficiary received a clearly identifiable MH service. Months receiving an SA service are those in which the beneficiary had at least one nonprescription medication claim on which the primary diagnosis was a substance use disorder.

[3] Expenditures are claims-based Medicaid payments, including both Federal and State shares. Expenditures for FFS months are defined as expenditures for services during FFS months minus expenditures for capitation premium payments.

[4] Eligibility groups are mutually exclusive. All individuals aged 65 or older are in the aged group; all remaining individuals who qualify for Medicaid due to disability are in the disabled group; remaining individuals are categorized as adults or children according to their classification in State enrollment files. Children who qualify for Medicaid through receipt of Supplemental Security Income payments are included in the disabled category.

NOTES: This study identified Medicaid beneficiaries using MH or SA services in FFS plans in 13 States in 2003 (n = 1,380,190) and examined their use of medical services.

The States included in this table are Arkansas, Georgia, Idaho, Illinois, Indiana, Kansas, Maine, Montana, North Carolina, South Carolina, Texas, Vermont, and Wyoming. Table originally published in Substance Abuse and Mental Health Services Administration (SAMHSA). (2010). *Mental Health, United States, 2008* (DHHS Publication No. SMA 10-4590). Rockville, MD: Center for Mental Health Services, SAMHSA. The study analyzed Medicaid Analytic eXtract (MAX) files of all 50 States and the District of Columbia for the year 2003. This table displays data for 13 States that were selected after examining the completeness and quality of their MAX data. "Data completeness" refers to the extent to which FFS data were available (States with a greater proportion of beneficiaries in FFS are considered to have more complete data than States with a greater proportion of beneficiaries in managed care). "Data quality" refers to technical problems, such as missing diagnosis codes, missing eligibility data, duplicate records, and missing claims. Each State's data were assigned a score from 1 to 4; scores were developed specifically for purposes of the analysis presented in *Mental Health and Substance Abuse Services in Medicaid, 2003: Charts and State Tables*, strictly to assist readers in understanding how to interpret the data presented, and were not intended to reflect the quality of the States' overall MAX data.

SOURCE: Substance Abuse and Mental Health Services Administration (SAMHSA). (2010). *Mental health and substance abuse services in Medicaid, 2003: Charts and state tables* (DHHS Publication No. SMA 10-4608). Rockville, MD: Center for Mental Health Services, SAMHSA.

Table 79. Medicaid fee-for-service (FFS) mental health and substance abuse beneficiaries, by diagnostic category and age group in 13 States, 2003

[Data are based on Medicaid claims from 13 States]

Diagnostic category	All ages		Aged 21 or younger		Aged 22 to 64		Aged 65 or older	
	Number	Percent	Number	Percent	Number	Percent	Number	Percent
Mental health[1]								
Schizophrenia	116,116	9.0	3,636	0.6	97,050	18.1	15,430	13.5
Major depression and affective psychoses	254,669	19.7	55,423	8.6	170,967	31.9	28,279	24.7
Other psychoses	38,199	3.0	3,648	0.6	17,649	3.3	16,902	14.8
Childhood psychoses	20,965	1.6	17,241	2.7	3,414	0.6	310	0.3
Neurotic and other depressive disorders	280,681	21.7	84,048	13.1	160,043	29.9	36,590	31.9
Personality disorders	6,953	0.5	1,515	0.2	4,679	0.9	759	0.7
Special symptoms or syndromes	42,436	3.3	21,402	3.3	16,954	3.2	4,080	3.6
Stress and adjustment reactions	158,617	12.3	113,030	17.6	39,488	7.4	6,099	5.3
Conduct disorders	57,902	4.5	48,831	7.6	7,997	1.5	1,074	0.9
Emotional disturbances	57,894	4.5	57,383	8.9	447	0.1	64	0.1
Hyperkinetic syndrome	234,093	18.1	229,542	35.7	4,477	0.8	74	0.1
Mental disorders associated with childbirth	7,799	0.6	2,686	0.4	5,111	1.0	*	*
Other mental disorders	16,311	1.3	4,090	0.6	7,475	1.4	4,746	4.1
No diagnosis	218	0.0	29	0.0	16	0.0	173	0.2
Total	1,292,853	100.0	642,504	100.0	535,767	100.0	114,582	100.0
Substance abuse[2]								
Alcohol-induced mental disorders	3,672	4.2	178	0.8	2,475	4.0	1,019	27.5
Alcohol dependence or nondependent abuse	29,939	34.3	4,080	18.3	24,087	39.3	1,772	47.8
Drug psychoses	4,830	5.5	743	3.3	3,534	5.8	553	14.9
Drug dependence or nondependent abuse	45,847	52.5	15,647	70.1	29,842	48.7	358	9.7
Substance abuse associated with childbirth	3,048	3.5	1,668	7.5	1,377	2.2	*	*
Total	87,336	100.0	22,316	100.0	61,315	100.0	3,705	100.0

See notes on page 210.

Table 79 notes

*Estimates are considered unreliable.

[1] Schizophrenia (ICD-9-CM diagnosis codes beginning with 295) includes both chronic and acute schizophrenic disorders. Major depression and affective psychoses (ICD-9-CM diagnosis codes beginning with 296) includes manic, depressive, and bipolar disorders. Other psychoses (ICD-9-CM diagnosis codes beginning with 297 or 298) includes paranoid states, delusional disorders, depressive psychosis, and reactive psychoses. Childhood psychoses (ICD-9-CM diagnosis codes beginning with 299) includes infantile autism, disintegrative disorders, and childhood type schizophrenia. Neurotic and other depressive disorders (ICD-9-CM diagnosis codes beginning with 300 or 311) includes anxiety states; phobic, obsessive compulsive, and other neurotic disorders; and unspecified depressive disorders. Personality disorders (ICD-9-CM diagnosis codes beginning with 301) includes affective, schizoid, explosive, histrionic, antisocial, dependent, and other personality disorders. Other mental disorders (ICD-9-CM diagnosis codes beginning with 302, 306, or 310) includes sexual deviations, physiological malfunction arising from mental factors, and nonpsychotic mental disorders due to organic brain damage. Special symptoms or syndromes (ICD-9-CM diagnosis codes beginning with 307) includes eating disorders, tics and repetitive movement disorders, sleep disorders, and enuresis. Stress and adjustment reactions (ICD-9-CM diagnosis codes beginning with 308 or 309) includes acute reaction to stress, depressive reaction, separation disorders, and conduct disturbance. Conduct disorders (ICD-9-CM diagnosis codes beginning with 312) includes aggressive outbursts, truancy, delinquency, kleptomania, impulse control disorder, and other conduct disorders. Emotional disturbances (ICD-9-CM diagnosis codes beginning with 313) includes overanxious disorder; shyness; relationship problems; and other mixed emotional disturbances of childhood or adolescence, such as oppositional disorder. Hyperkinetic syndrome (ICD-9-CM diagnosis codes beginning with 314) includes attention deficit with and without hyperactivity and hyperkinesis with or without developmental delay. Mental disorders associated with childbirth (ICD-9-CM diagnosis codes 648.40 through 648.44) includes mental disorders of the mother associated with pregnancy, delivery, and postpartum periods.

[2] Alcohol-induced mental disorders includes conditions with ICD-9-CM diagnosis codes beginning with 291. Alcohol dependence or nondependent abuse (ICD-9-CM diagnosis codes beginning with 303 and 305.0) includes alcohol dependence syndrome, acute alcoholic intoxication, and nondependent alcohol abuse. Drug psychoses (ICD-9-CM diagnosis codes beginning with 292) includes drug-induced mental disorders and drug withdrawal. Drug dependence or nondependence abuse (ICD-9-CM diagnosis codes beginning with 304, 305.2–305.9, and 965.0) includes all drug dependence and nondependent abuse, except for those relating to alcohol or nicotine, and poisoning by opiates and related narcotics. Substance abuse associated with childbirth (ICD-9-CM diagnosis codes 648.3, 760.71, and 779.5) includes drug dependence complicating pregnancy, childbirth, or the puerperium; fetal alcohol syndrome or alcohol withdrawal in a newborn; and drug withdrawal syndrome in a newborn.

NOTES: This study identified Medicaid beneficiaries using mental health (MH) or substance abuse (SA) services in fee-for-service (FFS) plans in 13 States in 2003 (n = 1,380,190) and examined their use of medical services.

FFS beneficiaries include beneficiaries enrolled in Medicaid, but not in comprehensive managed care or a behavioral health managed care plan, for at least 1 month during the year. FFS MH beneficiaries include FFS beneficiaries who, during the year, had at least one claim on which one of the MH or SA disorders shown in the table was the primary diagnosis or who received a clearly identifiable MH or SA service. FFS SA beneficiaries include all FFS beneficiaries who, during the year, had at least one claim on which one of the substance use disorders shown in this table was the primary diagnosis. The specific diagnoses and services used to define these beneficiaries are listed in SAMHSA (2010). If beneficiaries had multiple diagnoses on different claims during the year, they are included in the category that represents the most frequent diagnosis.

The States included in this table are Arkansas, Georgia, Idaho, Illinois, Indiana, Kansas, Maine, Montana, North Carolina, South Carolina, Texas, Vermont, and Wyoming. Table originally published in Substance Abuse and Mental Health Services Administration (SAMHSA). (2010). *Mental Health, United States, 2008* (DHHS Publication No. SMA 10-4590). Rockville, MD: Center for Mental Health Services, SAMHSA.

SOURCE: Substance Abuse and Mental Health Services Administration (SAMHSA). (2010). *Mental health and substance abuse services in Medicaid, 2003: Charts and state tables* (DHHS Publication No. SMA 10-4608). Rockville, MD: Center for Mental Health Services, SAMHSA.

Table 80. Prescription medication use for Medicaid fee-for-service (FFS) beneficiaries in 13 States, 2003

[Data are based on Medicaid claims from 13 States]

Age group	Total FFS beneficiaries[1] with any psychotropic[2] medication use		FFS mental health (MH) beneficiaries with any psychotropic medication use		FFS substance abuse (SA) beneficiaries with any psychotropic medication use		FFS non-MH/non-SA beneficiaries with any psychotropic medication use	
	Number	Percent	Number	Percent	Number	Percent	Number	Percent
0–5	95,506	3.4	19,986	24.8	60	4.9	75,460	2.7
6–12	277,173	12.4	193,350	65.7	160	29.7	83,663	4.3
13–18	205,765	13.5	141,065	62.3	3,963	25.7	60,737	4.7
19–21	55,017	11.1	27,098	65.7	1,502	29.4	26,417	5.9
22–44	526,965	23.3	262,080	79.6	21,243	50.1	243,642	12.9
45–64	399,802	41.0	174,611	84.5	11,198	59.3	213,993	28.6
65 or older[3]	441,565	29.9	92,456	80.7	2,154	58.1	346,955	25.6
All ages	2,001,793	16.9	910,646	70.4	40,280	46.1	1,050,867	10.1

[1] Fee-for-service (FFS) beneficiaries include beneficiaries enrolled in Medicaid, but not in comprehensive managed care or a behavioral health managed care plan, for at least 1 month during the year. FFS mental health (MH) beneficiaries include FFS beneficiaries who, during the year, (1) had at least one claim on which an MH disorder was the primary diagnosis or (2) received a clearly identifiable MH service. FFS substance abuse (SA) beneficiaries include FFS beneficiaries who, during the year, had at least one claim on which a substance use disorder was the primary diagnosis. If beneficiaries had at least one claim on which an MH disorder was the primary diagnosis and at least one claim on which a substance use disorder was the primary diagnosis, they are included in the category that represents the diagnosis most frequently listed during the year.

[2] Psychotropic drugs include antidepressants, antipsychotics, antianxiety agents, and stimulants.

[3] Beneficiaries dually eligible for Medicaid and Medicare may have received MH treatment under Medicare that is not reported in Medicaid coinsurance claims, so diagnoses that would classify them as MH beneficiaries may be missing.

NOTES: This study identified Medicaid beneficiaries using MH or SA services in FFS plans in 13 States in 2003 (n = 1,380,190) and examined their use of medical services.

The States included in this table are Arkansas, Georgia, Idaho, Illinois, Indiana, Kansas, Maine, Montana, North Carolina, South Carolina, Texas, Vermont, and Wyoming. Table originally published in Substance Abuse and Mental Health Services Administration (SAMHSA). (2010). *Mental Health, United States, 2008* (DHHS Publication No. SMA 10-4590). Rockville, MD: Center for Mental Health Services, SAMHSA.

SOURCE: Substance Abuse and Mental Health Services Administration (SAMHSA). (2010). *Mental health and substance abuse services in Medicaid, 2003: Charts and state tables* (DHHS Publication No. SMA 10-4608). Rockville, MD: Center for Mental Health Services, SAMHSA.

Table 81. Utilization and expenditures, by service type for Medicaid fee-for-service (FFS) beneficiaries in 13 States, 2003

[Data are based on Medicaid claims from 13 States]

Service type[1]	All FFS beneficiaries[2]		FFS mental health (MH) beneficiaries		FFS substance abuse (SA) beneficiaries		Average annual expenditures[3] (dollars)		
	Number	Percent	Number	Percent	Number	Percent	FFS beneficiaries	FFS MH beneficiaries	FFS SA beneficiaries
Inpatient hospital	**1,595,061**	**13.5**	**235,921**	**18.2**	**29,220**	**33.5**	**$5,015**	**$7,156**	**$9,268**
Institutional long-term care									
Nursing facility	374,040	3.2	94,768	7.3	3,330	3.8	20,385	21,781	17,890
Inpatient psychiatric facility for individuals younger than age 21	21,372	0.2	20,967	1.6	383	0.4	16,824	16,931	9,479
Intermediate care facility for the mentally retarded	38,341	0.3	10,670	0.8	27	0.0	71,378	55,404	66,255
Mental hospital for the aged	6,418	0.1	5,913	0.5	173	0.2	13,139	11,516	6,195
Prescription medication	**7,708,085**	**65.2**	**1,171,956**	**90.6**	**72,467**	**83.0**	**1,046**	**2,339**	**1,598**
Other services									
Physician or other practitioner	7,832,280	66.3	1,134,155	87.7	73,567	84.2	443	581	762
Lab and X-ray	6,033,229	51.1	907,440	70.2	68,159	78.0	264	371	538
Psychiatric services	1,357,677	11.5	823,597	63.7	46,174	52.9	1,040	1,474	1,457
Outpatient hospital	3,942,545	33.4	650,990	50.4	55,827	63.9	509	688	912
Dental	2,828,533	23.9	450,478	34.8	21,136	24.2	318	344	414
Clinic	2,455,735	20.8	441,794	34.2	26,503	30.3	505	1,048	715
Durable medical equipment	2,202,692	18.6	389,390	30.1	27,657	31.7	426	547	380
Transportation services	1,262,649	10.7	297,714	23.0	23,417	26.8	270	413	471
Targeted case management	1,054,170	8.9	204,754	15.8	7,520	8.6	574	1,299	1,004
Rehabilitation services	159,683	1.4	97,611	7.6	17,438	20.0	2,419	2,617	2,591
Physical therapy, occupational therapy, speech, or hearing services	233,369	2.0	61,847	4.8	1,559	1.8	737	734	485
Nurse practitioner services	343,725	2.9	59,746	4.6	3,268	3.7	102	111	122

(continued)

Table 81. Utilization and expenditures, by service type for Medicaid fee-for-service (FFS) beneficiaries in 13 States, 2003
(continued)

Service type[1]	All FFS beneficiaries[2]		FFS mental health (MH) beneficiaries		FFS substance abuse (SA) beneficiaries		Average annual expenditures[3] (dollars)		
	Number	Percent	Number	Percent	Number	Percent	FFS beneficiaries	FFS MH beneficiaries	FFS SA beneficiaries
Personal care services	140,979	1.2	36,155	2.8	1,975	2.3	$4,537	$4,231	$3,987
Residential care	57,607	0.5	26,775	2.1	1,633	1.9	23,773	27,834	9,160
Adult day care	60,463	0.5	25,008	1.9	760	0.9	5,183	5,359	3,948
Home health	105,914	0.9	21,739	1.7	1,900	2.2	3,682	3,205	1,855
Sterilizations	61,761	0.5	7,556	0.6	1,040	1.2	1,156	971	1,100
Hospice benefits	32,108	0.3	5,316	0.4	280	0.3	8,551	8,757	7,792
Private duty nursing	17,459	0.1	4,012	0.3	277	0.3	4,549	2,052	654
Nurse midwife services	40,204	0.3	2,527	0.2	505	0.6	459	362	336
Abortions	7,097	0.1	689	0.1	71	0.1	417	360	300
Religious nonmedical health care institutions	*	*	*	*	*	*	*	*	*
Other services	1,121,163	9.5	269,586	20.9	15,822	18.1	2,947	3,879	1,695

*Estimates are considered unreliable.

[1] Fee-for-service (FFS) beneficiaries include beneficiaries enrolled in Medicaid, but not in comprehensive managed care or a behavioral health managed care plan, for at least 1 month during the year. FFS mental health (MH) beneficiaries include FFS beneficiaries who, during the year, (1) had at least one claim on which an MH disorder was the primary diagnosis or (2) received a clearly identifiable MH service. FFS substance abuse (SA) beneficiaries include FFS beneficiaries who, during the year, had at least one claim on which a substance use disorder was the primary diagnosis. If beneficiaries had at least one claim on which an MH disorder was the primary diagnosis and at least one claim on which a substance use disorder was the primary diagnosis, they are included in the category that represents the diagnosis most frequently listed during the year.

[2] Claims in the Medicaid Analytic eXtract (MAX) files are classified into 1 of 31 types of service (TOS) categories based on State and local service or procedure codes. States may vary in how they categorize similar claims into TOS categories. The psychiatric TOS includes both MH and SA services. In some cases, treatments classified in the psychiatric TOS in the MAX may be received by beneficiaries who are not identified as MH or SA beneficiaries in these tables.

[3] Expenditures are claims-based Medicaid payments, including both Federal and State share.

Table 81 notes *(continued)*

NOTES: This study identified Medicaid beneficiaries using MH or SA services in FFS plans in 13 States in 2003 (*n* = 1,380,190) and examined their use of medical services.

The States included in this table are Arkansas, Georgia, Idaho, Illinois, Indiana, Kansas, Maine, Montana, North Carolina, South Carolina, Texas, Vermont, and Wyoming. Table originally published in Substance Abuse and Mental Health Services Administration (SAMHSA). (2010). *Mental Health, United States, 2008* (DHHS Publication No. SMA 10-4590). Rockville, MD: Center for Mental Health Services, SAMHSA. Services are rank ordered within groups by MH utilization as a percentage of all FFS MH beneficiaries.

SOURCE: Substance Abuse and Mental Health Services Administration. (2010). *Mental health and substance abuse services in Medicaid, 2003: Charts and state tables* (DHHS Publication No. SMA 10-4608). Rockville, MD: Center for Mental Health Services, SAMHSA.

7. TABLES

7.3 Payers and Payment Mechanisms: Tables

7.3.1 Mental Health Expenditures: Overview

7.3.2 Revenues and Expenditures by Public Funding Source

Medicaid

Medicare
Tables 82–84

Veterans Mental Health

State Mental Health Agencies

7.3.3 Private Employer-Sponsored Mental Health Benefits

7.3.4 Mental Health Prescription Medication Use

Table 82. Percentage distribution of and expenditures for Medicare fee-for-service (FFS) claimants, by demographic characteristics: all health and mental health, 2007

[Data are from national Medicare claims]

Characteristic	All claimants		Mental health claimants[1]	
	Claimants (*N* = 34,600,780)	Expenditures ($288,024,000)	Claimants (*N* = 4,500,900)	Expenditures ($76,591,000)
Percent distribution by age				
0–64	20.0	19.0	39.0	27.0
65+	80.0	81.0	61.0	73.0
Percent distribution by sex				
Male	43.0	44.0	37.0	40.0
Female	57.0	56.0	63.0	60.0
Percent distribution by race/ethnicity				
White	85.0	82.0	84.0	81.0
Black	10.0	13.0	11.0	13.0
Hispanic	2.0	3.0	3.0	3.0
Other	1.0	1.0	1.0	1.0

[1] Mental health claimants are defined by having at least one of the following ICD-9-CM diagnosis codes as a primary diagnosis on at least one Medicare claim during 2007: 293–302, 306–314, and 316.

NOTES: The Medicare Standard Analytical Files (SAF) is a nationally representative claims database that consists of a randomly selected 5 percent sample of U.S. Medicare beneficiaries. The database includes claims across various care settings, including inpatient, outpatient, skilled nursing, home health, and hospice, as well as for durable medical equipment. Estimates do not include expenditures on prescription medications.

Data include all 50 U.S. States, U.S. territories, and foreign/unknown.

SOURCE: Medicare 5 Percent Standard Analytical Files, 2007, Centers for Medicare & Medicaid Services.

Table 83. Percentage distribution of and expenditures for Medicare fee-for-service (FFS) mental health (MH) claimants, by treatment modality, 1998 and 2007

[Data are from national Medicare claims]

Treatment modality	1998				2007			
	FFS MH claimants for MH services (*N* = 3,486,000) (percent share)[1]	FFS MH claimants for any health services (*N* = 3,486,000) (percent share)	Expenditures for MH services ($4,887,000) (percent share)[1]	Expenditures for all health services ($39,348,000) (percent share)[1]	FFS MH claimants for MH services (*N* = 4,500,900) (percent share)[1]	FFS MH claimants for any health services (*N* = 4,500,900) (percent share)	Expenditures for MH services ($6,764,000) (percent share)[1]	Expenditures for all health services ($76,591,000) (percent share)[1]
Inpatient	9.3	40.4	57.3	53.5	7.2	39.4	50.1	45.9
Outpatient	24.8	81.4	14.2	9.2	24.0	82.2	13.7	10.3
Physician/supplier	90.4	99.0	20.0	19.6	90.7	99.2	20.3	20.6
Home health agency/ hospice/skilled nursing facility	3.4	26.0	8.5	17.7	2.9	28.4	15.9	23.2

[1] Mental health claimants are defined by having at least one of the following ICD-9-CM diagnosis codes as a primary diagnosis on at least one Medicare claim during 2004: 293–302, 306–314, and 316. The number of mental health claimants is the unique number of patients who had a mental health claim in each calendar year. The sum of claimants across settings is greater than this number because a patient could have claims in more than one setting.

NOTES: The Medicare Standard Analytical Files (SAF) is a nationally representative claims database that consists of a randomly selected 5 percent sample of U.S. Medicare beneficiaries. The database includes claims across various care settings, including inpatient, outpatient, skilled nursing, home health, and hospice, as well as for durable medical equipment. Estimates do not include expenditures on prescription medications.

Data include all 50 U.S. States, U.S. territories, and foreign/unknown.

SOURCE: Medicare 5 Percent Standard Analytical Files, 2007, Centers for Medicare & Medicaid Services.

Table 84. Percentage distribution of and expenditures for Medicare fee-for-service (FFS) mental health (MH) claimants, by mutually exclusive diagnostic categories, 1998 and 2007

[Data are from national Medicare claims]

Diagnostic category[1]	1998			2007		
	FFS MH claimants (N = 3,486,000) (percent share)	Expenditures for MH services ($4,887,000) (percent share)	Expenditures for all health services ($39,348,000) (percent share)	FFS MH claimants (N = 4,500,900) (percent share)	Expenditures for MH services ($6,764,000) (percent share)	Expenditures for all health services ($76,591,000) (percent share)
Schizophrenia	10.8	27.4	6.8	10.0	28.0	6.0
Major depression	17.7	28.7	20.8	19.0	20.0	19.0
Bipolar disorders and manic disorders	5.5	12.5	4.3	9.0	15.0	6.0
Other psychoses	21.7	15.1	29.7	25.0	24.0	36.0
Anxiety disorders and other mood disorders	28.5	10.8	21.9	25.0	10.0	20.0
Stress and adjustment disorders	6.5	2.7	9.2	6.0	2.0	9.0
All other mental disorders	7.9	1.9	6.0	6.0	2.0	4.0

[1] Diagnostic category for each claimant was selected based on the most frequent diagnosis category in the year across all treatment settings.

NOTES: The Medicare Standard Analytical Files (SAF) is a nationally representative claims database that consists of a randomly selected 5 percent sample of U.S. Medicare beneficiaries. The database includes claims across various care settings, including inpatient, outpatient, skilled nursing, home health, and hospice, as well as for durable medical equipment. Estimates do not include expenditures on prescription medications.

ICD-9 diagnostic codes for each of the categories are as follows: schizophrenia (295), major depression (296.2, 296.3), bipolar disorders and manic disorders (296.0, 296.1, 296.4–296.99), other psychoses (293, 294, 297, 298, 299), anxiety disorders and other mood disorders (300, 301.13, 311), stress and adjustment disorders (308, 309), and all other mental disorders (302, 306, 307, 310, 312, 313, 314, 316, 301 w/o 301.13).

Data include all 50 U.S. States, U.S. territories, and foreign/unknown; as a result, the cumulative estimates shown here may differ from national estimates reported in Tables 129 and 130.

SOURCE: Medicare 5 Percent Standard Analytical Files, 2007, Centers for Medicare & Medicaid Services.

7. TABLES

7.3 Payers and Payment Mechanisms: Tables

Table 85. Volume and cost of mental health (MH) and substance abuse (SA) services in the Veterans Health Administration, United States, FY 2008 and FY 2009

[Data are based on cost and utilization records from the Veterans Health Administration]

Treatment modality	Mental health FY 2008		Mental health FY 2009		Substance abuse FY 2008		Substance abuse FY 2009		Combined FY 2008		Combined FY 2009	
	Count[1]	Dollars[2] (millions)	Count[1]	Dollars[2] (millions)	Count[1]	Dollars[2] (millions)	Count[1]	Dollars[2] (millions)	Count[1]	Dollars[2] (millions)	Count[1]	Dollars[2] (millions)
Inpatient days	994,669	$1,121	1,128,036	$1,360	17,454	$16	18,580	$17	1,012,123	$1,137	1,146,616	$1,377
Residential days	1,824,377	678	1,775,337	638	515,900	216	519,951	237	2,340,277	894	2,295,288	874
Outpatient visits	8,644,630	—	9,124,644	—	2,043,944	—	2,166,063	—	10,688,574	—	11,290,707	—
Outpatient except pharmacy	—	1,765	—	2,091	—	259	—	276	—	2,024	—	2,368
Outpatient pharmacy[3]	—	—	—	—	—	—	—	—	—	1,068	—	1,138

— Data not available.

[1] Volume of services is for specialized mental health (MH) facilities/units only; it excludes any MH care in primary care, for instance.

[2] Expenditures are in nominal dollars.

[3] Outpatient pharmacy is for all MH and SA users, including those treated outside specialty MH/SA facilities. MH and SA prescriptions are not separated. Inpatient and residential include pharmacy items dispensed through those facilities, such as IV medications or ward stock, but exclude items dispensed directly to the patient. The latter items are covered under outpatient pharmacy.

NOTE: The Veterans Health Administration (VHA) Decision Support System is a managerial cost accounting system that interacts with Veterans Affairs national databases to provide data elements on VHA costs to VHA products (goods and services provided during patient care).

SOURCE: Decision Support System, 2010, Department of Veterans Affairs.

7. TABLES

7.3 Payers and Payment Mechanisms: Tables

7.3.1 Mental Health Expenditures: Overview

7.3.2 Revenues and Expenditures by Public Funding Source

Medicaid

Medicare

Veterans Mental Health

State Mental Health Agencies
Tables 86–88

7.3.3 Private Employer-Sponsored Mental Health Benefits

7.3.4 Mental Health Prescription Medication Use

Table 86. Percentage distribution of revenue for State mental health agencies, by source, United States, FY 2001–FY 2008

[Data are based on State mental health revenues and expenditures studies]

Source	FY 2001 ($23,265,000) (percent)	FY 2002 ($25,112,000) (percent)	FY 2003 ($26,694,000) (percent)	FY 2004 ($27,916,000) (percent)	FY 2005 ($29,583,000) (percent)	FY 2006 ($31,231,000) (percent)	FY 2007 ($34,216,000) (percent)	FY 2008 ($37,380,000) (percent)
State general funds	52.0	48.7	48.7	46.1	47.0	45.9	42.3	42.9
Medicaid	36.6	38.3	39.1	42.1	42.2	43.3	47.3	45.8
Medicare/block grant/other Federal/local/other	11.4	13.0	12.2	11.8	10.8	10.8	10.3	11.3

NOTE: NRI's Revenues and Expenditures Study describes the major expenditures and funding sources of the State mental health agencies. NRI has conducted this survey every year since 1981.

SOURCE: Revenues and Expenditures Study, 2011, NRI Inc.

Table 87. Percentage distribution of expenditures for State mental health agencies, by source, United States, FY 2001–FY 2008

[Data are based on State mental health revenues and expenditures studies]

Source	FY 2001 ($23,060,000) (percent)	FY 2002 ($25,156,000) (percent)	FY 2003 ($26,411,000) (percent)	FY 2004 ($27,802,000) (percent)	FY 2005 ($29,397,000) (percent)	FY 2006 ($30,978,000) (percent)	FY 2007 ($33,995,000) (percent)	FY 2008 ($37,295,000) (percent)
State psychiatric hospital—inpatient	31.6	30.4	28.6	27.5	27.5	27.6	26.4	25.7
Community mental health	65.8	67.1	68.9	70.1	69.9	70.1	71.4	71.5
State mental health agency central office[1]	2.6	2.5	2.4	2.4	2.2	2.3	2.2	2.2

[1] Central office includes administration, research, training, prevention, and other central and regional office expenditures.

NOTE: NRI's Revenues and Expenditures Study describes the major expenditures and funding sources of the State mental health agencies. NRI has conducted this survey every year since 1981.

SOURCE: Revenues and Expenditures Study, 2011, NRI Inc.

Table 88. Number of State mental health agencies reporting cuts to budgets for adult, child, and forensic mental health programs, FY 2010 and FY 2011

[Data are based on reports from State mental health agencies]

Type of program	State made cuts in FY 2010 (number)	State anticipates making cuts in FY 2011 (number)
Adult programs		
State inpatient: acute care	19	17
State inpatient: long-term care	20	15
Other inpatient	9	8
Clinic services	12	12
Day services	9	8
Targeted case management	4	8
Housing	8	8
Employment	5	8
Prescriptions	6	5
Crisis services	4	7
Workforce development/training	13	13
Self-help/peer supports	6	6
Evidence-based practices	8	4
Other	9	6
Child programs		
State inpatient: acute care	11	5
Other inpatient	4	3
Clinic services	7	7
Day services	4	6
Targeted case management	3	5
Housing	4	3
Crisis services	0	0
Managed care waiver(s)	1	1
Workforce development/training	4	6
Prescriptions	1	2
Other	7	4
Forensic programs		
Forensic (nonsexually violent persons) inpatient	6	6
Sexually violent persons inpatient	4	4
Outreach to jails and prisons	4	5
Other	0	1

NOTES: The State Mental Health Agency (SMHA) Budget Reductions Survey is conducted by the National Association of State Mental Health Program Directors and NRI Inc. The survey is a semiannual series on the impact of State budget shortages on SMHA systems. The above estimates are from the summer 2010 survey.

This table includes data from reports from 42 States and the District of Columbia.

SOURCE: State Mental Health Agency Budget Reductions Survey, 2010, NRI Inc.

7. TABLES

7.3 Payers and Payment Mechanisms: Tables

7.3.1 Mental Health Expenditures: Overview

7.3.2 Revenues and Expenditures by Public Funding Source

Medicaid

Medicare

Veterans Mental Health

State Mental Health Agencies

7.3.3 Private Employer-Sponsored Mental Health Benefits
Tables 89–94

7.3.4 Mental Health Prescription Medication Use

Table 89. Proportion of private sector health plans with separate benefit limits for mental health care, United States, selected years 1997–2005

[Data are based on a survey of employers]

Coverage limitation	Private industry				Prepaid plans in private industry				Indemnity plans in private industry			
	1997 (percent)	2000 (percent)	2002 (percent)	2005 (percent)	1997 (percent)	2000 (percent)	2002 (percent)	2005 (percent)	1997 (percent)	2000 (percent)	2002 (percent)	2005 (percent)
Inpatient care												
Total with mental health care benefits	**100**	**100**	**100**	**—**	**100**	**100**	**100**	**100**	**100**	**100**	**100**	**100**
No separate limits[1]	14	15	15	—	10	15	16	23	16	15	14	18
Subject to separate limits[2]	86	85	85	—	90	85	84	77	84	85	86	82
Days[3]	61	76	77	—	84	77	77	68	50	75	77	74
Maximum dollar[4]	41	10	7	—	12	7	4	4	55	11	9	8
Coinsurance[5]	13	13	11	—	10	10	8	4	15	15	13	9
Co-payment[6]	7	3	12	—	16	5	14	24	3	2	10	8
Other[7]	1	4	4	—	1	2	3	1	2	5	5	3
Outpatient care[8]												
Total with mental health care benefits	**100**	**100**	**100**	**—**	**100**	**100**	**100**	**100**	**100**	**100**	**100**	**100**
No separate limits[1]	4	7	10	—	3	9	7	10	4	7	12	10
Subject to separate limits[2]	96	93	90	—	97	91	93	90	96	93	88	90
Visits[9]	53	72	75	—	83	77	84	78	38	70	70	74
Maximum dollar[4]	55	15	7	—	19	8	4	3	74	19	9	9
Coinsurance[5]	36	20	18	—	13	6	10	5	47	28	22	18
Co-payment[6]	30	30	29	—	61	44	44	54	14	20	21	24
Other[7]	2	16	9	—	1	8	7	1	2	22	11	7

See notes on page 227.

Table 89 notes

— Data not available.

[1] Plans that provide coverage without any separate limits may include plans that provide coverage subject to only the major medical limits of the plans.

[2] Separate limitations indicate that mental health care benefits are more restrictive than benefits for other treatments. For example, if a plan limits inpatient mental health care to 30 days per year, but the limit on inpatient care for any other type of illness is more than 30 days per year, the plan contains separate limits. The total is less than the sum of the individual items because many plans had more than one type of limitation.

[3] Days is the maximum number of inpatient days covered by a plan in a policy year.

[4] Maximum dollar is the highest amount of spending authorized and paid for by the medical plan.

[5] Coinsurance is the percentage of authorized expenses paid by the medical plan. For example, the plan may have a coinsurance rate of 80 percent. In this case, the plan pays 80 percent of covered medical expenses, and the participant (employee) pays the remaining 20 percent. In some plans, the coinsurance rate is lower for outpatient mental health care than for other services.

[6] Co-payment is the out-of-pocket expense paid by the participant at the time of service.

[7] Separate limits mean that patient contributions are structured differently for mental health and other health care. For example, outpatient mental health care may have a 50 percent coinsurance payment, whereas outpatient care for other illnesses has a $10 co-payment.

[8] Outpatient care includes treatment in one or more of the following: outpatient department of a hospital, residential treatment center, organized outpatient clinic, day-night treatment center, or doctor's office. If benefits differed by location of treatment, the location offering the most beneficial coverage was tabulated.

[9] Visits is the maximum number of visits covered by a plan in a policy year.

NOTES: The Bureau of Labor Statistics' National Compensation Survey provides comprehensive measures of occupational wages, employment cost trends, benefit incidence, and detailed plan provisions from more than 361 metropolitan statistical areas and 573 micropolitan statistical areas in the United States, as defined by the Office of Management and Budget. The 1997 Employee Benefits Survey reports on benefits provided to employees in establishments with 100 or more workers in all private nonfarm industries. The survey included a national sample of 1,945 U.S. employers with more than 100 workers. Because smaller employers generally offer less generous health benefits packages, the estimates likely represent the upper limits on rates of mental health coverage by employer-based health insurance in the United States. Between 1979 and 1986, the survey provided benefits data on full-time employees in medium and large establishments, those with either 100 or 250 employees or more, depending on the industry; coverage in the service industries was limited.

Sum of individual items is greater than total because some of the participants were in plans with more than one type of limit.

SOURCES: Morton, J. D., & Aleman, P. (April 2005). Trends in employer-provided mental health and substance abuse benefits. *Monthly Labor Review*, 25–35.

Employee Benefits Survey, 1997, Bureau of Labor Statistics.

National Compensation Survey, 2000, 2002, 2005, Bureau of Labor Statistics.

Table 90. Private health plan coverage of mental health (MH) and/or substance abuse (SA) services, by plan-vendor contracting arrangement, United States, 2003

[Data are based on a survey of private health plans]

Service covered	Total (*N* = 7,469) (percent)[1]	Vendor provides MH/SA services only (MBHO)[2] (*N* = 5,405) (percent)	Vendor provides both MH/SA and general medical services[3] (*N* = 920) (percent)	Plan (not vendor) provides or manages MH/SA services directly[4] (*N* = 1,143) (percent)
Mental health services				
Inpatient hospital care	100.0	100.0	100.0	100.0
Residential treatment	80.4	88.9	76.9	41.7
Intensive outpatient treatment	98.5	99.2	96.3	96.1
Outpatient visits	100.0	100.0	100.0	100.0
Substance abuse services				
Inpatient or residential detoxification	99.5	100.0	95.1	100.0
Inpatient hospital	97.7	97.4	99.6	98.0
Residential rehabilitation	86.0	93.9	76.9	52.4
Intensive outpatient treatment	98.0	98.7	93.6	97.3
Outpatient detoxification	95.1	96.5	92.4	89.6
Outpatient methadone maintenance	64.8	68.2	84.1	35.8
Outpatient rehabilitation	97.7	98.2	95.8	96.5

[1] Percentages are based on nonmissing responses.

[2] The plan contracts with a vendor that provides mental health/substance abuse (MH/SA) care; that type of vendor is often known as a managed behavioral health organization (MBHO). General medical care is provided either by the plan or another vendor.

[3] The plan contracts with one vendor that provides both general medical and behavioral health care.

[4] Plan (not vendor) provides or manages MH/SA directly. The plan employs providers or manages the provider network itself.

Table 90 notes *(continued)*

NOTES: The Brandeis Health Plan Survey on Alcohol, Drug Abuse, and Mental Health Services is a nationally representative survey that tracks trends in how alcohol, drug abuse, and MH services are provided for the more than 200 million privately insured individuals in 1999 (*n* = 434, 92 percent response) and 2003 (*n* = 368, 83 percent response).

In this table, the unit of analysis is an insurance product, not an employer or person. The Brandeis Health Plan Survey defined insurance products as market-specific health plan offerings that differ in out-of-network coverage, referrals, or primary care physicians. For example, if Health Plan X offers a health maintenance organization (HMO) in two market areas, those are two products; and if Plan X also offers a preferred provider organization (PPO) in each market, those are two more products. Only commercial managed care products were included in the survey (unweighted *n* = 808 products).

SOURCES: Brandeis Health Plan Survey on Alcohol, Drug Abuse, and Mental Health Services, 2003, Brandeis University.

Horgan, C. M., Garnick, D. W., Merrick, E. L., & Hodgkin, D. (2009). Changes in how health plans provide behavioral health services. *The Journal of Behavioral Health Services & Research, 36*(1), 11–24. Table 2 adapted with kind permission from Springer Science+Business Media B.V.

Table 91. Prior authorization requirements among private health plans for mental health (MH) and/or substance abuse (SA) services, United States, 2003

[Data are based on a survey of private health plans]

Prior authorization requirement[1]	Total products[2] (number)	Total products (percent[3])	Vendor provides MH/SA services only (MBHO)[4] (percent)	Vendor provides both MH/SA and general medical services[5] (percent)	Plan (not vendor) provides or manages MH/SA services directly[6] (percent)
Mental health services					
Inpatient hospital care	7,103	92.3	96.4	82.7	77.7
Residential treatment	3,778	88.2	99.5	30.4	73.2
Intensive outpatient treatment	6,921	89.3	96.8	43.3	78.1
Outpatient counseling	7,156	58.1	62.8	14.7	62.6
Substance abuse services					
Inpatient or residential detoxification	7,124	95.2	99.8	86.6	77.6
Inpatient or residential rehabilitation	6,744	94.7	99.9	84.0	70.6
Intensive outpatient treatment	6,777	90.9	98.0	40.8	85.6
Outpatient detoxification	6,792	55.6	60.8	41.1	37.1
Outpatient methadone maintenance	3,990	79.1	94.0	1.4	57.3
Outpatient rehabilitation	6,932	57.5	62.7	11.8	60.3

[1] Prior authorization means that the health plan or primary care provider must approve certain treatments, procedures, or prescribed medications before they are provided. The data report on prior authorization requirements for initiating outpatient visits for specialty behavioral health care with in-network providers.

[2] In this table, the unit of analysis is an insurance product, not an employer or person. The Brandeis Health Plan Survey defined insurance products as market-specific health plan offerings that differ in out-of-network coverage, referrals, or primary care physicians. For example, if Health Plan X offers a health maintenance organization (HMO) in two market areas, those are two products; and if Plan X also offers a preferred provider organization (PPO) in each market, those are two more products. Only commercial managed care products were included in the survey (unweighted n = 808 products).

[3] Percentages are based on nonmissing responses.

[4] The plan contracts with a vendor that provides MH/SA care; that type of vendor is often known as a managed behavioral health organization (MBHO). General medical care is provided either by the plan or another vendor.

[5] The plan contracts with one vendor that provides both general medical and behavioral health care.

[6] The plan employs providers or manages the provider network itself.

NOTE: The Brandeis Health Plan Survey on Alcohol, Drug Abuse, and Mental Health Services is a nationally representative survey that tracks trends in how alcohol, drug abuse, and mental health services are provided for the more than 200 million privately insured individuals in 1999 (n = 434; 92 percent response) and 2003 (n = 368; 83 percent response).

SOURCES: Brandeis Health Plan Survey on Alcohol, Drug Abuse, and Mental Health Services, 2003, Brandeis University.

Horgan, C. M., Garnick, D. W., Merrick, E. L., & Hodgkin, D. (2009). Changes in how health plans provide behavioral health services. *The Journal of Behavioral Health Services & Research, 36*(1), 11–24. Table 3 adapted with kind permission from Springer Science+Business Media B.V.

Table 92. Percentage of employers covering specific mental health services in primary plans, by employer size, United States, 1997 and 2003

[Data are based on a survey of employer-sponsored health plans]

Mental health service	Less than 500 employees		500 or more employees	
	1997 (*N* = 1,356) (percent)	2003 (*N* = 772) (percent)	1997 (*N* = 1,315) (percent)	2003 (*N* = 1,299) (percent)
Inpatient psychiatric care	94	88	98	98
Nonhospital residential care	52	48	54	40
Intensive outpatient treatment	64	72	71	76
Outpatient psychotherapy	85	80	93	91
Crisis services	49	46	48	32

NOTES: Established in 1986, the Mercer National Survey of Employer-Sponsored Health Plans is an annual survey that collects information on a wide range of health care issues regarding employer health plans, including costs, strategic planning, and the scope and limitations of coverage. Nearly 3,000 employers participated in the 2003 survey.

Data are from the Mercer National Survey of Employer-Sponsored Health Plans in 1997 and 2003. The survey includes only employers that sponsor health insurance. A primary plan represents the employer's single plan with the largest enrollment, regardless of plan type. Small employers with fewer than 10 employees are not included in the survey. Table originally published in Substance Abuse and Mental Health Services Administration (SAMHSA). (2010). *Mental Health, United States, 2008* (DHHS Publication No. SMA 10-4590). Rockville, MD: Center for Mental Health Services, SAMHSA.

SOURCE: Teich, J. L., & Buck, J. A. (2007). Mental health benefits in employer-sponsored health plans, 1997–2003. *Journal of Behavioral Health Services Research, 34*(3), 343–348. Table 1 adapted with kind permission from Springer Science+Business Media B.V.

Table 93. Percentage of covered workers with various outpatient and inpatient mental health visit limits, annual maximums/days covered, by plan type, 2000 and 2008

[Data are based on employer-sponsored health benefits]

Mental health coverage limit	Conventional		HMO		PPO		POS		HDHP/SO		All plans	
	2000 (percent)	2008 (percent)	2000 (percent)	2008 (percent)	2000 (percent)	2008 (percent)	2000 (percent)	2008 (percent)	2000 (percent)	2008 (percent)	2000 (percent)	2008 (percent)
Number of annual outpatient mental health visits covered												
20 visits or less	24	—	41	49	27	29	30	38	—	41	29	34
21–30 visits	14	—	29	22	25	30	25	20	—	27	26	27
31–50 visits	13	—	7	10	13	11	8	16	—	14	13	11
More than 50 visits	5	—	3	5	5	11	5	9	—	6	7	9
No limit	25	—	9	15	17	19	18	18	—	12	14	18
Don't know	20	—	11	—	13	—	15	—	—	—	12	—
Number of annual inpatient mental health days covered												
10 days or less	6	—	4	12	5	5	6	8	—	10	5	7
11–20 days	3	—	9	12	8	11	6	17	—	11	7	11
21–30 days	21	—	47	46	38	44	39	35	—	49	38	44
31 or more days	22	—	14	14	14	17	13	21	—	15	18	16
No limit	29	—	11	17	19	24	17	19	—	16	17	22
Don't know	19	—	15	—	16	—	19	—	—	—	15	—

— Data not available.

NOTES: The Henry J. Kaiser Family Foundation and Health Research & Educational Trust Employer Health Benefits Survey is an annual survey of employers that provides a detailed look at trends in employer-sponsored health coverage, including premiums, employee contributions, cost-sharing provisions, and other relevant information. The 2008 survey included 2,832 randomly selected public and private firms with three or more employees, and the 2000 survey included 1,887 randomly selected public and private firms with three or more employees.

HMO = health maintenance organization, PPO = preferred provider organization, POS = point of service, HDHP/SO = high deductible health plan with savings option.

In 2008, 2 percent of covered workers did not have outpatient or inpatient mental health coverage. Given the decline in conventional health plan enrollment and the addition of HDHP/SO as a plan type option, nearly all questions pertaining to conventional coverage were removed from the survey instrument, and thus information for the conventional plan type is not included in 2008. In 2006, the survey began asking questions about HDHP/SO as a separate plan type, equal to the other plan types. In prior years, data on HDHP/SO plans were collected as part of one of the other types of plans, and some differences between years in HMO, PPO, and POS plan types may be a result of this reclassification. Table originally published in Substance Abuse and Mental Health Services Administration (SAMHSA). (2010). *Mental Health, United States, 2008* (DHHS Publication No. SMA 10-4590). Rockville, MD: Center for Mental Health Services, SAMHSA.

Table 93 notes *(continued)*

SOURCES: Kaiser Family Foundation/Health Research & Educational Trust (2008). *Employer health benefits, 2008*. Menlo Park, CA: Kaiser Family Foundation. Retrieved from http://ehbs.kff.org/pdf/7790.pdf

Kaiser Family Foundation/Health Research & Educational Trust (2000). *Employer health benefits, 2000*. Menlo Park, CA: Kaiser Family Foundation. Retrieved from http://www.kff.org/insurance/loader.cfm?url=/commonspot/security/getfile.cfm&PageID=13512

Table 94. Percentage of employers reporting various changes as a result of the Mental Health Parity and Addiction Equity Act of 2008, by firm size and region, 2010

[Data are based on a survey of employer-sponsored health plans]

Employer characteristic	Changed mental health benefits (percent)	Eliminated limits on coverage[1] (percent)	Dropped mental health coverage[1] (percent)	Increased utilization management of mental health benefits[1] (percent)	Other[1] (percent)
Firm size					
51–199 workers	26	61	7	18	20
200–999 workers	35	70	4	13	30
1,000–4,999 workers	58	79	1	15	24
5,000 or more workers	71	85	1	11	16
All small firms (51–199 workers)	26	61	7	18	20
All large firms (200 or more workers)	43	75	2	13	26
Region					
Northeast	21	68	<1	11	30
Midwest	35	77	1	8	19
South	36	68	1	27	20
West	29	51	18	11	26
All firms (51 or more workers)	**31**	**66**	**5**	**16**	**23**

[1] Among firms reporting that they made changes to the mental health benefits they offer as a result of the Mental Health Parity and Addiction Equity Act of 2008.

NOTES: The Henry J. Kaiser Family Foundation and Health Research & Educational Trust Employer Health Benefits Survey is an annual survey of employers that provides a detailed look at trends in employer-sponsored health coverage, including premiums, employee contributions, cost-sharing provisions, and other relevant information. The 2010 survey included 3,143 randomly selected public and private firms with three or more employees.

Asked of firms with more than 50 workers. An employer may have more than one response.

SOURCE: Kaiser Family Foundation/Health Research & Educational Trust (2010). *Employer health benefits, 2010 annual survey.* Menlo Park, CA: Kaiser Family Foundation. Retrieved from http://ehbs.kff.org/pdf/2010/8085.pdf

7. TABLES

7.3 Payers and Payment Mechanisms: Tables

7.3.1 Mental Health Expenditures: Overview

7.3.2 Revenues and Expenditures by Public Funding Source

Medicaid

Medicare

Veterans Mental Health

State Mental Health Agencies

7.3.3 Private Employer-Sponsored Mental Health Benefits

7.3.4 ***Mental Health Prescription Medication Use***
Tables 95–97

Table 95. Number of users and annual expenditures on selected mental health/ substance abuse (MH/SA) medications for an MH/SA condition among persons aged 18 or older, by insurance status and selected therapeutic categories, United States, 1998, 2003, and 2008

[Data are based on a nationally representative survey of households, medical providers, and employers]

Coverage group/ medication category	Users (millions)			Expenditures (millions of dollars)[1]		
	1998	2003	2008	1998	2003	2008
All coverage groups	**15.1**	**22.5**	**27.2**	**$10,077**	**$18,966**	**$25,449**
Antianxiety, all classes[2]	5.4	6.8	9.3	1,341	2,258	1,825
Antidepressants, all classes	11.2	18.0	21.5	6,584	11,793	12,243
Antipsychotics, all classes	1.4	1.8	2.8	1,418	2,609	6,788
Antimanics, anticonvulsants	1.0	1.6	2.3	560	1,494	2,609
Private insurance (total)	**7.9**	**12.5**	**14.3**	**$4,704**	**$9,304**	**$12,003**
Antianxiety, all classes[2]	2.3	3.1	4.2	558	896	560
Antidepressants, all classes	6.4	10.7	11.6	3,640	6,843	6,845
Antipsychotics, all classes	0.4	0.4	0.9	*	559	1,971
Antimanics, anticonvulsants	0.4	0.6	1.0	*	480	1,275
Medicare, aged 65 or older (total)	**3.3**	**4.4**	**5.5**	**$1,485**	**$2,912**	**$2,694**
Antianxiety, all classes[2]	1.5	1.9	2.2	340	521	320
Antidepressants, all classes	2.1	3.1	4.1	1,030	2,015	1,821
Antipsychotics, all classes	0.2	0.3	0.2	*	*	*
Antimanics, anticonvulsants	*	*	*	*	*	*
Medicare, aged 18 to 64 (total)	**1.2**	**2.0**	**2.3**	**$1,753**	**$3,040**	**$4,115**
Antianxiety, all classes[2]	0.6	0.8	1.1	204	450	554
Antidepressants, all classes	0.8	1.4	1.8	728	1,123	1,374
Antipsychotics, all classes	0.3	0.5	0.6	*	893	1,602
Antimanics, anticonvulsants	*	*	*	*	*	*
Medicaid/other public (total)	**1.8**	**2.3**	**2.9**	**$1,623**	**$2,747**	**$4,658**
Antianxiety, all classes[2]	0.8	0.7	1.1	179	296	180
Antidepressants, all classes	1.2	1.8	2.1	818	1,336	1,147
Antipsychotics, all classes	0.5	0.5	0.7	430	828	2,521
Antimanics, anticonvulsants	0.3	0.3	0.6	*	259	649
Uninsured (total)	**0.9**	**1.3**	**2.2**	**$512**	**$963**	**$1,979**
Antianxiety, all classes[2]	0.3	0.3	0.8	*	95	210
Antidepressants, all classes	0.7	1.0	1.8	369	476	1,055
Antipsychotics, all classes	*	0.2	0.3	*	*	*
Antimanics, anticonvulsants	*	*	*	*	*	*

*Estimates are considered unreliable.

[1] Adjusted to constant 2008 dollars using the gross domestic product implicit price deflator.

[2] Antianxiety medications include sedative and hypnotic medications.

Table 95 notes *(continued)*

NOTES: The Medical Expenditure Panel Survey (MEPS) is a set of large-scale surveys of families and individuals, their medical providers (e.g., doctors, hospitals, pharmacies), and employers across the United States. Since 1996, MEPS has collected data on the specific health services that Americans use, how frequently they use them, the cost of these services, and how they are paid for, as well as data on the cost, scope, and breadth of health insurance held by and available to U.S. workers.

See Appendix C for complete list of medications. Categorization of medications follows that of the National Institute of Mental Health (http://www.nimh.nih.gov/health/publications/mental-health-medications/alphabetical-list-of-medications.shtml).

SOURCES: Medical Expenditure Panel Survey, 1996–2008, Center for Financing, Access, and Cost Trends, Agency for Healthcare Research and Quality.

Zuvekas, S. H. (2005). Prescription drugs and the changing patterns of treatment for mental disorders, 1996–2001. *Health Affairs, 24*(1), 195–205.

Table 96. Number of users and annual expenditures on selected mental health/ substance abuse (MH/SA) medications for an MH/SA condition among persons aged 17 or younger, by insurance status and selected therapeutic categories, United States, 1998, 2003, and 2008

[Data are based on a nationally representative survey of households, medical providers, and employers]

Coverage group/ medication category	Users (millions)			Expenditures (millions of 2008 dollars)[1]		
	1998	2003	2008	1998	2003	2008
All coverage groups[2]	**2.6**	**3.3**	**3.5**	**$1,082**	**$2,906**	**$4,094**
Antianxiety, all classes[3]	*	*	*	*	*	*
Antidepressants, all classes	0.6	1.2	0.8	248	732	192
Antipsychotics, all classes	0.1	0.3	0.7	*	334	1,065
Stimulants	2.0	2.3	2.8	653	1,539	2,584
Private insurance (total)	**2.0**	**2.2**	**2.1**	**$850**	**$1,877**	**$2,322**
Antianxiety, all classes[3]	*	*	*	*	*	*
Antidepressants, all classes	0.5	0.8	0.5	207	516	123
Antipsychotics, all classes	*	*	*	*	*	*
Stimulants	1.5	1.6	1.6	498	987	1,503
Medicaid/other public (total)	**0.5**	**1.0**	**1.2**	**$194**	**$954**	**$1,619**
Antianxiety, all classes[3]	*	*	*	*	*	*
Antidepressants, all classes	0.1	0.3	0.2	*	*	*
Antipsychotics, all classes	*	0.1	0.3	*	*	510
Stimulants	0.4	0.7	1.0	120	522	1,012

*Estimates are considered unreliable.

[1] Adjusted to constant 2008 dollars using the gross domestic product implicit price deflator.

[2] Coverage group of uninsured people aged 17 or younger is omitted because all of the estimates in this group are considered unreliable.

[3] Antianxiety medications include sedative and hypnotic medications.

NOTES: The Medical Expenditure Panel Survey (MEPS) is a set of large-scale surveys of families and individuals, their medical providers (e.g., doctors, hospitals, pharmacies), and employers across the United States. Since 1996, MEPS has collected data on the specific health services that Americans use, how frequently they use them, the cost of these services, and how they are paid for, as well as data on the cost, scope, and breadth of health insurance held by and available to U.S. workers.

See Appendix C for complete list of medications. Categorization of medications follows that of the National Institute of Mental Health (http://www.nimh.nih.gov/health/publications/mental-health-medications/alphabetical-list-of-medications.shtml).

SOURCES: Medical Expenditure Panel Survey, 1996–2008, Center for Financing, Access, and Cost Trends, Agency for Healthcare Research and Quality.

Zuvekas, S. H. (2005). Prescription drugs and the changing patterns of treatment for mental disorders, 1996–2001. *Health Affairs, 24*(1), 195–205.

Table 97. Clubhouse costs, United States, 2010

[Data are from an annual survey of clubhouses]

Funding and costs	ICCD certified		Non-ICCD certified	
	Number of clubhouses responding	Dollars	Number of clubhouses responding	Dollars
Annual budget (excluding housing)	63	$704,276	26	$482,490
Cost per member per year	61	4,436	25	4,985
Cost per day	62	40	24	39

NOTE: The International Survey of Clubhouses was conducted by the International Center for Clubhouse Development (ICCD). The survey gathers information about clubhouse characteristics, governance and administration, membership, staffing and staff credentials, unit structure, employment, housing activities, services, and participation in clubhouse training. In 2010, there were 197 ICCD clubhouses in the United States; however, data were only available for 114 of them.

SOURCE: International Survey of Clubhouses, 2010, ICCD.

7. TABLES

7.4 State-Level Estimates

Table 98. Number and percentage of persons aged 18 or older with past year any mental illness (AMI) and serious mental illness (SMI), United States and by State, 2008–2009

[Data are based on a survey of a representative sample of the national population]

State	Total adult population (1,000s)	Past year AMI		Past year SMI	
		Number (1,000s)	Percent	Number (1,000s)	Percent
Alabama	3,480	706	20.3	157	4.5
Alaska	487	92	18.8	20	4.1
Arizona	4,736	889	18.8	199	4.2
Arkansas	2,114	451	21.3	146	6.9
California	26,898	5,279	19.6	1,157	4.3
Colorado	3,681	764	20.8	193	5.2
Connecticut	2,641	521	19.7	116	4.4
Delaware	658	129	19.6	29	4.4
District of Columbia	472	99	21.0	18	3.8
Florida	14,066	2,551	18.1	660	4.7
Georgia	6,977	1,343	19.3	287	4.1
Hawaii	959	187	19.5	34	3.5
Idaho	1,095	246	22.5	63	5.8
Illinois	9,530	1,727	18.1	418	4.4
Indiana	4,714	1,037	22.0	281	6.0
Iowa	2,245	427	19.0	111	4.9
Kansas	2,046	421	20.6	91	4.4
Kentucky	3,200	640	20.0	172	5.4
Louisiana	3,240	639	19.7	154	4.8
Maine	1,028	215	20.9	48	4.7
Maryland	4,223	706	16.7	154	3.6
Massachusetts	5,021	1,014	20.2	211	4.2
Michigan	7,490	1,539	20.5	390	5.2
Minnesota	3,918	751	19.1	210	5.3
Mississippi	2,110	411	19.5	87	4.1
Missouri	4,413	921	20.9	229	5.2
Montana	735	149	20.2	37	5.0
Nebraska	1,309	267	20.4	61	4.7
Nevada	1,916	413	21.6	88	4.6
New Hampshire	1,014	198	19.6	46	4.6
New Jersey	6,530	1,193	18.3	269	4.1
New Mexico	1,459	277	19.0	64	4.4
New York	14,837	2,949	19.9	675	4.5
North Carolina	6,826	1,341	19.6	293	4.3
North Dakota	484	87	18.0	17	3.6
Ohio	8,615	1,759	20.4	447	5.2
Oklahoma	2,663	575	21.6	136	5.1
Oregon	2,894	595	20.6	155	5.4
Pennsylvania	9,535	1,691	17.7	358	3.8
Rhode Island	807	195	24.2	58	7.2
South Carolina	3,342	632	18.9	137	4.1

(continued)

Table 98. Number and percentage of persons aged 18 or older with past year any mental illness (AMI) and serious mental illness (SMI), United States and by State, 2008–2009 *(continued)*

State	Total adult population (1,000s)	Past year AMI		Past year SMI	
		Number (1,000s)	Percent	Number (1,000s)	Percent
South Dakota	592	107	18.1	21	3.5
Tennessee	4,672	1,004	21.5	235	5.0
Texas	17,260	3,377	19.6	741	4.3
Utah	1,876	452	24.1	116	6.2
Vermont	488	96	19.7	23	4.7
Virginia	5,765	1,064	18.5	225	3.9
Washington	4,948	1,048	21.2	233	4.7
West Virginia	1,406	310	22.0	86	6.1
Wisconsin	4,248	900	21.2	211	5.0
Wyoming	399	87	21.8	21	5.2
United States	**226,065**	**44,471**	**19.7**	**10,388**	**4.6**

NOTES: The National Survey on Drug Use and Health (NSDUH) is a nationally representative survey of the civilian, noninstitutionalized population of the United States aged 12 or older. The survey interviews approximately 67,500 persons each year.

Mental illness among persons aged 18 or older is defined according to two dimensions: (1) the presence of a diagnosable mental, behavioral, or emotional disorder in the past year (excluding developmental and substance use disorders) of sufficient duration to meet diagnostic criteria specified in the *Diagnostic and Statistical Manual of Mental Disorders, Fourth Edition* (DSM-IV) (APA, 1994); and (2) the level of interference with or limitation of one or more major life activities resulting from a disorder (functional impairment). Adult NSDUH respondents' mental illness was determined based on modeling their responses to questions on distress (K6 scale) and impairment (truncated version of the World Health Organization Disability Assessment Schedule). Serious mental illness (SMI) among adults is defined as persons aged 18 or older who currently or at any time in the past year had a diagnosable mental, behavioral, or emotional disorder as defined above and resulting in substantial impairment in carrying out major life activities, based on Global Assessment of Functioning (GAF) scores of 50 or less. Any mental illness (AMI) among adults is defined as persons aged 18 or older who currently or at any time in the past year had a diagnosable mental, behavioral, or emotional disorder as defined above, regardless of the level of impairment in carrying out major life activities. AMI includes persons with mental illness having serious, moderate, or mild functional impairment; SMI is a subset of the AMI group.

Data from more than one year were combined to ensure statistically precise estimates.

SOURCE: National Survey on Drug Use and Health, 2008–2009, Substance Abuse and Mental Health Services Administration, Office of Applied Studies.

Table 99. Percentage of persons aged 18 or older with a past year major depressive episode (MDE), United States and by State, 2005–2009

[Data are based on a survey of a representative sample of the national population]

State	2005–2006 (percent)	2006–2007 (percent)	2007–2008 (percent)	2008–2009 (percent)
Alabama	6.3	6.0	5.8	6.4
Alaska	6.1	6.7	6.2	5.8
Arizona	6.4	6.7	7.1	7.0
Arkansas	7.6	7.5	7.4	7.9
California	5.5	5.8	6.1	6.0
Colorado	7.1	6.6	6.9	7.5
Connecticut	6.3	6.3	6.8	5.9
Delaware	7.2	6.6	6.1	6.4
District of Columbia	7.8	7.5	6.6	5.8
Florida	6.0	6.2	6.5	6.4
Georgia	6.5	6.9	6.5	6.2
Hawaii	4.6	4.6	5.9	6.2
Idaho	7.2	7.3	7.5	7.5
Illinois	6.0	5.9	5.8	6.1
Indiana	7.4	7.6	8.2	8.2
Iowa	6.3	6.9	6.2	5.8
Kansas	7.0	6.7	7.3	6.6
Kentucky	7.8	8.3	7.7	7.2
Louisiana	6.6	7.1	6.2	5.7
Maine	7.6	8.2	7.4	6.7
Maryland	6.0	5.9	5.9	5.9
Massachusetts	7.4	7.1	6.5	6.7
Michigan	7.4	7.3	6.6	6.6
Minnesota	6.3	6.3	7.1	7.6
Mississippi	6.9	5.7	5.3	5.7
Missouri	7.7	7.8	7.1	7.1
Montana	7.3	7.0	6.7	6.8
Nebraska	6.9	6.3	5.5	6.3
Nevada	7.9	8.0	7.0	6.9
New Hampshire	7.4	8.4	7.8	7.6
New Jersey	6.2	5.7	5.8	5.9
New Mexico	6.4	6.7	7.4	6.5
New York	6.3	6.1	6.6	6.7
North Carolina	6.5	6.8	7.1	6.8
North Dakota	7.0	7.4	6.5	6.2
Ohio	7.3	7.0	6.6	6.2
Oklahoma	7.2	8.2	8.0	7.4
Oregon	7.0	6.6	7.1	7.6
Pennsylvania	5.8	6.1	5.6	5.2
Rhode Island	8.4	7.3	7.6	9.5
South Carolina	7.1	7.0	6.2	7.1
South Dakota	5.7	5.5	6.0	5.7
Tennessee	7.9	8.7	7.6	6.8
Texas	6.3	6.2	6.1	6.0

(continued)

Table 99. Percentage of persons aged 18 or older with a past year major depressive episode (MDE), United States and by State, 2005–2009 *(continued)*

State	2005–2006 (percent)	2006–2007 (percent)	2007–2008 (percent)	2008–2009 (percent)
Utah	7.7	6.9	7.0	7.5
Vermont	7.6	7.8	6.5	6.5
Virginia	6.6	7.1	6.9	6.4
Washington	6.3	6.5	7.6	7.2
West Virginia	7.8	8.5	8.5	7.7
Wisconsin	7.1	6.8	7.4	7.3
Wyoming	7.4	7.7	7.9	7.4
United States	**6.5**	**6.6**	**6.6**	**6.5**

NOTES: The National Survey on Drug Use and Health is a nationally representative survey of the civilian, noninstitutionalized population of the United States aged 12 or older. The survey interviews approximately 67,500 persons each year.

Major depressive episode (MDE) is defined as a period of at least 2 weeks when a person experienced a depressed mood or loss of interest or pleasure in daily activities and had a majority of specified depression symptoms. According to the *Diagnostic and Statistical Manual of Mental Disorders, Fourth Edition* (DSM-IV) (APA, 1994), two or more MDEs are necessary to meet the criteria for recurrent major depressive disorder.

Data from more than one year were combined to ensure statistically precise estimates.

SOURCE: National Survey on Drug Use and Health, 2005–2009, Substance Abuse and Mental Health Services Administration, Office of Applied Studies.

7. TABLES

7.4 State-Level Estimates: Tables

Table 100. Percentage of persons aged 12 to 17 with a past year major depressive episode (MDE), United States and by State, 2005–2009

[Data are based on a survey of a representative sample of the national population]

State	2005–2006 (percent)	2006–2007 (percent)	2007–2008 (percent)	2008–2009 (percent)
Alabama	7.6	7.7	8.3	8.0
Alaska	8.7	8.0	7.6	7.5
Arizona	8.7	8.1	9.0	9.1
Arkansas	8.4	8.2	8.9	9.2
California	8.1	7.6	7.9	8.2
Colorado	9.7	9.0	8.8	9.2
Connecticut	8.3	7.6	8.1	8.0
Delaware	9.0	8.9	8.1	7.8
District of Columbia	7.5	7.4	7.2	6.8
Florida	8.9	7.6	7.7	8.5
Georgia	8.3	8.5	8.2	7.8
Hawaii	8.6	8.3	8.3	8.1
Idaho	9.4	8.8	8.6	9.0
Illinois	7.6	7.3	7.5	7.5
Indiana	8.0	8.4	9.0	9.4
Iowa	8.3	7.9	7.7	8.0
Kansas	8.6	9.3	8.9	8.5
Kentucky	9.5	9.7	9.4	8.4
Louisiana	8.2	8.3	8.0	7.5
Maine	9.0	8.7	8.4	8.1
Maryland	8.4	7.7	7.0	7.1
Massachusetts	8.0	8.0	8.4	8.0
Michigan	8.3	8.1	8.3	8.2
Minnesota	8.4	8.9	9.5	8.6
Mississippi	7.9	7.5	7.3	7.1
Missouri	9.3	9.1	8.7	9.0
Montana	9.0	8.8	8.6	9.1
Nebraska	8.5	7.5	7.5	8.1
Nevada	8.2	8.1	8.2	7.4
New Hampshire	9.4	9.1	8.9	8.9
New Jersey	8.1	8.0	7.8	7.3
New Mexico	8.9	9.1	8.9	9.0
New York	7.8	7.3	8.0	8.2
North Carolina	8.4	8.5	9.0	8.4
North Dakota	8.5	8.4	8.7	8.9
Ohio	8.3	8.0	8.3	8.3
Oklahoma	9.1	8.6	8.4	8.1
Oregon	8.1	7.9	9.3	10.3
Pennsylvania	7.7	7.9	7.4	6.8
Rhode Island	7.9	7.3	8.5	9.6
South Carolina	7.9	8.5	8.7	8.9
South Dakota	7.6	7.8	8.2	8.3
Tennessee	8.2	8.5	8.8	8.5
Texas	8.6	7.9	7.6	7.4

(continued)

Table 100. Percentage of persons aged 12 to 17 with a past year major depressive episode (MDE), United States and by State, 2005–2009 *(continued)*

State	2005–2006 (percent)	2006–2007 (percent)	2007–2008 (percent)	2008–2009 (percent)
Utah	8.2	8.3	9.1	8.4
Vermont	8.7	8.6	8.1	8.1
Virginia	8.9	9.2	9.7	8.9
Washington	9.1	7.7	8.6	9.4
West Virginia	8.3	8.4	9.1	8.4
Wisconsin	9.0	8.5	9.2	8.9
Wyoming	8.9	9.7	10.0	8.6
United States	**8.4**	**8.0**	**8.2**	**8.2**

NOTES: The National Survey on Drug Use and Health is a nationally representative survey of the civilian, noninstitutionalized population of the United States aged 12 or older. The survey interviews approximately 67,500 persons each year. In 2009, 22,626 youth aged 12 to 17 were interviewed.

Major depressive episode (MDE) is defined as a period of at least 2 weeks when a person experienced a depressed mood or loss of interest or pleasure in daily activities and had a majority of specified depression symptoms. According to the *Diagnostic and Statistical Manual of Mental Disorders, Fourth Edition* (DSM-IV) (APA, 1994), two or more MDEs are necessary to meet the criteria for recurrent major depressive disorder.

Data from more than one year were combined to ensure statistically precise estimates.

SOURCE: National Survey on Drug Use and Health, 2005–2009, Substance Abuse and Mental Health Services Administration, Office of Applied Studies.

7. TABLES

7.4 State-Level Estimates: Tables

Table 101. Number and death rates for suicide, United States and by State, 2005 and 2007

[Data are based on death certificate records]

State	2005			2007		
	Number	Age-adjusted[1] death rate	Crude death rate[2]	Number	Age-adjusted[1] death rate	Crude death rate[2]
Alabama	535	11.5	11.7	592	12.5	12.8
Alaska	131	20.2	19.7	149	22.1	21.8
Arizona	945	16.2	15.9	1,016	16.1	16.0
Arkansas	400	14.2	14.4	402	14.3	14.2
California	3,206	9.1	8.9	3,602	9.8	9.9
Colorado	800	17.3	17.1	811	16.4	16.7
Connecticut	295	8.1	8.4	271	7.4	7.7
Delaware	83	9.6	9.8	95	10.7	11.0
District of Columbia	33	5.5	6.0	36	5.8	6.1
Florida	2,347	12.6	13.2	2,587	13.3	14.2
Georgia	924	10.5	10.2	997	10.7	10.4
Hawaii	107	8.3	8.4	133	9.7	10.4
Idaho	228	16.2	16.0	223	15.1	14.9
Illinois	1,086	8.5	8.5	1,108	8.5	8.6
Indiana	745	11.9	11.9	790	12.4	12.5
Iowa	333	10.9	11.2	322	10.6	10.8
Kansas	362	13.1	13.2	382	13.7	13.8
Kentucky	566	13.3	13.6	649	15.1	15.3
Louisiana	505	11.1	11.2	522	12.2	12.2
Maine	175	12.3	13.2	191	13.7	14.5
Maryland	472	8.4	8.4	518	9.0	9.2
Massachusetts	480	7.2	7.5	516	7.6	8.0
Michigan	1,108	10.8	10.9	1,131	11.0	11.2
Minnesota	547	10.3	10.7	572	10.8	11.0
Mississippi	363	12.6	12.4	396	13.8	13.6
Missouri	727	12.4	12.5	808	13.5	13.7
Montana	206	21.5	22.0	196	19.4	20.5
Nebraska	187	10.8	10.6	181	10.2	10.2
Nevada	480	20.1	19.9	471	18.3	18.4
New Hampshire	162	11.8	12.4	158	11.1	12.0
New Jersey	536	6.0	6.1	596	6.7	6.9
New Mexico	342	17.7	17.7	401	20.4	20.4
New York	1,189	6.0	6.2	1,396	7.0	7.2
North Carolina	1,009	11.5	11.6	1,077	11.7	11.9
North Dakota	92	13.7	14.5	95	14.4	14.9
Ohio	1,341	11.4	11.7	1,295	11.0	11.3
Oklahoma	522	14.7	14.7	531	14.7	14.7
Oregon	560	14.8	15.4	594	15.2	15.9
Pennsylvania	1,430	11.1	11.5	1,441	11.2	11.6
Rhode Island	71	6.3	6.6	96	8.7	9.1
South Carolina	510	11.8	12.0	530	11.7	12.0

(continued)

Table 101. Number and death rates for suicide, United States and by State, 2005 and 2007 *(continued)*

State	2005			2007		
	Number	Age-adjusted[1] death rate	Crude death rate[2]	Number	Age-adjusted[1] death rate	Crude death rate[2]
South Dakota	121	15.3	15.6	102	12.5	12.8
Tennessee	856	14.0	14.4	844	13.3	13.7
Texas	2,418	10.9	10.6	2,433	10.4	10.2
Utah	348	15.1	14.1	378	15.4	14.3
Vermont	78	12.2	12.5	89	13.8	14.3
Virginia	866	11.2	11.4	880	11.2	11.4
Washington	822	12.7	13.1	865	13.0	13.4
West Virginia	255	13.2	14.0	300	15.9	16.6
Wisconsin	643	11.5	11.6	729	12.7	13.0
Wyoming	90	17.2	17.7	101	19.7	19.3
United States	**32,637**	**10.9**	**11.0**	**34,598**	**11.3**	**11.5**

[1] Estimates are age-adjusted to the year 2000 standard population using 11 age groups: younger than 1 year (3,794,901 persons), 1 to 4 years (15,191,619), 5 to 14 years (39,976,619), 15 to 24 years (38,076,743), 25 to 34 years (37,233,437), 35 to 44 years (44,659,185), 45 to 54 years (37,030,152), 55 to 64 years (23,961,506), 65 to 74 years (18,135,514), 75 to 84 years (12,314,793), and 85 years or older (4,259,173).

[2] Crude death rate equals total number of deaths in the State divided by total number in the population of the State multiplied by 100,000.

NOTE: The National Vital Statistics Report presents detailed data on the deaths and death rates according to a number of social, demographic, and medical characteristics. In 2007, 2,423,712 deaths were reported in the United States.

SOURCE: Xu, J. Q., Kochanek, K. D., Murphy, S. L., & Tejada-Vera, B. (2010). Deaths: Final data for 2007. *National Vital Statistics Reports, 58*(19). Hyattsville, MD: National Center for Health Statistics.

7. TABLES

7.4 State-Level Estimates: Tables

Table 102. Number and percentage of inmates in State correctional facilities receiving mental health treatment, United States and by State, 2000

[Data are based on a survey of correctional facilities]

State	24-hour mental health care		Therapy/ counseling		Psychotropic medication	
	Number	Percent	Number	Percent	Number	Percent
Alabama	556	2.5	1,768	8.4	1,078	4.9
Alaska	93	2.9	286	10.8	238	9.0
Arizona	378	1.4	3,874	14.7	2,194	8.3
Arkansas	82	0.8	1,117	10.7	424	4.1
California	3,144	2.1	18,863	12.5	15,831	10.5
Colorado	274	1.8	2,213	14.9	2,180	14.2
Connecticut	341	2.3	2,596	17.8	1,659	11.4
Delaware	2	0.0	801	14.5	739	12.5
District of Columbia	38	1.6	503	21.1	213	8.9
Florida	191	0.3	10,689	14.9	7,764	10.8
Georgia	2,070	4.8	5,302	12.1	4,659	10.6
Hawaii	120	3.2	100	2.7	746	19.8
Idaho	1	0.0	547	14.3	728	19.1
Illinois	672	1.5	4,374	9.9	2,954	6.7
Indiana	354	1.9	4,281	23.5	2,392	13.1
Iowa	134	1.5	1,293	14.3	1,122	12.4
Kansas	218	2.4	2,075	23.1	1,518	16.9
Kentucky	126	1.0	2,626	21.9	2,296	18.5
Louisiana	201	1.2	5,062	27.0	1,626	8.7
Maine	26	2.8	538	33.0	367	23.5
Maryland	253	1.3	2,829	14.9	2,344	12.4
Massachusetts	309	3.0	2,271	21.8	1,331	12.7
Michigan	760	1.7	4,678	10.5	2,161	4.8
Minnesota	32	0.4	1,222	16.4	1,312	17.6
Mississippi	580	3.9	1,607	10.9	1,935	13.1
Missouri	12	0.0	3,331	11.9	1,054	3.8
Montana	13	0.6	268	12.0	478	21.4
Nebraska	84	2.4	982	28.0	691	19.7
Nevada	54	0.8	599	10.6	529	7.7
New Hampshire	92	4.9	387	20.7	228	12.2
New Jersey	467	1.8	2,308	9.2	2,541	9.4
New Mexico	138	2.7	803	15.6	427	8.5
New York	262	0.4	6,888	10.2	4,539	6.7
North Carolina	715	2.5	3,747	13.2	2,783	10.2
North Dakota	—	—	—	—	247	39.3
Ohio	1,042	2.2	7,165	15.0	4,921	10.3
Oklahoma	187	0.8	3,349	14.6	2,716	11.8
Oregon	65	0.8	2,032	21.8	1,796	19.6
Pennsylvania	178	0.5	4,761	13.0	3,891	10.6
Rhode Island	10	0.3	—	—	—	—
South Carolina	39	0.2	1,122	5.3	28	1.1
South Dakota	43	1.7	577	22.3	420	16.2

(continued)

Table 102. Number and percentage of inmates in State correctional facilities receiving mental health treatment, United States and by State, 2000 *(continued)*

State	24-hour mental health care		Therapy/ counseling		Psychotropic medication	
	Number	Percent	Number	Percent	Number	Percent
Tennessee	399	2.2	430	6.5	1,811	9.9
Texas	1,638	1.5	9,599	7.7	7,838	6.2
Utah	22	1.8	306	29.0	239	19.8
Vermont	30	3.0	350	34.9	284	28.3
Virginia	0	0.0	3,215	10.6	2,540	8.4
Washington	381	2.6	—	—	1,925	13.1
West Virginia	29	1.0	353	12.6	486	16.1
Wisconsin	492	3.2	2,483	20.4	2,735	18.0
Wyoming	7	0.3	815	37.3	378	17.3
United States	**17,354**	**1.6**	**137,385**	**12.8**	**105,336**	**9.7**

— Data not available.

NOTES: The 2000 Census of State and Federal Adult Correctional Facilities provides information on facilities, inmates, programs, and staff of State and Federal correctional facilities throughout the United States, and of private correctional facilities housing State or Federal inmates. Data were gathered from 1,668 separate institutions (prisons; prison boot camps; reception, diagnostic, and classification centers; prison forestry camps and farms; prison hospitals; youthful offender facilities [except in California]; facilities for alcohol and drug treatment; work release and prerelease; and State-operated local detention facilities in Alaska, Connecticut, Delaware, Hawaii, Rhode Island, and Vermont).

Percentages are based on the number of inmates held in facilities reporting data. Total inmates (denominators for the percentages) vary by category of treatment: 1,073,455 for 24-hour mental health care; 1,069,605 for therapy/ counseling; and 1,088,023 for use of psychotropic medications.

SOURCE: Beck, A. J., & Maruschak, L. M. (2001). *Mental health treatment in State prisons, 2000* (NCJ 188215). Washington, DC: U.S. Department of Justice, Office of Justice Programs, Bureau of Justice Statistics. Retrieved from http://bjs.ojp.usdoj.gov/content/pub/pdf/mhtsp00.pdf

7. TABLES

7.4 State-Level Estimates: Tables

7.4.1 Populations by State: People's Mental Health

Mental Health of Adults

Mental Health of Children

Suicide

Special Populations

7.4.2 Populations by State: Providers and Settings for Mental Health Services

Mental Health of Adults
Tables 103–105

Mental Health of Children

Mental Health Service Capacity

7.4.3 Populations by State: Payers and Payment Mechanisms

Revenues and Expenditures by Public Funding Source

Table 103. Total adult population and percentage of persons aged 18 or older who received outpatient specialty mental health treatment, by treatment setting, United States and by State, 2005–2009

[Data are based on a survey of a representative sample of the national population]

State	Total adult population (1,000s)	Any outpatient specialty treatment (percent)	Outpatient mental health clinic or center (percent)	Office of a private therapist, psychologist, psychiatrist, social worker, or counselor—not part of a clinic (percent)	Partial day hospital or day treatment program (percent)
Alabama	3,439	3.6	1.5	2.3	0.1
Alaska	473	4.4	1.7	2.8	0.1
Arizona	4,557	5.2	1.1	4.2	0.2
Arkansas	2,087	4.3	1.9	2.5	0.2
California	26,534	5.1	1.3	3.8	0.2
Colorado	3,571	6.9	1.9	5.4	0.1
Connecticut	2,630	7.9	1.9	6.5	0.2
Delaware	646	5.8	0.9	4.9	0.2
District of Columbia	458	8.7	1.3	7.5	0.1
Florida	13,837	4.2	1.1	3.3	0.1
Georgia	6,799	3.5	0.9	2.7	0.1
Hawaii	947	3.0	0.5	2.6	0.0
Idaho	1,067	4.3	0.7	3.8	0.1
Illinois	9,459	4.4	1.0	3.5	0.1
Indiana	4,665	4.7	1.8	3.1	0.2
Iowa	2,238	4.6	2.4	2.4	0.2
Kansas	2,027	5.7	2.2	3.7	*
Kentucky	3,159	4.3	1.6	2.8	0.0
Louisiana	3,194	4.0	1.6	2.2	0.3
Maine	1,026	7.2	2.6	5.2	0.1
Maryland	4,174	5.1	1.0	4.2	0.1
Massachusetts	4,947	8.0	1.6	6.7	0.2
Michigan	7,490	4.9	1.8	3.4	0.1
Minnesota	3,879	5.9	2.5	3.9	0.1
Mississippi	2,100	3.3	2.1	1.3	0.0
Missouri	4,362	5.2	1.2	4.2	0.2
Montana	724	5.4	2.0	3.7	0.0
Nebraska	1,301	5.2	1.7	3.8	0.5
Nevada	1,860	4.4	1.5	2.9	0.0
New Hampshire	1,005	7.9	1.9	6.2	0.1
New Jersey	6,507	4.6	1.2	3.5	0.4
New Mexico	1,435	4.8	1.7	3.4	*
New York	14,655	7.0	1.9	5.1	0.2
North Carolina	6,627	4.7	1.8	2.8	0.2
North Dakota	481	4.8	1.9	3.3	0.1
Ohio	8,570	5.0	1.5	3.8	0.0
Oklahoma	2,632	5.0	1.6	3.3	0.2
Oregon	2,838	5.6	1.9	4.0	0.0
Pennsylvania	9,465	4.7	1.7	3.2	0.1

(continued)

Table 103. Total adult population and percentage of persons aged 18 or older who received outpatient specialty mental health treatment, by treatment setting, United States and by State, 2005–2009 *(continued)*

State	Total adult population (1,000s)	Any outpatient specialty treatment (percent)	Outpatient mental health clinic or center (percent)	Office of a private therapist, psychologist, psychiatrist, social worker, or counselor—not part of a clinic (percent)	Partial day hospital or day treatment program (percent)
Rhode Island	810	9.5	2.5	7.1	0.6
South Carolina	3,250	3.8	1.7	2.3	0.2
South Dakota	581	3.7	1.6	2.4	0.0
Tennessee	4,580	4.3	1.8	2.6	*
Texas	16,782	3.4	0.8	2.7	0.0
Utah	1,798	5.9	1.4	4.9	0.2
Vermont	486	8.1	1.3	7.3	0.1
Virginia	5,659	4.5	1.3	3.5	0.0
Washington	4,837	5.4	1.5	4.1	0.1
West Virginia	1,406	5.8	2.5	3.5	0.2
Wisconsin	4,204	5.9	2.3	3.8	0.0
Wyoming	391	5.3	2.2	3.2	0.1
United States	**222,646**	**5.0**	**1.5**	**3.7**	**0.1**

*Estimates are considered unreliable.

NOTES: The National Survey on Drug Use and Health is a nationally representative survey of the civilian, noninstitutionalized population of the United States aged 12 or older. The survey interviews approximately 67,500 persons each year.

Respondents could indicate multiple service sources; thus, these response categories are not mutually exclusive.

Data from more than one year were combined to ensure statistically precise estimates.

SOURCE: National Survey on Drug Use and Health, 2005–2009, Substance Abuse and Mental Health Services Administration, Office of Applied Studies.

Table 104. Percentage of persons aged 18 or older who received outpatient nonspecialty mental health treatment, by treatment setting, United States and by State, 2005–2009

[Data are based on a survey of a representative sample of the national population]

State	Total adult population (1,000s)	Any outpatient nonspecialty treatment[1] (percent)	Doctor's office—not part of a clinic[1] (percent)	Outpatient medical clinic[1] (percent)	School or university setting/ clinic/ center[1,2] (percent)	Some other place[1,3] (percent)
Alabama	3,439	2.7	2.0	0.6	0.0	0.1
Alaska	473	2.0	0.9	0.9	*	0.4
Arizona	4,557	2.5	1.6	0.8	0.1	0.2
Arkansas	2,087	2.8	2.0	0.7	0.0	0.3
California	26,534	1.5	1.0	0.5	0.0	0.0
Colorado	3,571	2.0	1.3	0.5	0.0	0.2
Connecticut	2,630	1.8	1.4	0.5	0.0	0.0
Delaware	646	2.4	2.0	0.2	0.1	0.3
District of Columbia	458	1.7	0.8	0.8	0.0	0.1
Florida	13,837	2.0	1.4	0.5	0.0	0.2
Georgia	6,799	2.7	1.8	0.7	0.1	0.1
Hawaii	947	1.1	0.5	0.5	0.0	0.0
Idaho	1,067	2.2	1.6	0.5	0.0	0.1
Illinois	9,459	1.4	1.0	0.3	0.0	0.1
Indiana	4,665	2.9	2.2	0.8	0.0	0.0
Iowa	2,238	2.1	1.1	0.8	0.1	0.2
Kansas	2,027	2.2	1.3	0.6	0.1	0.2
Kentucky	3,159	3.0	2.3	0.6	*	0.0
Louisiana	3,194	2.8	1.5	1.2	0.1	0.1
Maine	1,026	2.9	2.0	0.5	0.1	0.4
Maryland	4,174	2.1	1.8	0.3	0.0	0.1
Massachusetts	4,947	2.2	1.4	0.6	0.1	0.1
Michigan	7,490	2.3	1.7	0.5	0.0	0.1
Minnesota	3,879	2.1	0.6	1.4	0.0	0.1
Mississippi	2,100	1.6	1.1	0.5	0.0	0.0
Missouri	4,362	2.3	1.5	0.6	0.0	0.3
Montana	724	2.6	1.6	0.7	0.1	0.3
Nebraska	1,301	2.0	1.2	0.8	0.0	0.1
Nevada	1,860	1.3	1.0	0.3	0.0	0.0
New Hampshire	1,005	2.7	1.9	0.8	0.0	0.1
New Jersey	6,507	2.1	1.6	0.3	0.1	0.2
New Mexico	1,435	1.8	1.1	0.6	0.0	0.1
New York	14,655	1.8	1.2	0.5	0.0	0.1
North Carolina	6,627	2.7	2.0	0.6	0.0	0.0
North Dakota	481	2.2	0.4	1.4	0.1	0.3
Ohio	8,570	2.4	1.9	0.4	0.0	0.2
Oklahoma	2,632	2.5	1.6	0.7	*	0.2
Oregon	2,838	2.3	1.4	0.6	0.1	0.1
Pennsylvania	9,465	2.1	1.8	0.3	0.0	0.1

(continued)

Table 104. Percentage of persons aged 18 or older who received outpatient nonspecialty mental health treatment, by treatment setting, United States and by State, 2005–2009 *(continued)*

State	Total adult population (1,000s)	Any outpatient nonspecialty treatment[1] (percent)	Doctor's office—not part of a clinic[1] (percent)	Outpatient medical clinic[1] (percent)	School or university setting/ clinic/ center[1,2] (percent)	Some other place[1,3] (percent)
Rhode Island	810	3.6	2.4	0.9	*	0.3
South Carolina	3,250	2.2	1.6	0.4	0.0	0.2
South Dakota	581	1.8	0.6	1.0	0.0	0.2
Tennessee	4,580	2.4	1.9	0.5	*	0.0
Texas	16,782	1.9	1.2	0.6	0.0	0.1
Utah	1,798	3.7	2.6	0.7	0.2	0.2
Vermont	486	2.9	2.3	0.7	0.1	0.0
Virginia	5,659	2.4	1.7	0.7	0.0	0.0
Washington	4,837	2.4	1.5	0.7	0.0	0.1
West Virginia	1,406	3.3	2.5	0.6	0.1	0.1
Wisconsin	4,204	1.8	0.6	1.1	0.1	0.1
Wyoming	391	2.6	1.4	0.7	0.0	0.5
United States	**222,646**	**2.1**	**1.4**	**0.6**	**0.0**	**0.1**

*Estimates are considered unreliable.

[1] This does not exclude contact with a medical provider for prescription medication.

[2] Respondents were permitted to specify other locations for receiving outpatient mental health treatment/ counseling. This location was the most commonly reported other location for receiving outpatient treatment/ counseling.

[3] Respondents with unknown or invalid responses to the location "some other place received outpatient mental health treatment/counseling" were excluded.

NOTES: The National Survey on Drug Use and Health is a nationally representative survey of the civilian, noninstitutionalized population of the United States aged 12 or older. The survey interviews approximately 67,500 persons each year.

Respondents could indicate multiple service sources; thus, these response categories are not mutually exclusive.

Data from more than one year were combined to ensure statistically precise estimates.

SOURCE: National Survey on Drug Use and Health, 2005–2009, Substance Abuse and Mental Health Services Administration, Office of Applied Studies.

Table 105. Clinical, rehabilitation, and evidence-based practices services under Medicaid available for adults, United States and by State, 2008

[Data are based on a study of States' policies on Medicaid programs]

State	Clinical services									
	Crisis intervention	Mobile crisis response	Crisis stabilization	Substance abuse outpatient	Substance abuse intensive outpatient	Substance abuse ambulatory detox	Methadone maintenance	Partial hospitalization	Day treatment (mental health)	Day treatment (substance abuse)
Alabama	Y	N	Y	Y	Y	N	Y	Y	Y	Y
Alaska	Y	N	Y	Y	Y	N	Y	N	Y	Y
Arizona	Y	Y	Y	Y	N	N	Y	Y	Y	N
Arkansas	Y	N	N	N	N	N	N	N	Y	N
California	Y	N	Y	Y	Y	N	N	N	Y	N
Colorado	Y	N	N	N	N	N	N	Y	N	N
Connecticut	Y	N	N	Y	Y	N	Y	Y	Y	N
Delaware	Y	N	N	N	N	N	N	N	N	N
District of Columbia	Y	N	Y	N	N	N	N	N	Y	N
Florida	Y	N	Y	Y	N	N	Y	Y	N	Y
Georgia	Y	N	Y	Y	Y	Y	N	Y	N	Y
Hawaii	Y	Y	Y	Y	Y	Y	Y	Y	Y	N
Idaho	Y	N	Y	N	N	N	N	Y	N	N
Illinois	Y	N	N	Y	N	Y	N	N	N	Y
Indiana	Y	N	Y	Y	Y	Y	N	Y	N	N
Iowa[1]	Y	Y	N	Y	Y	N	N	Y	Y	Y
Kansas	Y	N	Y	Y	N	N	N	N	N	N
Kentucky	Y	N	N	Y	N	N	N	Y	Y	N
Louisiana	N	N	Y	Y	N	N	N	N	N	N
Maine	Y	Y	Y	Y	Y	N	Y	N	Y	N
Maryland	Y	Y	Y	Y	N	N	Y	Y	Y	N
Massachusetts	Y	Y	Y	Y	Y	Y	Y	Y	Y	Y
Michigan	Y	N	Y	Y	Y	Y	Y	Y	Y	N
Minnesota	Y	Y	Y	Y	Y	N	N	Y	Y	N
Mississippi	Y	N	N	N	N	N	N	Y	Y	N
Missouri	Y	N	Y	Y	N	N	N	N	Y	N

(continued)

Table 105. Clinical, rehabilitation, and evidence-based practices services under Medicaid available for adults, United States and by State, 2008 *(continued)*

State	Clinical services									
	Crisis intervention	Mobile crisis response	Crisis stabilization	Substance abuse outpatient	Substance abuse intensive outpatient	Substance abuse ambulatory detox	Methadone maintenance	Partial hospitalization	Day treatment (mental health)	Day treatment (substance abuse)
Montana	Y	N	N	Y	Y	Y	N	Y	Y	Y
Nebraska	Y	N	Y	Y	N	N	N	N	N	N
Nevada[1]	Y	Y	Y	Y	N	N	N	Y	Y	Y
New Hampshire	Y	N	N	N	N	N	N	Y	N	N
New Jersey	Y	N	N	Y	N	N	N	Y	N	N
New Mexico	Y	N	Y	Y	N	N	N	Y	N	N
New York	Y	N	N	Y	N	N	N	Y	Y	N
North Carolina	N	Y	Y	Y	Y	Y	N	Y	N	N
North Dakota	Y	N	Y	Y	N	N	N	N	Y	Y
Ohio	Y	Y	Y	Y	Y	Y	Y	Y	N	N
Oklahoma	Y	Y	Y	Y	Y	N	N	N	N	N
Oregon	Y	Y	Y	Y	Y	Y	Y	Y	Y	N
Pennsylvania	Y	Y	Y	Y	Y	Y	Y	Y	Y	Y
Rhode Island	Y	Y	N	Y	Y	Y	Y	Y	N	Y
South Carolina	Y	N	Y	N	N	N	N	N	Y	N
South Dakota	Y	N	N	N	N	N	N	N	N	N
Tennessee	Y	Y	Y	Y	Y	Y	N	Y	Y	N
Texas	Y	Y	N	N	N	N	N	N	Y	N
Utah	Y	N	Y	Y	N	N	N	N	Y	N
Vermont	Y	Y	Y	Y	Y	N	N	Y	N	N
Virginia	Y	Y	Y	Y	Y	N	N	Y	Y	Y
Washington	Y	N	N	Y	N	N	Y	N	Y	N
West Virginia	Y	N	Y	N	N	N	N	N	N	N
Wisconsin	Y	Y	N	Y	N	N	Y	N	Y	Y
Wyoming	Y	N	Y	Y	Y	N	N	N	Y	N
Total number of States offering services	**49**	**19**	**34**	**40**	**23**	**13**	**16**	**30**	**31**	**14**

(continued)

Table 105. Clinical, rehabilitation, and evidence-based practices services under Medicaid available for adults, United States and by State, 2008 *(continued)*

State	Rehabilitation services									
	Site-based rehabilitation	Drop-in centers	Clubhouses	Employment skills	Services at job site	Housing skills	Education skills	Recreation-based services	Socialization	Natural supports[2]
Alabama	Y	N	N	Y	N	N	Y	Y	N	N
Alaska	N	N	N	N	N	N	N	N	N	N
Arizona	N	N	N	Y	N	N	Y	N	N	N
Arkansas	N	N	N	N	N	N	N	N	N	N
California	Y	N	N	N	N	N	N	N	N	N
Colorado	N	N	N	Y	N	N	N	N	N	N
Connecticut	N	N	N	Y	N	Y	Y	N	N	N
Delaware	Y	N	N	N	N	Y	N	N	N	N
District of Columbia	N	N	N	N	N	N	N	N	N	N
Florida	Y	N	Y	N	N	N	N	N	N	N
Georgia	Y	N	N	Y	N	Y	N	N	N	N
Hawaii	Y	N	Y	Y	Y	N	Y	Y	Y	N
Idaho	Y	N	N	Y	N	Y	Y	N	N	N
Illinois	N	N	N	N	N	N	N	N	N	Y
Indiana	N	N	N	N	N	N	N	N	N	N
Iowa[1]	Y	N	N	Y	N	N	Y	N	N	N
Kansas	Y	N	N	N	Y	N	Y	N	N	N
Kentucky	Y	N	N	Y	N	N	N	N	N	N
Louisiana	Y	N	N	Y	N	N	N	N	N	N
Maine	N	N	N	Y	N	N	Y	N	N	N
Maryland	Y	N	N	N	N	Y	N	N	N	N
Massachusetts	Y	N	N	Y	N	N	N	N	N	N
Michigan	Y	Y	Y	Y	Y	Y	Y	Y	Y	Y
Minnesota	Y	Y	Y	Y	Y	Y	N	N	N	N
Mississippi	Y	N	N	N	N	N	N	N	N	N
Missouri	Y	N	N	Y	N	Y	N	N	N	N

(continued)

Table 105. Clinical, rehabilitation, and evidence-based practices services under Medicaid available for adults, United States and by State, 2008 *(continued)*

State	Rehabilitation services									
	Site-based rehabilitation	Drop-in centers	Clubhouses	Employment skills	Services at job site	Housing skills	Education skills	Recreation-based services	Socialization	Natural supports[2]
Montana	Y	N	N	Y	Y	N	Y	N	N	N
Nebraska	Y	N	N	Y	N	N	N	Y	Y	N
Nevada[1]	Y	N	N	N	N	N	N	Y	Y	N
New Hampshire	N	N	N	N	N	N	N	N	N	Y
New Jersey	N	N	N	Y	N	N	N	N	N	N
New Mexico	Y	N	N	N	N	Y	Y	N	N	N
New York	Y	N	N	Y	Y	Y	Y	N	N	Y
North Carolina	Y	N	N	Y	N	N	Y	N	N	N
North Dakota	Y	N	N	Y	N	N	N	N	N	N
Ohio	N	N	N	Y	N	Y	N	Y	Y	N
Oklahoma	Y	N	N	N	N	N	N	N	Y	Y
Oregon	N	N	N	Y	N	Y	Y	N	N	N
Pennsylvania	Y	N	Y	Y	N	N	N	N	N	N
Rhode Island	Y	N	N	N	N	N	N	N	N	N
South Carolina	Y	N	N	Y	N	Y	N	N	N	N
South Dakota	N	N	N	N	N	N	N	N	N	N
Tennessee	Y	N	Y	Y	Y	Y	Y	N	N	Y
Texas	Y	N	N	Y	N	Y	N	N	N	N
Utah	Y	N	N	N	N	N	N	N	N	N
Vermont	Y	N	N	Y	Y	Y	Y	Y	Y	N
Virginia	Y	N	N	N	N	N	N	N	N	N
Washington	N	N	N	Y	N	N	N	N	N	N
West Virginia	N	N	N	Y	N	N	Y	N	N	N
Wisconsin	Y	N	N	Y	Y	N	N	Y	Y	N
Wyoming	Y	N	N	N	N	N	N	N	N	N
Total number of States offering services	**35**	**2**	**6**	**31**	**9**	**16**	**17**	**8**	**8**	**6**

(continued)

Table 105. Clinical, rehabilitation, and evidence-based practices services under Medicaid available for adults, United States and by State, 2008 *(continued)*

State	Evidence-based practices						
	Supported employment	Supported housing	Supported education	Family psychoeducation	Illness/disability self-management	Integrated mental health/substance abuse treatment	Assertive community treatment
Alabama	N	N	N	N	Y	N	Y
Alaska	N	N	N	N	Y	N	Y
Arizona	Y	N	N	N	N	N	N
Arkansas	N	N	N	N	N	Y	N
California	N	N	N	N	N	Y	N
Colorado	N	N	N	N	N	N	N
Connecticut	N	N	N	N	Y	N	Y
Delaware	N	N	N	Y	N	N	Y
District of Columbia	N	N	N	N	Y	Y	Y
Florida	N	N	N	N	N	N	Y
Georgia	Y	Y	N	Y	N	Y	Y
Hawaii	N	N	N	N	Y	N	Y
Idaho	N	N	N	Y	N	N	N
Illinois	Y	Y	N	N	Y	Y	Y
Indiana	N	N	N	N	N	N	Y
Iowa[1]	Y	N	N	N	N	Y	Y
Kansas	N	N	N	N	Y	N	N
Kentucky	N	N	N	N	N	N	N
Louisiana	N	N	N	N	N	N	N
Maine	Y	N	N	Y	Y	Y	Y
Maryland	Y	Y	N	N	Y	Y	Y
Massachusetts	N	N	N	Y	N	Y	Y
Michigan	Y	Y	N	Y	N	Y	Y
Minnesota	N	N	N	N	Y	N	Y
Mississippi	N	N	N	N	N	N	N
Missouri	N	N	N	N	N	N	N

(continued)

Table 105. Clinical, rehabilitation, and evidence-based practices services under Medicaid available for adults, United States and by State, 2008 *(continued)*

State	Evidence-based practices						
	Supported employment	Supported housing	Supported education	Family psychoeducation	Illness/disability self-management	Integrated mental health/substance abuse treatment	Assertive community treatment
Montana	N	N	N	N	N	N	Y
Nebraska	N	N	N	N	N	N	Y
Nevada[1]	N	N	N	N	N	N	Y
New Hampshire	Y	N	N	N	N	N	N
New Jersey	N	N	N	N	N	N	Y
New Mexico	N	N	N	N	Y	N	Y
New York	Y	Y	N	Y	Y	Y	Y
North Carolina	N	N	N	Y	N	N	Y
North Dakota	N	N	N	N	N	Y	N
Ohio	N	N	N	Y	N	N	N
Oklahoma	N	N	N	Y	Y	N	Y
Oregon	Y	Y	N	N	Y	Y	Y
Pennsylvania	Y	N	Y	Y	Y	Y	Y
Rhode Island	Y	Y	N	N	N	N	Y
South Carolina	N	N	N	N	N	N	N
South Dakota	N	N	N	N	N	N	Y
Tennessee	Y	Y	N	N	Y	Y	Y
Texas	N	N	N	N	N	N	N
Utah	N	N	N	N	N	N	N
Vermont	Y	Y	N	Y	Y	Y	Y
Virginia	Y	N	N	N	Y	Y	Y
Washington	N	N	N	N	N	N	Y
West Virginia	N	N	N	N	N	N	Y
Wisconsin	N	N	N	Y	N	Y	Y
Wyoming	N	N	N	N	Y	Y	N
Total number of States offering services	**15**	**9**	**1**	**13**	**19**	**19**	**33**

See notes on page 270.

Table 105 notes

[1] Iowa and Nevada adjusted Medicaid coverage under the Federal Deficit Reduction Act of 2005. See Bazelon Center for Mental Health Law (2008) for details.

[2] Natural supports refers to relationships that occur in everyday life.

NOTE: In 2007, the Judge David L. Bazelon Center for Mental Health Law reviewed States' written policies for their Medicaid programs, namely coverage of mental health services under the Clinic, Rehabilitation, and Home- and Community-Based State Plan service categories and their definitions of eligibility groups under targeted case management. Data from this study indicate the degree to which 50 States and the District of Columbia have been able to include in their Medicaid programs the range of effective interventions covered under Federal policy in force today.

SOURCE: Bazelon Center for Mental Health Law. (2008). *Following the rules: A report on Federal rules and State actions to cover mental health services under Medicaid*. Washington, DC: Judge David L. Bazelon Center for Mental Health Law. Retrieved from http://www.bazelon.org/LinkClick.aspx?fileticket=zeqlTk_ltSk%3D&tabid=104

7. TABLES

7.4 State-Level Estimates: Tables

Table 106. Total youth population and percentage of persons aged 12 to 17 who received specialty and nonspecialty mental health treatment, by treatment setting, United States and by State, 2005–2009

[Data are based on a survey of a representative sample of the national population]

State	Total youth population (1,000s)	Specialty inpatient or residential treatment[1] (percent)	Specialty outpatient treatment[2] (percent)	Nonspecialty mental health services from a medical pediatrician or other family doctor (percent)
Alabama	382	3.4	10.3	3.3
Alaska	64	3.0	9.7	1.5
Arizona	532	2.4	10.1	2.2
Arkansas	233	3.7	11.3	2.6
California	3,224	1.9	10.5	2.3
Colorado	387	2.5	14.1	3.1
Connecticut	294	2.2	14.5	3.0
Delaware	69	2.6	12.5	3.5
District of Columbia	36	5.2	14.8	2.8
Florida	1,378	2.5	11.2	2.8
Georgia	814	2.1	9.0	3.7
Hawaii	97	3.5	10.0	2.0
Idaho	132	2.2	11.0	3.8
Illinois	1,085	2.8	10.9	2.5
Indiana	538	3.0	12.1	3.4
Iowa	243	2.5	12.4	2.6
Kansas	232	3.6	11.7	3.2
Kentucky	339	3.5	11.2	3.6
Louisiana	376	3.3	9.1	2.6
Maine	104	2.4	14.3	3.0
Maryland	474	2.6	13.1	3.0
Massachusetts	506	2.7	15.0	3.2
Michigan	874	2.5	12.0	2.7
Minnesota	430	2.8	13.5	2.4
Mississippi	256	3.4	8.5	2.5
Missouri	488	3.0	12.3	3.0
Montana	77	2.2	11.4	3.2
Nebraska	147	2.4	11.9	3.1
Nevada	211	2.4	8.0	1.7
New Hampshire	110	2.2	16.9	4.4
New Jersey	722	3.2	13.2	2.8
New Mexico	169	3.9	12.4	2.4
New York	1,563	2.4	13.2	2.4
North Carolina	727	2.4	10.6	2.9
North Dakota	50	2.6	11.8	2.4
Ohio	960	3.0	12.0	3.4
Oklahoma	295	3.6	11.4	3.2
Oregon	295	2.4	14.3	3.7
Pennsylvania	1,006	2.0	10.8	2.4
Rhode Island	84	2.2	13.5	2.9

(continued)

Table 106. Total youth population and percentage of persons aged 12 to 17 who received specialty and nonspecialty mental health treatment, by treatment setting, United States and by State, 2005–2009 *(continued)*

State	Total youth population (1,000s)	Specialty inpatient or residential treatment[1] (percent)	Specialty outpatient treatment[2] (percent)	Nonspecialty mental health services from a medical pediatrician or other family doctor (percent)
South Carolina	360	2.5	10.0	3.5
South Dakota	66	3.6	11.3	2.3
Tennessee	492	2.3	11.2	3.4
Texas	2,100	2.1	9.5	2.7
Utah	243	1.8	11.8	4.0
Vermont	50	2.4	15.5	3.1
Virginia	614	2.5	12.0	2.6
Washington	528	3.0	12.7	2.7
West Virginia	135	3.3	12.2	4.5
Wisconsin	461	2.8	12.5	3.1
Wyoming	42	2.8	13.5	3.0
United States	**25,098**	**2.5**	**11.4**	**2.8**

[1] Inpatient treatment includes a stay of overnight or longer in a hospital or other facility for mental health problems.

[2] Outpatient treatment includes treatment/counseling from a (1) private therapist, psychologist, psychiatrist, social worker, or counselor; (2) mental health clinic or center; (3) partial day hospital or day treatment program; or (4) in-home therapist, counselor, or family preservation worker.

NOTES: The National Survey on Drug Use and Health is a nationally representative survey of the civilian, noninstitutionalized population of the United States aged 12 or older. The survey interviews approximately 67,500 persons each year. In 2009, 22,626 youth aged 12 to 17 were interviewed.

Respondents could indicate multiple service sources; thus, these response categories are not mutually exclusive.

Data from more than one year were combined to ensure statistically precise estimates.

SOURCE: National Survey on Drug Use and Health, 2005–2009, Substance Abuse and Mental Health Services Administration, Office of Applied Studies.

Table 107. Clinical, rehabilitation, and evidence-based practices services under Medicaid available for children, United States and by State, 2008

[Data are based on a study of States' policies on Medicaid programs]

State	Clinical services									
	Crisis intervention	Mobile crisis response	Crisis stabilization	Substance abuse outpatient	Substance abuse intensive outpatient	Substance abuse ambulatory detox	Methadone maintenance	Partial hospitalization	Day treatment (mental health)	Day treatment (substance abuse)
Alabama	Y	N	N	Y	N	N	Y	N	Y	N
Alaska	Y	N	Y	Y	Y	N	N	Y	Y	N
Arizona	Y	Y	Y	Y	N	N	N	N	Y	N
Arkansas	Y	N	Y	N	N	N	N	N	Y	N
California	Y	N	Y	Y	Y	N	N	N	Y	N
Colorado	Y	N	N	N	N	N	N	Y	N	N
Connecticut	Y	Y	Y	Y	Y	N	Y	Y	Y	N
Delaware	Y	Y	Y	Y	Y	N	N	Y	Y	Y
District of Columbia	Y	N	Y	N	N	N	N	N	Y	N
Florida	Y	N	N	Y	N	N	Y	N	Y	N
Georgia	Y	N	N	Y	Y	Y	Y	N	Y	Y
Hawaii	Y	Y	Y	Y	Y	Y	N	Y	Y	N
Idaho	Y	N	Y	N	N	N	N	Y	N	N
Illinois	Y	N	Y	Y	Y	N	N	N	N	Y
Indiana	Y	N	Y	Y	Y	N	N	Y	Y	N
Iowa[1]	Y	Y	N	Y	Y	N	N	N	Y	N
Kansas	Y	N	N	Y	N	N	N	N	N	N
Kentucky	Y	N	Y	Y	Y	N	N	N	Y	N
Louisiana	Y	N	N	Y	N	N	N	N	N	N
Maine	Y	Y	Y	Y	Y	N	Y	N	Y	N
Maryland	Y	Y	Y	Y	Y	N	Y	Y	Y	N
Massachusetts	Y	Y	Y	Y	Y	N	N	Y	Y	Y
Michigan	Y	N	Y	Y	Y	N	Y	Y	Y	N
Minnesota	Y	Y	Y	Y	N	N	N	Y	Y	N
Mississippi	Y	N	N	N	N	N	N	Y	Y	N
Missouri	Y	N	Y	Y	N	N	N	N	Y	N

(continued)

Table 107. Clinical, rehabilitation, and evidence-based practices services under Medicaid available for children, United States and by State, 2008 *(continued)*

State	Clinical services									
	Crisis intervention	Mobile crisis response	Crisis stabilization	Substance abuse outpatient	Substance abuse intensive outpatient	Substance abuse ambulatory detox	Methadone maintenance	Partial hospitalization	Day treatment (mental health)	Day treatment (substance abuse)
Montana	Y	N	N	Y	Y	Y	N	Y	Y	N
Nebraska	Y	Y	Y	Y	Y	N	N	N	Y	Y
Nevada[1]	Y	Y	Y	Y	N	N	N	Y	Y	N
New Hampshire	Y	N	N	N	N	N	N	Y	Y	N
New Jersey	Y	Y	Y	Y	N	N	N	Y	Y	Y
New Mexico	Y	N	Y	Y	N	N	N	Y	Y	Y
New York	Y	N	N	Y	N	N	N	Y	Y	N
North Carolina	N	Y	Y	Y	Y	Y	N	Y	Y	N
North Dakota	Y	N	Y	Y	N	N	N	N	N	N
Ohio	Y	Y	Y	Y	Y	Y	Y	Y	N	N
Oklahoma	Y	Y	Y	Y	Y	N	N	N	N	N
Oregon	Y	Y	Y	Y	Y	Y	Y	Y	Y	N
Pennsylvania	Y	Y	Y	Y	Y	Y	N	Y	Y	N
Rhode Island	Y	Y	N	Y	N	N	N	Y	Y	N
South Carolina	Y	N	Y	N	N	N	N	N	Y	N
South Dakota	Y	N	N	N	N	N	N	N	N	N
Tennessee	Y	Y	N	Y	Y	Y	Y	Y	Y	N
Texas	Y	Y	N	N	N	N	N	N	N	N
Utah	Y	N	N	Y	N	N	N	N	Y	N
Vermont	Y	N	Y	Y	N	N	N	N	Y	N
Virginia	Y	Y	Y	Y	Y	N	N	Y	Y	Y
Washington	Y	N	N	Y	N	N	N	N	Y	N
West Virginia	Y	N	N	N	N	N	N	N	N	N
Wisconsin	Y	Y	N	Y	N	N	Y	N	Y	Y
Wyoming	Y	N	Y	Y	Y	N	N	N	Y	N
Total number of States offering services	**50**	**22**	**32**	**41**	**24**	**8**	**11**	**25**	**40**	**9**

(continued)

Table 107. Clinical, rehabilitation, and evidence-based practices services under Medicaid available for children, United States and by State, 2008 *(continued)*

State	Rehabilitation services												
	Natural supports[2]	Employ-ment skills	Education skills	Services in schools	School day treatment	After-school	Summer programs	Recre-ation-based services	Social-ization	Housing skills	Thera-peutic nursery	Early in-tervention services (0–3)	Transition services (child to adult)
Alabama	N	N	N	Y	Y	N	N	N	N	N	N	N	N
Alaska	N	N	Y	Y	N	N	N	N	N	N	N	N	N
Arizona	N	Y	N	Y	N	Y	N	N	N	N	Y	N	N
Arkansas	N	N	N	N	N	N	N	N	N	N	N	N	N
California	N	N	N	N	N	N	N	N	N	N	N	N	N
Colorado	N	Y	N	Y	N	N	N	N	N	N	N	N	N
Connecticut	Y	Y	Y	Y	N	Y	Y	Y	N	Y	N	N	N
Delaware	N	N	N	Y	Y	N	N	N	N	N	N	Y	Y
District of Columbia	N	N	N	Y	N	N	N	N	N	N	N	N	N
Florida	N	N	N	Y	N	N	N	N	N	N	N	Y	N
Georgia	N	Y	Y	Y	N	N	N	N	N	N	N	N	N
Hawaii	Y	Y	Y	Y	N	N	N	Y	Y	N	N	N	N
Idaho	N	Y	Y	Y	N	N	N	N	N	N	N	N	N
Illinois	N	N	N	Y	N	N	N	N	N	N	N	N	Y
Indiana	N	N	N	N	N	N	N	N	N	N	N	N	N
Iowa[1]	N	N	N	N	N	N	N	N	N	N	N	N	N
Kansas	N	N	N	Y	N	N	N	N	N	N	N	N	Y
Kentucky	N	N	N	N	N	Y	Y	N	N	N	N	Y	Y
Louisiana	N	Y	N	Y	N	N	N	N	N	N	N	N	N
Maine	N	N	N	Y	Y	N	N	N	N	N	N	Y	N
Maryland	N	N	N	N	N	Y	N	N	N	Y	Y	N	N
Massachusetts	N	Y	N	Y	N	N	N	N	N	N	N	N	Y
Michigan	Y	N	N	Y	N	N	N	N	N	N	N	Y	N
Minnesota	N	Y	N	Y	N	N	N	N	N	N	N	N	N
Mississippi	N	N	N	Y	Y	N	N	N	N	N	N	N	N
Missouri	N	Y	N	Y	N	N	N	N	N	N	N	N	N

(continued)

Table 107. Clinical, rehabilitation, and evidence-based practices services under Medicaid available for children, United States and by State, 2008 *(continued)*

State	Rehabilitation services												
	Natural supports[2]	Employment skills	Education skills	Services in schools	School day treatment	After-school	Summer programs	Recreation-based services	Socialization	Housing skills	Therapeutic nursery	Early intervention services (0–3)	Transition services (child to adult)
Montana	N	Y	Y	Y	N	N	N	N	N	N	N	N	N
Nebraska	N	Y	N	Y	N	N	N	Y	N	N	Y	N	N
Nevada[1]	N	N	Y	Y	N	N	N	Y	Y	N	N	N	N
New Hampshire	N	N	N	Y	N	N	N	N	N	N	N	N	N
New Jersey	N	N	Y	Y	N	N	N	N	N	N	N	N	N
New Mexico	Y	Y	Y	Y	Y	N	N	N	N	N	N	Y	N
New York	N	N	N	Y	N	N	N	N	N	N	N	N	N
North Carolina	N	Y	Y	Y	N	N	N	N	N	N	N	Y	N
North Dakota	N	Y	N	Y	N	N	N	N	N	N	N	N	N
Ohio	N	Y	N	Y	N	N	N	Y	Y	N	N	N	N
Oklahoma	N	N	Y	Y	N	N	N	N	N	N	N	Y	N
Oregon	N	Y	Y	Y	N	N	N	Y	N	Y	N	N	N
Pennsylvania	Y	N	N	Y	Y	Y	Y	Y	Y	N	Y	N	N
Rhode Island	N	N	N	N	N	N	N	N	N	N	N	Y	N
South Carolina	N	N	Y	Y	N	N	N	N	N	N	N	Y	N
South Dakota	N	N	N	N	N	N	N	N	N	N	N	N	N
Tennessee	N	N	N	N	N	N	N	N	N	N	N	N	Y
Texas	N	N	Y	Y	N	N	N	N	N	N	N	N	N
Utah	N	N	N	Y	N	N	N	N	N	N	N	N	N
Vermont	N	Y	Y	Y	N	N	N	N	N	N	N	N	N
Virginia	N	N	N	Y	Y	N	N	N	N	N	N	Y	N
Washington	N	N	Y	Y	N	N	N	N	N	N	N	N	N
West Virginia	N	N	Y	N	N	N	N	N	N	N	N	N	N
Wisconsin	N	Y	N	Y	N	N	N	Y	Y	N	N	N	N
Wyoming	N	N	N	N	N	N	N	N	N	N	N	N	N
Total number of States offering services	**5**	**19**	**17**	**40**	**7**	**5**	**3**	**8**	**5**	**3**	**4**	**11**	**6**

(continued)

Table 107. Clinical, rehabilitation, and evidence-based practices services under Medicaid available for children, United States and by State, 2008 *(continued)*

State	Evidence-based practices										
	Intensive in-home services	Thera-peutic foster care	Multi-systemic therapy	Wrap-around	Family psycho-education	Integrated mental health/ substance abuse treatment	Illness/ disability self-man-agement	Supported education	Supported employ-ment	Supported housing	Assertive community treatment
Alabama	Y	N	N	N	Y	N	Y	N	N	N	N
Alaska	N	Y	N	N	Y	N	N	N	N	N	N
Arizona	Y	Y	Y	N	Y	N	N	N	N	N	N
Arkansas	Y	Y	N	N	N	N	N	N	N	N	N
California	N	N	Y	N	N	N	N	N	N	N	N
Colorado	Y	N	N	N	N	N	N	N	N	N	N
Connecticut	Y	Y	Y	Y	Y	Y	Y	N	N	Y	Y
Delaware	Y	Y	N	N	Y	N	N	N	N	N	N
District of Columbia	Y	N	Y	N	Y	Y	N	N	N	N	N
Florida	Y	Y	N	N	Y	N	N	N	N	N	N
Georgia	Y	Y	N	Y	Y	Y	N	N	N	N	N
Hawaii	Y	Y	Y	N	Y	Y	N	N	N	N	N
Idaho	N	N	N	N	N	N	N	N	N	N	N
Illinois	Y	Y	N	N	N	N	Y	N	N	N	N
Indiana	N	N	Y	N	N	N	N	N	N	N	N
Iowa[1]	N	N	N	N	Y	N	N	N	N	N	N
Kansas	Y	Y	N	N	Y	N	N	N	N	N	N
Kentucky	Y	Y	Y	N	N	N	N	N	N	N	N
Louisiana	Y	N	N	N	N	N	N	N	N	N	N
Maine	Y	Y	Y	Y	Y	N	N	N	N	N	Y
Maryland	Y	Y	Y	N	N	Y	Y	N	Y	Y	N
Massachusetts	Y	N	N	N	Y	Y	N	N	N	N	Y
Michigan	Y	N	Y	Y	Y	N	N	N	N	N	N
Minnesota	N	Y	N	N	N	N	N	N	N	N	N
Mississippi	Y	N	N	Y	N	N	N	N	N	N	N
Missouri	Y	Y	N	Y	Y	N	N	N	N	N	N

(continued)

Table 107. Clinical, rehabilitation, and evidence-based practices services under Medicaid available for children, United States and by State, 2008 *(continued)*

State	Evidence-based practices										
	Intensive in-home services	Thera-peutic foster care	Multi-systemic therapy	Wrap-around	Family psycho-education	Integrated mental health/ substance abuse treatment	Illness/ disability self-man-agement	Supported education	Supported employ-ment	Supported housing	Assertive community treatment
Montana	N	Y	N	N	N	N	N	N	N	N	N
Nebraska	Y	Y	N	N	Y	Y	N	N	N	N	N
Nevada[1]	Y	Y	Y	Y	Y	N	N	N	N	N	N
New Hampshire	N	N	N	N	N	N	N	N	Y	N	N
New Jersey	N	Y	Y	Y	Y	Y	Y	N	N	N	N
New Mexico	Y	Y	Y	N	Y	N	Y	N	N	N	Y
New York	N	N	N	N	N	N	N	N	N	N	N
North Carolina	Y	Y	Y	N	Y	N	N	N	N	N	N
North Dakota	Y	Y	N	N	N	N	N	N	N	N	N
Ohio	Y	N	N	N	Y	N	N	N	N	N	N
Oklahoma	N	Y	N	N	Y	N	N	N	N	N	N
Oregon	Y	Y	Y	Y	Y	Y	Y	N	Y	Y	Y
Pennsylvania	Y	Y	Y	Y	Y	Y	N	N	N	N	N
Rhode Island	N	Y	N	N	N	N	N	N	N	N	N
South Carolina	Y	Y	N	N	Y	N	N	N	N	N	N
South Dakota	Y	N	N	N	Y	N	N	N	N	N	N
Tennessee	Y	N	N	N	Y	Y	N	N	Y	N	Y
Texas	N	N	N	Y	Y	N	N	N	N	N	N
Utah	N	Y	N	N	Y	N	N	N	N	N	N
Vermont	Y	Y	N	N	Y	Y	N	N	N	N	N
Virginia	Y	Y	Y	Y	N	N	Y	N	Y	N	Y
Washington	N	N	N	N	N	N	N	N	N	N	N
West Virginia	N	N	N	N	N	N	N	N	N	N	N
Wisconsin	Y	N	N	N	Y	Y	N	N	N	N	Y
Wyoming	N	Y	N	Y	N	Y	N	N	N	N	N
Total number of States offering services	**34**	**31**	**17**	**13**	**31**	**14**	**8**	**0**	**5**	**3**	**8**

See notes on page 280.

Table 107 notes

[1] Services that may be covered under Medicaid are listed in several sections of the Federal law. Specifically, States may opt for Home- and Community-Based Services under Section 1915(i). Specifically allowable services for people with mental disorders under 1915(i) of Federal law are case management, personal care, respite, homemaker services, day treatment, partial hospitalization, psychosocial rehabilitation, and clinic services in any community setting. Section 1915(i) services can be limited to a specific number of individuals specified by the State (creating what are known as "slots") and can be available only to individuals with incomes at or below 150 percent of the Federal poverty level, which is a lower income threshold than for Section 1905(a) services. At this time, Home- and Community-Based State Plan services authorized by the Federal Deficit Reduction Act are covered in only two States: Iowa and Nevada.

[2] Natural supports refers to relationships that occur in everyday life.

NOTE: In 2007, the Judge David L. Bazelon Center for Mental Health Law reviewed States' written policies for their Medicaid programs, namely coverage of mental health services under the Clinic, Rehabilitation, and Home- and Community-Based State Plan service categories and their definitions of eligibility groups under targeted case management. Data from this study indicate the degree to which 50 States and the District of Columbia have been able to include in their Medicaid programs the range of effective interventions covered under Federal policy in force today.

SOURCE: Bazelon Center for Mental Health Law. (2008). *Following the rules: A report on Federal rules and State actions to cover mental health services under Medicaid*. Washington, DC: Judge David L. Bazelon Center for Mental Health Law. Retrieved from http://www.bazelon.org/LinkClick.aspx?fileticket=zeqlTk_ltSk%3D&tabid=104

Table 108. Number of youth aged 0 to 17 and number of child and adolescent psychiatrists, by State, 1990, 2000, and 2009

[Data are based on statistics from various government agencies]

State	Youth aged 0 to 17 in 2009 (number)	Youth living in poverty in 2009 (percent)	Child and adolescent psychiatrists			Child and adolescent psychiatrists per 100,000 youth[1]		
			1990 (number)	2000 (number)	2009 (number)	1990 (number)	2000 (number)	2009 (number)
Alabama	1,128,864	23.4	23	46	71	2.2	4.1	6.3
Alaska	183,546	12.9	7	4	11	4.1	2.1	6.0
Arizona	1,732,019	20.6	43	69	122	4.5	5.1	7.0
Arkansas	709,968	25.1	12	28	38	2.0	4.1	5.4
California	9,435,682	18.2	539	688	877	7.1	7.5	9.3
Colorado	1,227,763	15.7	80	122	149	9.4	11.1	12.1
Connecticut	807,919	11.6	121	153	176	16.4	18.2	21.8
Delaware	206,674	15.3	8	14	19	5.0	7.2	9.2
District of Columbia	113,854	26.5	39	45	57	34.7	39.4	50.1
Florida	4,057,773	18.2	150	232	302	5.3	6.4	7.4
Georgia	2,583,792	20.2	66	119	146	3.9	5.5	5.7
Hawaii	290,361	11.5	34	53	72	12.3	18.0	24.8
Idaho	419,190	17.2	9	17	21	3.0	4.6	5.0
Illinois	3,177,377	17.1	144	202	249	5.0	6.2	7.8
Indiana	1,589,153	17.8	44	76	90	3.1	4.8	5.7
Iowa	713,078	14.7	29	37	42	4.1	5.1	5.9
Kansas	704,951	15.4	65	71	68	10.0	10.0	9.6
Kentucky	1,014,323	23.2	46	78	86	4.9	7.8	8.5
Louisiana	1,123,133	25.6	49	79	66	4.0	6.5	5.9
Maine	271,113	17.1	20	34	56	6.6	11.3	20.7
Maryland	1,351,814	10.2	180	229	278	18.6	16.9	20.6
Massachusetts	1,432,698	12.7	252	299	348	18.9	20.0	24.3
Michigan	2,349,695	19.6	165	192	200	6.8	7.4	8.5
Minnesota	1,260,797	12.3	53	83	105	4.6	6.5	8.3
Mississippi	767,665	29.0	6	28	33	0.8	3.6	4.3
Missouri	1,431,338	18.8	63	91	118	5.3	6.4	8.2

(continued)

Table 108. Number of youth aged 0 to 17 and number of child and adolescent psychiatrists, by State, 1990, 2000, and 2009
(continued)

State	Youth aged 0 to 17 in 2009 (number)	Youth living in poverty in 2009 (percent)	Child and adolescent psychiatrists			Child and adolescent psychiatrists per 100,000 youth[1]		
			1990 (number)	2000 (number)	2009 (number)	1990 (number)	2000 (number)	2009 (number)
Montana	219,798	19.4	4	12	17	1.8	5.2	7.7
Nebraska	451,641	15.3	10	33	31	2.4	7.3	6.9
Nevada	681,033	15.2	7	16	31	2.5	3.1	4.6
New Hampshire	288,990	9.1	24	28	28	8.7	9.1	9.7
New Jersey	2,045,646	12.2	121	185	269	6.8	8.9	13.1
New Mexico	510,110	25.5	25	44	55	5.7	8.7	10.8
New York	4,424,083	19.1	626	778	931	15.0	16.6	21.0
North Carolina	2,277,967	20.8	75	158	221	4.7	8.1	9.7
North Dakota	143,926	13.8	5	14	19	2.9	8.7	13.2
Ohio	2,714,341	18.9	121	189	238	4.4	6.6	8.8
Oklahoma	918,849	22.9	22	28	42	2.7	3.1	4.6
Oregon	872,811	17.8	33	63	89	4.7	7.5	10.2
Pennsylvania	2,775,132	16.8	243	329	351	8.8	11.3	12.6
Rhode Island	226,706	16.0	21	39	44	9.4	15.8	19.4
South Carolina	1,080,732	22.2	43	91	111	4.7	9.0	10.3
South Dakota	199,505	17.1	3	9	16	1.5	4.4	8.0
Tennessee	1,493,252	22.1	45	83	88	3.8	5.9	5.9
Texas	6,895,969	23.6	249	370	447	5.2	6.3	6.5
Utah	868,824	11.3	23	33	46	3.7	4.6	5.3
Vermont	126,219	13.2	15	20	27	10.6	13.6	21.4
Virginia	1,847,182	13.0	114	158	188	9.5	9.1	10.2
Washington	1,569,592	15.4	57	96	120	4.6	6.4	7.6
West Virginia	386,449	23.8	12	17	22	2.7	4.2	5.7
Wisconsin	1,310,250	14.4	65	108	125	5.1	7.9	9.5
Wyoming	131,944	12.7	2	4	6	1.5	3.1	4.5

See notes on page 283.

Table 108 notes

[1] Ratio per 100,000 youth for 1990 used 1990 U.S. Census data, 2000 used 2000 U.S. Census data, and 2009 used data from the 2005–2009 American Community Survey.

NOTES: The Area Resource File of the U.S. Department of Health and Human Services is a database containing more than 6,000 variables for each U.S. county. It contains information on health facilities, health professions, measures of resource scarcity, health status, economic activity, health training programs, and socioeconomic and environmental characteristics.

For 2000, the number of youth aged 0 to 17 and the percent living in poverty are from the Public Use Microdata of the Decennial U.S. Census of 2000. For 2009, the number of youth aged 0 to 17 and the percent living in poverty are from the Public Use Microdata from the 2005–2009 American Community Survey of the U.S. Census, inflated to the 2000 U.S. Census estimates by age, sex, and race/ethnicity for 2009. With the exception of 2009, data on the number of child psychiatrists are from the Area Resource File. For 2009, the data on the number of child psychiatrists per State were provided by the American Medical Association to the American Association of Child and Adolescent Psychiatry. An earlier version of this table without 2009 was published in Thomas and Holzer (2006).

SOURCES: The American Medical Association and the American Association of Child and Adolescent Psychiatry.

Thomas, C. R., & Holzer, C. E. III (2006). The continuing shortage of child and adolescent psychiatrists. *Journal of the American Academy of Child and Adolescent Psychiatry, 45*(9), 1023–1031.

7. TABLES

7.4 State-Level Estimates: Tables

Table 109. Number and rate per 100,000 population of mental health personnel, by discipline, United States and by State, 2006 and 2008

[Data are based on association membership and certification data]

State	Psychiatry[1]		Psychology[2]		Advanced practice psychiatric nursing[3]		Counseling[4]		Marriage and family therapy[5]		Social work[6]	
	2006 (number)	2006 (rate per 100,000)	2006 (number)	2006 (rate per 100,000)	2006 (number)	2006 (rate per 100,000)	2008 (number)	2008 (rate per 100,000)	2006 (number)	2006 (rate per 100,000)	2008 (number)	2008 (rate per 100,000)
Alabama	378	8.2	546	11.9	71	1.6	1,662	35.9	194	4.2	1,301	28.3
Alaska	92	13.6	170	25.1	64	9.8	442	63.2	89	13.1	744	109.8
Arizona	629	10.2	1,392	22.6	175	3.0	3,272	51.6	336	5.4	3,365	54.6
Arkansas	238	8.5	679	24.2	34	1.2	1,227	43.3	91	3.2	1,157	41.2
California	5,977	16.5	16,279	44.9	345	1.0	8,125	22.2	27,874	76.9	19,359	53.4
Colorado	695	14.6	1,846	38.7	157	3.4	4,351	89.5	501	10.5	3,788	79.5
Connecticut	988	28.3	1,415	40.5	457	13.0	1,641	46.9	846	24.2	6,443	184.3
Delaware	99	11.6	312	36.6	28	3.4	476	55.0	3	0.4	673	78.9
District of Columbia	346	59.1	1,006	171.8	26	4.7	1,168	198.6	8	1.4	1,314	224.5
Florida	1,935	10.7	3,976	22.0	366	2.1	6,984	38.3	1,433	7.9	9,318	51.6
Georgia	983	10.5	1,783	19.1	229	2.6	4,139	43.3	561	6.0	4,111	44.0
Hawaii	285	22.3	479	37.5	52	4.1	190	14.8	139	10.9	1,806	141.2
Idaho	96	6.6	206	14.1	26	1.9	933	62.2	208	14.2	978	66.8
Illinois	1,602	12.5	4,031	31.5	201	1.6	5,986	46.6	415	3.2	11,547	90.4
Indiana	526	8.3	1,019	16.2	125	2.0	1,618	25.5	813	12.9	4,589	72.8
Iowa	220	7.4	431	14.5	85	2.9	953	31.9	163	5.5	1,835	61.7
Kansas	305	11.1	630	22.9	115	4.2	395	14.2	285	10.3	2,132	77.4
Kentucky	424	10.1	969	23.0	163	3.9	837	19.7	404	9.6	1,971	46.9
Louisiana	472	11.1	501	11.8	53	1.2	2,244	52.3	891	21.0	4,613	108.7
Maine	276	21.0	543	41.3	269	20.4	932	70.7	79	6.0	2,723	207.1
Maryland	1,536	27.4	2,047	36.5	429	7.7	2,367	42.1	158	2.8	8,459	151.0
Massachusetts	2,227	34.6	4,372	67.9	921	14.4	5,896	91.4	819	12.7	15,285	237.6
Michigan	1,156	11.4	2,660	26.3	211	2.1	5,804	57.6	780	7.7	12,535	124.1
Minnesota	590	11.4	2,866	55.6	268	5.3	576	11.1	994	19.3	2,639	51.2
Mississippi	208	7.2	255	8.8	93	3.2	1,115	38.2	396	13.7	852	29.4
Missouri	617	10.6	1,327	22.7	165	2.9	3,824	65.0	155	2.7	3,772	64.6

(continued)

Table 109. Number and rate per 100,000 population of mental health personnel, by discipline, United States and by State, 2006 and 2008 *(continued)*

State	Psychiatry[1]		Psychology[2]		Advanced practice psychiatric nursing[3]		Counseling[4]		Marriage and family therapy[5]		Social work[6]	
	2006 (number)	2006 (rate per 100,000)	2006 (number)	2006 (rate per 100,000)	2006 (number)	2006 (rate per 100,000)	2008 (number)	2008 (rate per 100,000)	2006 (number)	2006 (rate per 100,000)	2008 (number)	2008 (rate per 100,000)
Montana	150	15.8	218	23.0	31	3.3	944	98.6	31	3.3	878	92.7
Nebraska	177	10.0	342	19.4	74	4.2	1,087	61.3	84	4.8	923	52.3
Nevada	184	7.4	329	13.2	15	0.6	754	29.4	673	27.0	1,146	46.0
New Hampshire	196	14.9	588	44.8	145	11.2	572	43.5	68	5.2	1,653	126.0
New Jersey	1,543	17.8	2,737	31.6	360	4.1	2,740	31.5	699	8.1	13,971	161.2
New Mexico	301	15.5	501	25.8	99	5.2	2,532	128.6	212	10.9	1,761	90.7
New York	5,638	29.2	8,649	44.9	745	3.9	4,360	22.6	635	3.3	36,056	187.0
North Carolina	1,145	12.9	2,591	29.2	212	2.5	4,694	51.8	541	6.1	6,540	73.7
North Dakota	80	12.5	142	22.3	33	5.2	392	61.3	12	1.9	237	37.1
Ohio	1,249	10.9	3,125	27.3	338	2.9	4,004	34.9	140	1.2	5,615	49.0
Oklahoma	284	7.9	506	14.1	32	0.9	2,818	77.9	501	14.0	1,493	41.7
Oregon	527	14.3	1,055	28.6	120	3.3	1,771	47.3	342	9.3	3,472	94.1
Pennsylvania	2,081	16.8	5,018	40.5	432	3.5	4,514	36.3	347	2.8	9,823	79.2
Rhode Island	237	22.3	400	37.7	130	12.0	304	28.7	68	6.4	2,176	205.0
South Carolina	513	11.8	576	13.3	107	2.5	1,621	36.8	205	4.7	1,814	41.9
South Dakota	64	8.1	156	19.8	21	2.7	216	27.1	91	11.5	329	41.7
Tennessee	610	10.0	1,309	21.5	279	4.7	1,377	22.4	276	4.5	3,104	51.1
Texas	2,018	8.6	5,534	23.6	332	1.5	13,640	57.1	2,702	11.5	8,424	36.0
Utah	214	8.3	584	22.6	104	4.4	580	21.9	385	14.9	1,977	76.6
Vermont	169	27.2	502	80.9	57	9.2	572	92.1	29	4.7	1,088	175.3
Virginia	1,117	14.6	2,217	29.0	338	4.5	3,201	41.5	703	9.2	6,303	82.5
Washington	852	13.4	1,633	25.6	479	7.7	4,653	71.9	944	14.8	4,250	66.7
West Virginia	159	8.8	456	25.2	28	1.5	1,126	62.2	15	0.8	768	42.4
Wisconsin	668	12.0	1,213	21.8	112	2.0	2,583	46.1	274	4.9	3,330	59.8
Wyoming	44	8.6	106	20.7	13	2.6	674	128.9	54	10.5	463	90.2
United States	**43,120**	**14.4**	**92,227**	**30.9**	**9,764**	**3.3**	**128,886**	**54.4**	**48,666**	**16.3**	**244,900**	**82.0**

See notes on page 288.

Table 109 notes

[1] For psychiatry, the numerator of the rate is based on clinically active psychiatrists and does not include residents or fellows (see the American Medical Association's *Physician Characteristics and Distribution in the US, 2008*), and the denominator is from the U.S. Census Bureau population estimates as of July 1, 2006.

[2] For psychology, the estimates are based on clinically trained doctoral-level psychologists licensed by each State in 2007 reported from several sources, and the denominator is from the U.S. Census Bureau. Numbers for each State were reduced by the proportion of psychologists that are licensed in more than one State (8.5 percent) in an attempt to avoid counting psychologists more than once.

[3] Clinically active Advanced Practice Psychiatric Nurses may be underestimated by as much as 50 percent. The data source is the American Nurses Credentialing Center (ANCC) of all Advanced Practice Psychiatric Nurses who are certified in 2006. According to estimates from the National Survey of Registered Nurses (2004), there are an estimated 20,000 Advanced Practice Psychiatric Nurses in the United States. ANCC certification is only required if billing directly for services.

[4] 2008 National Board for Certified Counselors certification directory and national job analysis, American Counseling Association membership directory, and licensure data provided by individual States. The denominator is from the U.S. Census Bureau population estimates for 2007.

[5] The data for the numerator are based on information collected by the American Association of Marriage and Family Therapy (AAMFT) from State marriage and family therapy regulatory boards on the number of licensed marriage and family therapists in 2006. For those States that did not license marriage and family therapists in 2006, the numbers were obtained from the count of clinical members from the AAMFT Membership Database. The denominator is from the U.S. Census Bureau estimates as of July 1, 2006.

[6] For social work, the Association for Social Work Boards estimates the number of licensed social workers to be 310,000. This number excludes bachelor-level, doctorate-level, and nondegreed licensed social workers. An estimated 79 percent of this number, or 244,900, have MSWs, and are thus eligible to hold clinical licenses. The proportion of these MSWs that actually do hold clinical licenses is unknown. Hence, for purposes of this table, the total number of clinically trained social workers is considered to be 244,900. The MSW data were constructed as follows: The initial numerator was defined as 2 times the active National Association of Social Workers membership with an MSW degree in 2008 for the specified population aggregate. For the United States, this produced a total of 186,340. The denominator was defined as the population estimate for the aggregate from the U.S. Census Bureau population estimates for 2007. To adjust this ratio to the total of 244,900 MSW qualified social workers estimated above, each ratio was multiplied by 1.3142642 (or 244,900 divided by 186,340), and the final result was multiplied by 100,000 to produce a rate per 100,000.

NOTES: Originally published in Substance Abuse and Mental Health Services Administration (SAMHSA). (2010). *Mental Health, United States, 2008* (DHHS Publication No. SMA 10-4590). Rockville, MD: Center for Mental Health Services, SAMHSA.

Counts of mental health personnel are for clinically active and clinically trained personnel.

SOURCE: Data are drawn from multiple sources and are delineated in the footnotes.

Table 110. Number of community hospitals with specialty mental health/substance abuse units, United States and by State, selected years 1997–2007

[Data are from Medicare Cost Reports]

State	1997	2001	2005	2006	2007[1]
Alabama	29	24	25	26	30
Alaska	1	1	1	1	1
Arizona	16	12	16	15	13
Arkansas	30	31	27	22	23
California	98	87	75	71	66
Colorado	18	15	14	11	11
Connecticut	22	25	25	26	26
Delaware	5	3	2	2	1
District of Columbia	6	5	5	5	5
Florida	60	51	43	43	41
Georgia	24	24	23	23	23
Hawaii	1	3	3	2	2
Idaho	4	5	6	5	4
Illinois	80	69	58	56	53
Indiana	41	37	33	32	29
Iowa	24	25	24	19	20
Kansas	25	29	19	19	19
Kentucky	20	22	18	17	17
Louisiana	65	61	53	42	41
Maine	7	6	6	6	6
Maryland[2]	—	—	—	—	—
Massachusetts	48	40	40	39	39
Michigan	67	57	53	50	48
Minnesota	20	25	24	21	20
Mississippi	40	43	43	36	34
Missouri	47	43	39	34	33
Montana	3	3	3	2	2
Nebraska	9	5	7	7	7
Nevada	6	5	3	3	3
New Hampshire	15	12	9	10	10
New Jersey	34	38	37	37	34
New Mexico	10	7	7	8	8
New York	98	105	104	104	103
North Carolina	41	37	37	34	37
North Dakota	7	8	7	7	7
Ohio	83	83	65	58	56
Oklahoma	28	25	24	23	23
Oregon	12	12	10	10	10
Pennsylvania	94	100	84	82	82
Rhode Island	4	5	5	5	5
South Carolina	16	16	14	14	15
South Dakota	4	4	3	3	3
Tennessee	35	39	40	40	40
Texas	75	62	44	47	47

(continued)

Table 110. Number of community hospitals with specialty mental health/substance abuse units, United States and by State, selected years 1997–2007 *(continued)*

State	1997	2001	2005	2006	2007[1]
Utah	9	7	7	7	7
Vermont	4	4	4	2	2
Virginia	37	33	31	31	31
Washington	17	17	15	13	13
West Virginia	10	11	9	9	10
Wisconsin	25	26	20	18	16
Wyoming	4	4	4	4	4
United States	**1,478**	**1,411**	**1,268**	**1,201**	**1,180**

—Data not available.

[1] 2007 data are preliminary.

[2] Data for specialty units in Maryland are not available, because Maryland is exempt from the Medicare Prospective Payment System. As a result, Maryland hospitals do not provide specialty unit data on the Medicare Cost Report.

NOTE: The Medicare Cost Report is based on annual financial information reported to the Centers for Medicare & Medicaid Services. The Cost Report contains provider information, such as facility characteristics, utilization data, cost and charges by cost center (in total and for Medicare), Medicare settlement data, and financial statement data.

SOURCE: Medicare Cost Reports, 1997, 2001, 2005, 2006, 2007, Centers for Medicare & Medicaid Services.

Table 111. Percentage of State population living in counties with a shortage of mental health professionals in the United States, by State, 2006

[Data are based on estimates from multiple sources]

State	State population facing high shortage of mental health professionals[1] (percent)	State population living in counties with high shortage of prescribing professionals[1,2] (percent)	State population living in counties with high unmet need for other mental health professionals[1,3] (percent)
Alabama	29.0	81.0	3.3
Alaska	17.5	39.2	2.7
Arizona	25.4	82.3	0.0
Arkansas	28.5	67.7	6.5
California	11.1	25.2	0.0
Colorado	15.3	37.3	0.1
Connecticut	0.0	0.0	0.0
Delaware	11.4	22.2	0.0
District of Columbia	0.0	0.0	0.0
Florida	25.8	73.2	0.2
Georgia	24.3	50.9	1.1
Hawaii	11.3	11.3	0.0
Idaho	31.6	97.8	0.7
Illinois	20.2	27.9	0.0
Indiana	26.1	63.4	0.0
Iowa	27.8	78.2	0.2
Kansas	24.2	52.2	2.4
Kentucky	24.0	47.8	4.9
Louisiana	21.5	64.1	0.6
Maine	6.4	20.4	0.0
Maryland	0.0	10.5	0.0
Massachusetts	0.0	0.2	0.0
Michigan	21.2	48.2	0.0
Minnesota	21.0	42.9	2.4
Mississippi	29.0	69.2	0.3
Missouri	23.0	43.3	0.6
Montana	25.6	47.2	2.2
Nebraska	27.5	51.3	0.4
Nevada	29.9	81.6	0.6
New Hampshire	4.2	3.4	0.0
New Jersey	1.2	5.9	0.0
New Mexico	17.2	46.4	0.6
New York	0.0	7.1	0.0
North Carolina	20.9	58.0	0.1
North Dakota	22.4	38.6	11.5
Ohio	24.6	49.0	0.1
Oklahoma	26.0	51.1	0.2
Oregon	19.0	27.8	0.5
Pennsylvania	11.6	27.6	0.1
Rhode Island	5.0	0.0	0.0
South Carolina	24.6	65.0	2.4

(continued)

Table 111. Percentage of State population living in counties with a shortage of mental health professionals in the United States, by State, 2006 *(continued)*

State	State population facing high shortage of mental health professionals[1] (percent)	State population living in counties with high shortage of prescribing professionals[1,2] (percent)	State population living in counties with high unmet need for other mental health professionals[1,3] (percent)
South Dakota	28.0	54.1	10.7
Tennessee	25.4	62.7	2.6
Texas	28.5	75.1	3.1
Utah	26.3	58.7	0.6
Vermont	0.0	10.6	0.0
Virginia	8.9	25.7	0.3
Washington	19.1	38.2	0.0
West Virginia	26.9	85.0	1.0
Wisconsin	19.8	31.0	1.0
Wyoming	29.0	73.2	0.0

[1] Not all mental health professionals can prescribe medications. Typically, psychiatrists can prescribe medication, whereas advanced practice psychiatric nurses, licensed professional counselors, marriage and family therapists, psychologists, and social workers typically cannot prescribe medication.

[2] >50 percent shortage of prescribing mental health professionals.

[3] >50 percent shortage of nonprescribing mental health professionals.

NOTES: The National Comorbidity Survey Replication (NCS-R) is a nationally representative household survey of 9,282 English speakers aged 18 or older in the United States. The Medical Expenditure Panel Survey (MEPS) is a set of large-scale surveys of families and individuals, their medical providers (e.g., doctors, hospitals, pharmacies), and employers across the United States. Since 1996, MEPS has collected data on the specific health services that Americans use, how frequently they use them, the cost of these services, and how they are paid for, as well as data on the cost, scope, and breadth of health insurance held by and available to U.S. workers.

Estimates describe shortages of outpatient professional mental health services in the adult household population. County-level need was based on models using data from NCS-R, the U.S. Census, and MEPS. The supply of clinically active mental health professionals was estimated for each county using data from licensure and certification boards and professional associations. Shortage was estimated by smoothing the county-level need and supply estimates to account for travel within a defined radius and then calculating the percentage of need for mental health visits that was not met by available providers. Estimates measure relative need rather than absolute need. Details on estimate construction and limitations can be found in Ellis et al. (2009), Konrad et al. (2009), Morrissey et al. (2007), and Thomas et al. (2009, 2010).

SOURCES: Estimates provided by Cecil G. Sheps Center for Health Services Research, University of North Carolina at Chapel Hill.

Ellis, A. R., Konrad, T. R., Thomas, K. C., & Morrissey, J. P. (2009). County-level estimates of mental health professional supply in the United States. *Psychiatric Services, 60*(10), 1315–1322.

Konrad, T. R., Ellis, A. R., Holzer, C. E. III, Thomas, K. C., & Morrissey, J. (2009). County-level estimates of need for mental health professionals in the United States. *Psychiatric Services, 60*(10), 1307–1314.

Morrissey, J. P., Thomas, K. C., Ellis, A. R., & Konrad, T. R. (2007). *Development of a new method for designation of mental health professional shortage areas* (Contract No. HHSH-230200532038C). Prepared with the Bureau of Health Professions, Health Resources and Services Administration, U.S. Department of Health and Human Services.

Thomas, K. C., Ellis, A. R., Konrad, T. R., Holzer, C. E. III, & Morrissey, J. P. (2009). County-level estimates of mental health professional shortage in the United States. *Psychiatric Services, 60*(10), 1323–1328.

Thomas, K. C., Ellis, A. R., & Morrissey, J. P. (2010). Where are the psychiatric physician assistants? Reply. *Psychiatric Services, 61*(1), 95–96.

Table 112. Number of correctional facilities under State or Federal authority that provided psychological or psychiatric counseling to inmates, United States and by State, 2005

[Data are based on a census of State and Federal correctional facilities]

State	Total facilities	Any counseling	Drug dependency counseling or awareness	Alcohol dependency counseling or awareness	Psychological or psychiatric counseling
Alabama	33	30	29	28	8
Alaska	21	14	8	10	7
Arizona	21	19	19	19	14
Arkansas	26	25	25	25	25
California	100	85	80	80	64
Colorado	58	46	42	41	32
Connecticut	49	41	40	38	27
Delaware	12	12	11	12	10
District of Columbia[1]	5	4	4	4	3
Florida	109	109	9	9	60
Georgia	87	85	79	75	41
Hawaii	10	10	10	10	9
Idaho	15	14	13	14	9
Illinois[2]	44	40	33	33	22
Indiana	23	23	22	22	13
Iowa	31	29	24	25	21
Kansas	13	12	11	11	9
Kentucky	25	25	24	24	14
Louisiana	23	22	21	21	11
Maine	7	7	6	7	5
Maryland	29	26	19	21	16
Massachusetts[3]	17	16	14	15	13
Michigan	62	58	57	55	49
Minnesota	18	17	13	13	12
Mississippi	31	28	25	26	10
Missouri	28	26	22	23	24
Montana	11	11	10	9	6
Nebraska	9	9	8	8	6
Nevada	22	21	19	18	12
New Hampshire	8	8	6	6	6
New Jersey	42	36	33	34	22
New Mexico	11	9	9	9	7
New York	77	72	69	68	46
North Carolina	88	83	76	77	57
North Dakota	8	7	7	7	4
Ohio	59	55	54	54	42
Oklahoma	53	46	35	33	27
Oregon	15	14	11	11	7
Pennsylvania	52	42	42	42	39
Rhode Island	7	7	5	5	7
South Carolina	33	29	27	27	16

(continued)

Table 112. Number of correctional facilities under State or Federal authority that provided psychological or psychiatric counseling to inmates, United States and by State, 2005 *(continued)*

State	Total facilities	Any counseling	Drug dependency counseling or awareness	Alcohol dependency counseling or awareness	Psychological or psychiatric counseling
South Dakota	6	4	4	4	4
Tennessee	19	18	18	18	16
Texas	132	119	37	38	11
Utah	7	6	3	3	3
Vermont	9	9	6	6	7
Virginia	59	58	55	56	36
Washington	32	32	4	4	2
West Virginia	15	12	12	12	10
Wisconsin	41	39	28	27	27
Wyoming	7	7	7	7	6
United States[4]	**1,821**	**1,676**	**1,345**	**1,344**	**1,054**

[1] As of December 30, 2001, sentenced felons from the District of Columbia were the responsibility of the Federal Bureau of Prisons. Some inmates were housed in private facilities under contract to the District of Columbia on December 30, 2005.

[2] The total number of facilities reported by the Illinois Department of Corrections as of June 30, 2005.

[3] The total number of facilities reported by June 30, 2005.

[4] Includes facilities operated by both Federal and State authorities.

NOTES: The 2005 Census of State and Federal Adult Correctional Facilities provides information on facilities, inmates, programs, and staff of State and Federal correctional facilities throughout the United States and of private correctional facilities housing State or Federal inmates. Data were gathered from 1,821 separate institutions (prisons; prison boot camps; reception, diagnostic, and classification centers; prison forestry camps and farms; prison hospitals; youthful offender facilities [except in California]; facilities for alcohol and drug treatment; work release and prerelease; and State-operated local detention facilities in Alaska, Connecticut, Delaware, Hawaii, Rhode Island, and Vermont).

Information on counseling programs was not reported in 41 facilities.

SOURCE: Census of State and Federal Adult Correctional Facilities, December 30, 2005, Bureau of Justice Statistics.

Table 113. Number of inpatient State and local psychiatric beds in U.S. hospitals, United States and by State, FY 2007

[Data are based on a survey of hospitals]

State	FY 2007 adult population (1,000s)	Beds in State and local psychiatric hospitals		Beds in other State and local government hospitals	
		Number	Number per 100,000 adults	Number	Number per 100,000 adults
Alabama	3,510	990	28.2	399	11.4
Alaska	500	80	16.0	12	2.4
Arizona	4,674	338	7.2	199	4.3
Arkansas	2,139	202	9.4	26	1.2
California	26,799	4,885	18.2	1,521	5.7
Colorado	3,647	860	23.6	53	1.5
Connecticut	2,666	777	29.1	25	0.9
Delaware	659	323	49.0	0	0.0
District of Columbia	472	817	173.0	0	0.0
Florida	14,196	1,342	9.5	622	4.4
Georgia	6,997	2,539	36.3	129	1.8
Hawaii	986	202	20.5	28	2.8
Idaho	1,090	215	19.7	63	5.8
Illinois	9,585	1,830	19.1	56	0.6
Indiana	4,754	1,172	24.7	201	4.2
Iowa	2,267	223	9.8	210	9.3
Kansas	2,076	692	33.3	128	6.2
Kentucky	3,245	535	16.5	32	1.0
Louisiana	3,273	874	26.7	285	8.7
Maine	1,037	152	14.7	0	0.0
Maryland	4,267	1,230	28.8	0	0.0
Massachusetts	5,051	897	17.8	247	4.9
Michigan	7,605	625	8.2	101	1.3
Minnesota	3,926	1,147	29.2	134	3.4
Mississippi	2,155	1,553	72.1	225	10.4
Missouri	4,475	1,342	30.0	72	1.6
Montana	737	214	29.0	0	0.0
Nebraska	1,323	716	54.1	0	0.0
Nevada	1,900	401	21.1	0	0.0
New Hampshire	1,018	224	22.0	0	0.0
New Jersey	6,566	3,685	56.1	127	1.9
New Mexico	1,464	357	24.4	10	0.7
New York	14,923	6,071	40.7	1,628	10.9
North Carolina	6,844	1,611	23.5	382	5.6
North Dakota	495	140	28.3	0	0.0
Ohio	8,755	1,420	16.2	134	1.5
Oklahoma	2,710	450	16.6	77	2.8
Oregon	2,867	739	25.8	31	1.1
Pennsylvania	9,705	2,214	22.8	0	0.0
Rhode Island	821	0	0.0	0	0.0
South Carolina	3,358	506	15.1	179	5.3

(continued)

Table 113. Number of inpatient State and local psychiatric beds in U.S. hospitals, United States and by State, FY 2007 *(continued)*

State	FY 2007 adult population (1,000s)	Beds in State and local psychiatric hospitals		Beds in other State and local government hospitals	
		Number	Number per 100,000 adults	Number	Number per 100,000 adults
South Dakota	599	244	40.7	0	0.0
Tennessee	4,694	972	20.7	59	1.3
Texas	17,190	3,108	18.1	275	1.6
Utah	1,834	449	24.5	114	6.2
Vermont	489	54	11.0	0	0.0
Virginia	5,883	1,593	27.1	132	2.2
Washington	4,916	1,216	24.7	105	2.1
West Virginia	1,423	240	16.9	26	1.8
Wisconsin	4,277	1,225	28.6	0	0.0
Wyoming	397	166	41.8	31	7.8
United States	**227,240**	**53,857**	**23.7**	**8,078**	**3.6**

NOTES: The American Hospital Association Annual Survey is completed online by most U.S. hospitals and profiles more than 6,500 hospitals throughout the United States. The overall response rate for FY 2007 was 78 percent, but this rate varies among subgroups of hospitals depending on size, ownership, service, geographical location, and membership status. The survey covers hospital organization structure, service lines, staffing, expenses, physician organization structures, beds, and utilization.

The data exclude all children's hospitals. Data represent "staffed beds," beds regularly available (those set up and staffed for use) within the reporting period.

SOURCES: Aron, L., Honberg, R., Duckworth, K., Kimball, A., Edgar, E., Carolla, B., ... & Fitzpatrick, M. (2009). *Grading the States 2009: A report on America's health care system for adults with serious mental illness.* Arlington, VA: National Alliance on Mental Illness.

State Single Year of Age and Sex Resident Population Estimates: April 1, 2000 to July 1, 2009, U.S. Census Bureau.

Table 114. Number of inpatient private, not-for-profit, and for-profit psychiatric beds in U.S. hospitals, United States and by State, FY 2007

[Data are based on a survey of hospitals]

State	FY 2007 adult population (1,000s)	Beds in private, not-for-profit hospitals		Beds in private, for-profit hospitals		Beds in all private hospitals	
		Number	Number per 100,000 adults	Number	Number per 100,000 adults	Number	Number per 100,000 adults
Alabama	3,510	107	3.0	584	16.6	691	19.7
Alaska	500	49	9.8	74	14.8	123	24.6
Arizona	4,674	370	7.9	85	1.8	455	9.7
Arkansas	2,139	481	22.5	348	16.3	829	38.8
California	26,799	2,070	7.7	1,815	6.8	3,885	14.5
Colorado	3,647	300	8.2	140	3.8	440	12.1
Connecticut	2,666	810	30.4	0	0.0	810	30.4
Delaware	659	45	6.8	92	14.0	137	20.8
District of Columbia	472	131	27.7	104	22.0	235	49.8
Florida	14,196	1,235	8.7	1,261	8.9	2,496	17.6
Georgia	6,997	610	8.7	462	6.6	1,072	15.3
Hawaii	986	151	15.3	0	0.0	151	15.3
Idaho	1,090	70	6.4	237	21.7	307	28.2
Illinois	9,585	1,892	19.7	649	6.8	2,541	26.5
Indiana	4,754	886	18.6	386	8.1	1,272	26.8
Iowa	2,267	542	23.9	0	0.0	542	23.9
Kansas	2,076	337	16.2	0	0.0	337	16.2
Kentucky	3,245	695	21.4	463	14.3	1,158	35.7
Louisiana	3,273	188	5.7	675	20.6	863	26.4
Maine	1,037	359	34.6	0	0.0	359	34.6
Maryland	4,267	1,157	27.1	25	0.6	1,182	27.7
Massachusetts	5,051	1,300	25.7	598	11.8	1,898	37.6
Michigan	7,605	1,625	21.4	307	4.0	1,932	25.4
Minnesota	3,926	581	14.8	0	0.0	581	14.8
Mississippi	2,155	148	6.9	568	26.4	716	33.2
Missouri	4,475	983	22.0	702	15.7	1,685	37.7
Montana	737	92	12.5	0	0.0	92	12.5
Nebraska	1,323	259	19.6	0	0.0	259	19.6
Nevada	1,900	18	0.9	257	13.5	275	14.5
New Hampshire	1,018	182	17.9	84	8.2	266	26.1
New Jersey	6,566	1,747	26.6	210	3.2	1,957	29.8
New Mexico	1,464	10	0.7	302	20.6	312	21.3
New York	14,923	3,547	23.8	407	2.7	3,954	26.5
North Carolina	6,844	770	11.3	413	6.0	1,183	17.3
North Dakota	495	150	30.3	34	6.9	184	37.2
Ohio	8,755	1,560	17.8	206	2.4	1,766	20.2
Oklahoma	2,710	653	24.1	402	14.8	1,055	38.9
Oregon	2,867	349	12.2	0	0.0	349	12.2
Pennsylvania	9,705	2,785	28.7	971	10.0	3,756	38.7
Rhode Island	821	282	34.3	0	0.0	282	34.3

(continued)

Table 114. Number of inpatient private, not-for-profit, and for-profit psychiatric beds in U.S. hospitals, United States and by State, FY 2007 *(continued)*

State	FY 2007 adult population (1,000s)	Beds in private, not-for-profit hospitals		Beds in private, for-profit hospitals		Beds in all private hospitals	
		Number	Number per 100,000 adults	Number	Number per 100,000 adults	Number	Number per 100,000 adults
South Carolina	3,358	191	5.7	444	13.2	635	18.9
South Dakota	599	176	29.4	0	0.0	176	29.4
Tennessee	4,694	678	14.4	857	18.3	1,535	32.7
Texas	17,190	1,270	7.4	2,410	14.0	3,680	21.4
Utah	1,834	80	4.4	140	7.6	220	12.0
Vermont	489	137	28.0	0	0.0	137	28.0
Virginia	5,883	516	8.8	860	14.6	1,376	23.4
Washington	4,916	342	7.0	115	2.3	457	9.3
West Virginia	1,423	404	28.4	147	10.3	551	38.7
Wisconsin	4,277	813	19.0	0	0.0	813	19.0
Wyoming	397	0	0.0	86	21.7	86	21.7
United States	**227,240**	**34,133**	**15.0**	**17,920**	**7.9**	**52,053**	**22.9**

NOTES: The American Hospital Association Annual Survey is completed online by most U.S. hospitals and profiles more than 6,500 hospitals throughout the United States. The overall response rate for FY 2007 was 78 percent, but this rate varies among subgroups of hospitals depending on size, ownership, service, geographical location, and membership status. The survey covers hospital organization structure, service lines, staffing, expenses, physician organization structures, beds, and utilization.

The data exclude all children's hospitals. Data represent "staffed beds," beds regularly available (those set up and staffed for use) within the reporting period.

SOURCES: Aron, L., Honberg, R., Duckworth, K., Kimball, A., Edgar, E., Carolla, B., ... & Fitzpatrick, M. (2009). *Grading the States 2009: A report on America's health care system for adults with serious mental illness*. Arlington, VA: National Alliance on Mental Illness.

State Single Year of Age and Sex Resident Population Estimates: April 1, 2000 to July 1, 2009, U.S. Census Bureau.

Table 115. Number of inpatient Federal and non-Federal psychiatric beds in U.S. hospitals, United States and by State, FY 2007

[Data are based on a survey of hospitals]

State	FY 2007 adult population (1,000s)	Beds in all non-Federal hospitals[1]		Beds in Federal government hospitals		Beds in all (Federal and non-Federal) hospitals	
		Number	Number per 100,000 adults	Number	Number per 100,000 adults	Number	Number per 100,000 adults
Alabama	3,510	2,080	59.3	411	11.7	2,491	71.0
Alaska	500	215	43.0	0	0.0	215	43.0
Arizona	4,674	992	21.2	26	0.6	1,018	21.8
Arkansas	2,139	1,057	49.4	73	3.4	1,130	52.8
California	26,799	10,291	38.4	28	0.1	10,319	38.5
Colorado	3,647	1,353	37.1	8	0.2	1,361	37.3
Connecticut	2,666	1,612	60.5	0	0.0	1,612	60.5
Delaware	659	460	69.8	0	0.0	460	69.8
District of Columbia	472	1,052	222.7	0	0.0	1,052	222.7
Florida	14,196	4,460	31.4	31	0.2	4,491	31.6
Georgia	6,997	3,740	53.5	87	1.2	3,827	54.7
Hawaii	986	381	38.6	27	2.7	408	41.4
Idaho	1,090	585	53.7	0	0.0	585	53.7
Illinois	9,585	4,427	46.2	165	1.7	4,592	47.9
Indiana	4,754	2,645	55.6	0	0.0	2,645	55.6
Iowa	2,267	975	43.0	21	0.9	996	43.9
Kansas	2,076	1,157	55.7	125	6.0	1,282	61.8
Kentucky	3,245	1,725	53.2	19	0.6	1,744	53.7
Louisiana	3,273	2,022	61.8	82	2.5	2,104	64.3
Maine	1,037	511	49.3	16	1.5	527	50.8
Maryland	4,267	2,412	56.5	116	2.7	2,528	59.3
Massachusetts	5,051	3,042	60.2	732	14.5	3,774	74.7
Michigan	7,605	2,658	35.0	412	5.4	3,070	40.4
Minnesota	3,926	1,862	47.4	388	9.9	2,250	57.3
Mississippi	2,155	2,494	115.7	0	0.0	2,494	115.7
Missouri	4,475	3,099	69.3	106	2.4	3,205	71.6
Montana	737	306	41.5	0	0.0	306	41.5
Nebraska	1,323	975	73.7	0	0.0	975	73.7
Nevada	1,900	676	35.6	42	2.2	718	37.8
New Hampshire	1,018	490	48.1	0	0.0	490	48.1
New Jersey	6,566	5,769	87.9	0	0.0	5,769	87.9
New Mexico	1,464	679	46.4	30	2.0	709	48.4
New York	14,923	11,653	78.1	490	3.3	12,143	81.4
North Carolina	6,844	3,176	46.4	96	1.4	3,272	47.8
North Dakota	495	324	65.5	0	0.0	324	65.5
Ohio	8,755	3,320	37.9	370	4.2	3,690	42.1
Oklahoma	2,710	1,582	58.4	47	1.7	1,629	60.1
Oregon	2,867	1,119	39.0	0	0.0	1,119	39.0
Pennsylvania	9,705	5,970	61.5	175	1.8	6,145	63.3

(continued)

Table 115. Number of inpatient Federal and non-Federal psychiatric beds in U.S. hospitals, United States and by State, FY 2007 *(continued)*

State	FY 2007 adult population (1,000s)	Beds in all non-Federal hospitals[1]		Beds in Federal government hospitals		Beds in all (Federal and non-Federal) hospitals	
		Number	Number per 100,000 adults	Number	Number per 100,000 adults	Number	Number per 100,000 adults
Rhode Island	821	282	34.3	17	2.1	299	36.4
South Carolina	3,358	1,320	39.3	15	0.4	1,335	39.8
South Dakota	599	420	70.1	15	2.5	435	72.6
Tennessee	4,694	2,566	54.7	32	0.7	2,598	55.4
Texas	17,190	7,063	41.1	0	0.0	7,063	41.1
Utah	1,834	783	42.7	21	1.1	804	43.8
Vermont	489	191	39.0	10	2.0	201	41.1
Virginia	5,883	3,101	52.7	22	0.4	3,123	53.1
Washington	4,916	1,778	36.2	184	3.7	1,962	39.9
West Virginia	1,423	817	57.4	0	0.0	817	57.4
Wisconsin	4,277	2,038	47.6	18	0.4	2,056	48.1
Wyoming	397	283	71.3	203	51.1	486	122.4
United States	**227,240**	**113,988**	**50.2**	**4,660**	**2.1**	**118,648**	**52.2**

[1] "Beds in all non-Federal hospitals" is the sum of beds from Tables 113 and 114.

NOTES: The American Hospital Association Annual Survey is completed online by most U.S. hospitals and profiles more than 6,500 hospitals throughout the United States. The overall response rate for FY 2007 was 78 percent, but this rate varies among subgroups of hospitals depending on size, ownership, service, geographical location, and membership status. The survey covers hospital organization structure, service lines, staffing, expenses, physician organization structures, beds, and utilization.

The data exclude all children's hospitals. Data represent "staffed beds," beds regularly available (those set up and staffed for use) within the reporting period.

SOURCES: Aron, L., Honberg, R., Duckworth, K., Kimball, A., Edgar, E., Carolla, B., ... & Fitzpatrick, M. (2009). *Grading the States 2009: A report on America's health care system for adults with serious mental illness*. Arlington, VA: National Alliance on Mental Illness.

State Single Year of Age and Sex Resident Population Estimates: April 1, 2000 to July 1, 2009, U.S. Census Bureau.

Table 116. Number of mental health organizations, by organization type, United States and by State, 2008

[Data are based on a survey of mental health treatment facilities]

State	State and county psychiatric hospitals	Private psychiatric hospitals	General hospitals[1]	VA hospitals	RTCs for SEDs[2]	RTCs for adults	Outpatient clinics[3]	Multi-setting organizations
Alabama	5	3	22	2	7	2	6	25
Alaska	1	1	3	1	5	1	19	7
Arizona	1	8	12	3	7	1	18	10
Arkansas	1	6	25	3	4	—/0	11	7
California	11	24	75	8	47	8	172	46
Colorado	2	5	10	2	16	2	18	12
Connecticut	4	4	22	1	9	—/0	41	25
Delaware	1	3	2	1	3	—/0	3	3
District of Columbia	1	2	7	1	2	—/0	14	1
Florida	5	12	51	7	24	3	59	37
Georgia	8	7	19	3	9	—/0	13	28
Hawaii	1	1	6	1	1	—/0	8	2
Idaho	2	2	7	1	5	1	9	3
Illinois	10	7	64	6	23	2	67	55
Indiana	6	10	35	3	21	—/0	12	20
Iowa	5	—/0	27	3	10	—/0	23	10
Kansas	3	3	16	2	3	—/0	32	2
Kentucky	4	9	21	2	16	1	12	10
Louisiana	7	6	39	3	4	—/0	42	—/0
Maine	2	2	7	1	4	—/0	11	12
Maryland	7	3	29	2	7	3	28	18
Massachusetts	4	9	45	3	33	—/0	38	38
Michigan	6	7	48	5	13	2	80	27
Minnesota	12	—/0	28	2	11	5	45	13
Mississippi	4	5	28	2	4	1	6	12
Missouri	10	6	34	4	13	2	20	13
Montana	1	1	4	1	2	—/0	1	4
Nebraska	2	—/0	9	1	7	1	10	8
Nevada	2	3	2	2	1	—/0	4	1
New Hampshire	1	1	8	1	8	1	6	12
New Jersey	11	6	42	1	8	—/0	43	20
New Mexico	1	1	12	1	8	—/0	18	7
New York	26	8	103	9	33	1	113	35
North Carolina	5	6	37	4	12	1	35	12
North Dakota	1	2	7	—/0	4	—/0	2	6
Ohio	7	6	71	5	19	1	75	44
Oklahoma	4	8	25	1	3	—/0	36	9
Oregon	2	—/0	13	3	9	1	48	13
Pennsylvania	7	14	87	8	18	8	63	47
Rhode Island	—/0	2	6	1	2	—/0	4	9
South Carolina	4	5	14	2	9	—/0	14	6
South Dakota	1	—/0	4	3	3	—/0	7	7

(continued)

Table 116. Number of mental health organizations, by organization type, United States and by State, 2008 *(continued)*

State	State and county psychiatric hospitals	Private psychiatric hospitals	General hospitals[1]	VA hospitals	RTCs for SEDs[2]	RTCs for adults	Outpatient clinics[3]	Multi-setting organizations
Tennessee	6	10	31	4	10	—/0	20	5
Texas	11	22	52	8	22	—/0	41	10
Utah	1	2	8	1	18	2	7	6
Vermont	1	1	4	1	7	3	3	8
Virginia	10	4	33	3	15	1	29	21
Washington	5	2	19	3	10	—/0	44	14
West Virginia	2	4	9	3	2	—/0	4	11
Wisconsin	6	4	33	3	13	1	79	9
Wyoming	1	1	4	2	7	—/0	11	2
United States[4]	**241**	**258**	**1,319**	**143**	**551**	**55**	**1,524**	**762**

—/0 Data are not available, or the estimate is zero.

[1] Only includes general hospitals with separate psychiatric units.

[2] Residential treatment centers for children with severe emotional disturbance.

[3] Includes organizations formerly classified as partial care.

[4] U.S. territories are excluded.

NOTE: The 2008 National Survey of Mental Health Treatment Facilities includes approximately 15,000 point-of-contact facilities nationwide representing approximately 4,400 mental health organizations nationwide.

SOURCE: 2008 National Survey of Mental Health Treatment Facilities, Substance Abuse and Mental Health Services Administration.

Table 117. Number of mental health organizations providing 24-hour hospital or residential care, by organization type, United States and by State, 2008

[Data are based on a survey of mental health treatment facilities]

State	State and county psychiatric hospitals	Private psychiatric hospitals	General hospitals[1]	VA hospitals	RTCs for SEDs[2]	RTCs for adults	Outpatient clinics[3]	Multi-setting organizations
Alabama	5	3	22	1	7	2	—/0	21
Alaska	1	1	3	1	5	1	5	—/0
Arizona	1	8	12	3	7	1	3	7
Arkansas	1	6	24	3	4	—/0	—/0	3
California	11	24	73	7	46	8	8	33
Colorado	2	5	9	2	16	2	1	11
Connecticut	4	4	22	1	9	—/0	3	19
Delaware	1	3	2	1	3	—/0	—/0	3
District of Columbia	1	2	6	1	2	—/0	—/0	—/0
Florida	5	12	51	7	24	3	6	33
Georgia	8	7	18	3	9	—/0	—/0	24
Hawaii	1	1	6	1	—/0	—/0	—/0	2
Idaho	2	2	7	1	5	1	1	3
Illinois	10	7	61	6	22	2	5	40
Indiana	6	10	35	3	20	—/0	1	17
Iowa	5	—/0	26	3	10	—/0	—/0	7
Kansas	3	3	16	2	3	—/0	—/0	1
Kentucky	4	9	21	2	16	1	1	7
Louisiana	7	6	36	2	4	—/0	—/0	—/0
Maine	2	2	7	1	4	—/0	—/0	10
Maryland	7	3	29	2	7	3	3	8
Massachusetts	4	9	43	3	32	—/0	2	26
Michigan	6	7	48	3	13	2	2	17
Minnesota	12	—/0	28	2	10	5	—/0	12
Mississippi	4	5	28	2	4	1	—/0	7
Missouri	10	6	34	3	13	2	1	10
Montana	1	1	4	—/0	2	—/0	—/0	4
Nebraska	2	—/0	9	1	7	1	—/0	6
Nevada	2	2	2	1	1	—/0	—/0	1
New Hampshire	1	1	8	—/0	8	1	—/0	11
New Jersey	11	6	42	1	8	—/0	1	14
New Mexico	1	1	11	1	7	—/0	2	4
New York	26	8	100	8	33	1	4	22
North Carolina	5	6	37	4	12	1	3	8
North Dakota	1	2	7	—/0	4	—/0	—/0	5
Ohio	7	6	71	5	19	1	5	34
Oklahoma	4	8	25	1	3	—/0	2	4
Oregon	2	—/0	13	3	8	—/0	1	9
Pennsylvania	7	14	84	7	18	8	6	30
Rhode Island	—/0	2	6	1	2	—/0	—/0	6
South Carolina	4	5	14	2	9	—/0	—/0	2
South Dakota	1	—/0	4	3	3	—/0	—/0	4

(continued)

Table 117. Number of mental health organizations providing 24-hour hospital or residential care, by organization type, United States and by State, 2008 *(continued)*

State	State and county psychiatric hospitals	Private psychiatric hospitals	General hospitals[1]	VA hospitals	RTCs for SEDs[2]	RTCs for adults	Outpatient clinics[3]	Multi-setting organizations
Tennessee	6	10	31	3	10	—/0	3	3
Texas	11	21	52	7	20	—/0	2	6
Utah	1	2	8	1	18	2	—/0	5
Vermont	1	1	3	1	7	3	—/0	6
Virginia	10	4	31	3	15	1	2	10
Washington	5	2	18	3	8	—/0	3	11
West Virginia	2	4	9	3	2	—/0	—/0	9
Wisconsin	6	4	32	3	12	1	3	5
Wyoming	1	1	4	2	7	—/0	—/0	—/0
United States[4]	**241**	**256**	**1,292**	**130**	**538**	**54**	**79**	**540**

—/0 Data are not available, or the estimate is zero.

[1] Only includes general hospitals with separate psychiatric units.

[2] Residential treatment centers for children with severe emotional disturbance.

[3] Includes organizations formerly classified as partial care.

[4] U.S. territories are excluded.

NOTE: The 2008 National Survey of Mental Health Treatment Facilities includes approximately 15,000 point-of-contact facilities nationwide representing approximately 4,400 mental health organizations nationwide.

SOURCE: 2008 National Survey of Mental Health Treatment Facilities, Substance Abuse and Mental Health Services Administration.

Table 118. Number of mental health organizations providing less than 24-hour care, by organization type, United States and by State, 2008

[Data are based on a survey of mental health treatment facilities]

State	State and county psychiatric hospitals	Private psychiatric hospitals	General hospitals[1]	VA hospitals	RTCs for SEDs[2]	RTCs for adults	Outpatient clinics[3]	Multi-setting organiza-tions
Alabama	—/0	2	4	2	1	—/0	6	24
Alaska	—/0	1	2	1	4	—/0	19	7
Arizona	—/0	4	6	3	3	—/0	18	9
Arkansas	—/0	5	9	2	3	—/0	11	6
California	7	15	42	7	26	—/0	172	42
Colorado	2	5	8	2	8	1	18	12
Connecticut	2	4	18	1	4	—/0	41	24
Delaware	—/0	3	2	1	1	—/0	3	2
District of Columbia	1	2	5	1	—/0	—/0	14	1
Florida	2	8	17	7	12	—/0	57	36
Georgia	4	6	10	3	3	—/0	13	26
Hawaii	—/0	1	1	1	1	—/0	8	2
Idaho	—/0	1	6	1	—/0	—/0	9	—/0
Illinois	1	6	42	5	12	1	67	54
Indiana	—/0	10	22	2	6	—/0	11	20
Iowa	—/0	—/0	14	3	4	—/0	23	10
Kansas	—/0	3	3	2	1	—/0	32	2
Kentucky	—/0	6	7	2	—/0	1	12	10
Louisiana	3	3	11	3	—/0	—/0	42	—/0
Maine	1	1	3	1	3	—/0	11	11
Maryland	—/0	3	24	1	4	—/0	28	17
Massachusetts	—/0	8	29	3	12	—/0	38	34
Michigan	—/0	5	21	5	2	1	80	27
Minnesota	1	—/0	17	2	5	1	45	13
Mississippi	1	1	12	2	4	1	6	12
Missouri	—/0	3	11	4	4	—/0	20	12
Montana	—/0	1	3	1	1	—/0	1	4
Nebraska	1	—/0	6	1	4	1	10	8
Nevada	1	2	2	2	1	—/0	4	1
New Hampshire	—/0	—/0	4	1	1	—/0	6	12
New Jersey	1	6	27	1	2	—/0	43	19
New Mexico	1	—/0	5	1	4	—/0	18	7
New York	22	4	57	8	15	—/0	113	35
North Carolina	2	3	10	3	3	—/0	35	9
North Dakota	1	1	7	—/0	—/0	—/0	2	6
Ohio	2	4	33	5	15	—/0	75	43
Oklahoma	2	3	10	1	—/0	—/0	35	8
Oregon	—/0	—/0	5	3	7	1	47	12
Pennsylvania	—/0	8	44	8	8	—/0	62	46
Rhode Island	—/0	2	2	1	1	—/0	4	9
South Carolina	1	3	6	2	2	—/0	14	6
South Dakota	—/0	—/0	3	3	2	—/0	7	7

(continued)

Table 118. Number of mental health organizations providing less than 24-hour care, by organization type, United States and by State, 2008 *(continued)*

State	State and county psychiatric hospitals	Private psychiatric hospitals	General hospitals[1]	VA hospitals	RTCs for SEDs[2]	RTCs for adults	Outpatient clinics[3]	Multi-setting organiza-tions
Tennessee	2	8	11	4	2	—/0	20	5
Texas	1	19	26	7	4	—/0	41	10
Utah	—/0	—/0	4	1	4	1	7	6
Vermont	—/0	1	3	1	2	—/0	3	8
Virginia	1	4	19	2	1	—/0	29	20
Washington	2	1	8	3	5	—/0	44	14
West Virginia	—/0	2	5	3	1	—/0	4	11
Wisconsin	3	4	18	3	8	—/0	79	9
Wyoming	1	1	3	2	3	—/0	11	2
United States[4]	**69**	**183**	**667**	**134**	**219**	**9**	**1,518**	**730**

—/0 Data are not available, or the estimate is zero.

[1] Only includes general hospitals with separate psychiatric units.

[2] Residential treatment centers for children with severe emotional disturbance.

[3] Includes organizations formerly classified as partial care.

[4] U.S. territories are excluded.

NOTE: The 2008 National Survey of Mental Health Treatment Facilities includes approximately 15,000 point-of-contact facilities nationwide representing approximately 4,400 mental health organizations nationwide.

SOURCE: 2008 National Survey of Mental Health Treatment Facilities, Substance Abuse and Mental Health Services Administration.

7. TABLES

7.4 State-Level Estimates

7.4.1 Populations by State: People's Mental Health

Mental Health of Adults

Mental Health of Children

Suicide

Special Populations

7.4.2 Populations by State: Providers and Settings for Mental Health Services

Mental Health of Adults

Mental Health of Children

Mental Health Service Capacity

7.4.3 Populations by State: Payers and Payment Mechanisms

Revenues and Expenditures by Public Funding Source
Tables 119–132

Table 119. Source of revenue for State mental health agencies, by State, FY 2001, FY 2005, and FY 2008

[Data are based on reports from State mental health agencies]

State	Total (millions of dollars)			State general funds (percent of total)			Medicaid (percent of total)			Medicare/block grant (percent of total)		
	FY 2001	FY 2005	FY 2008	FY 2001	FY 2005	FY 2008	FY 2001	FY 2005	FY 2008	FY 2001	FY 2005	FY 2008
Alabama	$253	$274	$369	52.4	57.7	52.8	37.8	33.6	34.7	9.8	8.7	12.5
Alaska[1]	51	174	184	63.7	18.1	21.2	18.6	77.6	75.6	17.7	4.3	3.1
Arizona	472	867	1,127	49.3	15.7	16.7	37.0	77.6	78.1	13.7	6.7	5.2
Arkansas	76	99	115	69.5	61.3	60.1	20.4	26.1	26.9	10.1	12.6	13.0
California	3,148	4,270	5,504	37.7	38.2	43.4	44.1	42.4	38.4	18.2	19.4	18.2
Colorado	283	344	401	35.8	42.6	33.3	57.8	51.3	61.3	6.5	6.1	5.4
Connecticut	440	549	659	92.4	91.1	93.0	3.0	4.0	2.1	4.5	4.9	4.8
Delaware	74	75	97	76.3	79.5	78.3	15.3	19.1	16.3	8.4	1.4	5.4
District of Columbia	227	234	225	75.9	82.6	88.8	11.7	14.0	8.3	12.4	3.4	2.8
Florida	578	647	769	69.2	71.8	77.3	16.0	18.5	16.7	14.8	9.7	6.0
Georgia	381	444	472	91.2	80.5	83.6	0.7	12.5	—	8.0	7.1	16.4
Hawaii	214	193	260	95.6	95.2	88.9	1.7	2.0	8.3	2.7	2.8	2.8
Idaho	61	54	73	46.9	64.2	74.2	16.9	16.1	10.9	36.2	19.7	14.9
Illinois	790	1,022	1,110	75.1	57.9	56.8	22.6	39.3	40.0	2.3	2.8	3.3
Indiana	412	519	569	40.5	20.3	32.4	34.4	75.9	63.9	25.1	3.9	3.8
Iowa	152	236	374	—	32.6	15.3	—	41.2	54.4	—	26.2	30.3
Kansas	162	254	322	36.4	36.3	36.5	54.8	61.4	62.6	8.9	2.3	0.9
Kentucky	197	208	230	56.0	61.1	59.1	34.8	28.8	30.0	9.2	10.1	11.0
Louisiana	201	259	325	36.4	42.8	46.5	44.1	40.9	31.0	19.5	16.3	22.5
Maine[1]	138	180	448	39.7	27.3	11.5	57.7	68.7	87.8	2.6	4.0	0.7
Maryland	678	777	899	73.8	75.1	68.3	24.3	23.3	29.7	1.9	1.6	2.1
Massachusetts	682	686	792	83.5	81.7	81.6	14.3	15.7	15.3	2.3	2.6	3.1
Michigan	844	974	1,358	51.8	34.2	28.0	43.6	61.7	64.2	4.6	4.0	7.9
Minnesota	518	669	833	50.7	41.3	45.1	34.7	45.4	44.5	14.7	13.3	10.4
Mississippi	247	306	320	49.9	42.4	47.2	43.6	51.3	43.1	6.6	6.4	9.7
Missouri	336	414	482	68.4	48.4	52.1	26.2	45.7	41.9	5.4	5.9	6.0
Montana	112	125	147	30.7	30.9	34.4	66.4	68.1	63.3	2.9	1.1	2.3
Nebraska	87	106	119	68.2	86.0	71.7	15.3	8.4	14.3	16.5	5.7	14.0
Nevada	120	151	211	30.2	69.7	73.0	62.8	15.1	13.9	7.0	15.2	13.1

(continued)

Table 119. Source of revenue for State mental health agencies, by State, FY 2001, FY 2005, and FY 2008 *(continued)*

State	Total (millions of dollars)			State general funds (percent of total)			Medicaid (percent of total)			Medicare/block grant (percent of total)		
	FY 2001	FY 2005	FY 2008	FY 2001	FY 2005	FY 2008	FY 2001	FY 2005	FY 2008	FY 2001	FY 2005	FY 2008
New Hampshire	$140	$155	$178	31.2	28.9	7.6	58.6	58.8	79.3	10.2	12.3	13.2
New Jersey	763	1,216	1,707	78.7	64.5	60.5	13.3	18.9	26.7	8.0	16.6	12.8
New Mexico[1]	59	46	190	71.9	82.8	35.6	21.4	9.6	62.2	6.7	7.5	2.2
New York	3,332	3,978	4,493	21.3	28.2	27.8	60.0	55.6	54.3	18.7	16.2	17.9
North Carolina	440	1,028	1,808	74.0	30.8	20.3	12.1	60.0	73.0	13.8	9.2	6.6
North Dakota	50	47	48	54.7	47.4	45.8	24.3	21.9	20.2	21.1	30.7	33.9
Ohio	692	758	856	60.3	53.9	37.4	32.9	40.9	27.1	6.8	5.2	35.5
Oklahoma	136	157	199	84.7	76.8	77.9	3.9	12.4	13.0	11.3	10.7	9.1
Oregon[1]	202	435	473	36.8	28.2	34.7	47.1	68.9	62.7	16.1	2.9	2.7
Pennsylvania	1,860	2,541	3,396	65.3	63.5	28.2	25.2	27.9	67.4	9.6	8.5	4.4
Rhode Island	92	102	117	13.4	13.3	12.4	70.8	84.3	86.0	15.8	2.4	1.6
South Carolina	299	285	288	40.6	37.5	51.8	48.8	54.5	37.3	10.6	7.9	10.9
South Dakota	46	55	68	16.3	57.8	56.3	61.9	34.9	34.5	21.8	7.3	9.3
Tennessee	395	522	609	21.5	27.6	27.2	73.6	68.1	69.1	5.0	4.3	3.7
Texas	797	832	874	61.6	63.0	69.1	27.2	22.4	17.3	11.2	14.7	13.6
Utah	159	160	178	36.3	23.1	22.8	43.1	66.8	72.5	20.6	10.1	4.7
Vermont	80	109	139	7.8	18.0	16.1	87.5	78.6	81.5	4.7	3.4	2.4
Virginia	467	532	710	67.1	64.1	60.8	25.7	28.3	33.0	7.2	7.6	6.2
Washington	526	585	755	10.0	9.2	31.7	85.2	86.3	61.8	4.7	4.4	6.5
West Virginia	87	119	144	43.3	42.1	46.4	48.9	37.1	47.9	7.7	20.8	5.7
Wisconsin	405	580	589	60.4	52.0	46.8	31.3	23.4	27.0	8.3	24.6	26.3
Wyoming	30	50	75	79.7	83.4	83.4	15.8	14.9	12.7	4.5	1.7	4.0

—Data not available.

[1] Series may contain substantial changes due to the consolidation and/or restructuring of State agencies and funding streams. See NRI Inc. Revenues and Expenditures Study at http://www.nri-inc.org/projects/Profiles/RevenuesExpenditures.cfm for more details.

NOTES: NRI's Revenues and Expenditures Study describes the major expenditures and funding sources of the State mental health agencies. NRI has conducted this survey every year since 1981.

The estimates in Tables 119 and 120 correspond to the totals in Table 86.

SOURCE: Revenues and Expenditures Study, 2011, NRI Inc.

Table 120. Expenditures and categories of expenditures controlled by State mental health agencies, by State, FY 2001, FY 2005, and FY 2008

[Data are based on reports from State mental health agencies]

State	Total (millions of dollars)			State psychiatric hospital—inpatient (percent of total)			Community mental health (percent of total)			State mental health agency central office[1] (percent of total)		
	FY 2001	FY 2005	FY 2008	FY 2001	FY 2005	FY 2008	FY 2001	FY 2005	FY 2008	FY 2001	FY 2005	FY 2008
Alabama	$253	$274	$369	40.9	45.8	45.2	56.3	51.4	51.8	2.8	2.8	3.0
Alaska[2]	51	174	184	33.3	11.1	14.7	60.6	86.1	83.4	6.1	2.8	1.9
Arizona	472	867	1,127	9.8	7.2	6.9	87.9	91.2	90.9	2.2	1.5	2.2
Arkansas	76	99	115	30.7	28.6	34.4	65.0	64.4	62.0	4.3	7.0	3.5
California	3,148	4,270	5,504	18.1	17.9	21.3	80.9	81.4	77.5	1.0	0.7	1.2
Colorado	283	344	401	29.6	26.2	26.7	69.9	73.4	72.7	0.5	0.4	0.6
Connecticut	440	549	659	30.4	30.5	32.1	60.8	59.7	60.0	8.8	9.8	7.9
Delaware	74	75	97	64.5	52.2	47.6	33.5	45.7	49.9	2.0	2.2	2.4
District of Columbia	227	234	225	45.6	34.3	44.3	54.4	56.6	46.8	—	9.1	8.9
Florida	578	647	769	43.6	44.4	47.7	54.7	53.8	50.5	1.8	1.9	1.8
Georgia	381	444	472	45.6	45.5	43.5	48.6	54.5	54.6	5.8	0.0	2.0
Hawaii	214	193	260	15.8	27.4	22.4	71.4	68.1	72.4	12.8	4.5	5.1
Idaho	61	54	73	36.4	42.6	41.0	61.8	57.4	48.6	1.8	0.0	10.5
Illinois	790	1,022	1,110	38.8	28.6	29.3	59.0	69.6	68.9	2.2	1.8	1.8
Indiana	412	519	569	35.7	32.9	33.1	63.4	66.5	65.3	0.9	0.6	1.5
Iowa	152	236	374	23.7	11.6	9.5	75.9	86.7	89.3	0.4	1.7	1.1
Kansas	162	254	322	35.5	27.1	27.5	63.0	72.9	68.3	1.5	0.0	4.1
Kentucky	197	208	230	51.2	49.9	50.6	47.0	45.7	43.7	1.9	4.4	5.7
Louisiana	201	259	325	57.9	52.2	56.1	40.2	41.1	39.8	2.0	6.7	4.2
Maine[2]	138	180	448	30.1	28.8	12.5	65.1	—	84.6	4.8	2.3	3.0
Maryland	678	777	899	30.0	27.8	27.2	65.6	67.8	69.2	4.4	4.4	3.6
Massachusetts	682	686	792	18.0	16.4	16.8	78.9	80.6	80.3	3.1	3.0	2.9
Michigan	844	974	1,358	35.0	22.3	16.7	64.0	76.9	82.8	1.1	0.7	0.5
Minnesota	518	669	833	29.9	26.1	24.3	69.5	73.3	75.1	0.6	0.5	0.7
Mississippi	247	306	320	59.6	54.7	47.4	39.2	44.3	51.6	1.2	1.0	1.0
Missouri	336	414	482	50.4	46.8	49.1	45.0	50.6	48.3	4.6	2.6	2.6
Montana	112	125	147	17.4	17.2	18.4	79.2	79.7	79.1	3.5	3.1	2.5
Nebraska	87	106	119	63.4	59.3	39.2	34.7	37.7	59.8	1.9	3.0	1.0
Nevada	120	151	211	36.2	23.9	32.6	62.9	74.0	65.2	0.9	2.2	2.3

(continued)

Table 120. Expenditures and categories of expenditures controlled by State mental health agencies, by State, FY 2001, FY 2005, and FY 2008 *(continued)*

State	Total (millions of dollars)			State psychiatric hospital—inpatient (percent of total)			Community mental health (percent of total)			State mental health agency central office[1] (percent of total)		
	FY 2001	FY 2005	FY 2008	FY 2001	FY 2005	FY 2008	FY 2001	FY 2005	FY 2008	FY 2001	FY 2005	FY 2008
New Hampshire	$140	$155	$178	29.6	30.8	30.0	68.6	66.7	67.8	1.8	2.5	2.2
New Jersey	763	1,216	1,707	38.9	35.5	29.4	59.3	63.3	69.3	1.7	1.2	1.3
New Mexico[2]	59	46	190	37.1	46.8	11.5	62.3	53.2	88.3	0.6	0.0	0.2
New York	3,332	3,978	4,493	29.8	27.0	26.9	66.3	68.7	68.5	3.9	4.3	4.6
North Carolina	440	1,028	1,808	68.3	25.4	17.9	31.7	73.0	81.5	—	1.6	0.6
North Dakota	50	47	48	44.9	40.1	22.7	53.7	59.9	77.2	1.4	0.1	0.1
Ohio	692	758	856	28.0	26.0	26.7	67.8	70.1	69.6	4.2	3.9	3.7
Oklahoma	136	157	199	29.9	28.8	28.0	64.3	64.8	65.8	5.8	6.4	6.2
Oregon[2]	202	435	473	40.1	23.9	27.0	57.4	73.3	70.9	2.5	2.9	2.1
Pennsylvania	1,860	2,541	3,396	21.5	19.4	15.1	77.8	80.0	84.6	0.7	0.7	0.3
Rhode Island	92	102	117	25.6	25.6	28.1	72.1	72.7	70.2	2.3	1.7	1.6
South Carolina	299	285	288	36.3	28.9	30.8	58.2	65.8	62.8	5.5	5.3	6.3
South Dakota	46	55	68	67.0	63.3	63.1	31.3	36.7	34.6	1.7	0.0	2.3
Tennessee	395	522	609	32.1	31.4	29.0	65.2	66.1	68.0	2.7	2.5	3.0
Texas	797	832	874	38.4	37.9	40.0	58.0	60.5	58.3	3.6	1.6	1.7
Utah	159	160	178	25.9	28.6	30.4	73.4	70.7	68.7	0.7	0.7	0.8
Vermont	80	109	139	12.0	14.0	15.5	85.2	83.1	81.0	2.8	2.8	3.5
Virginia	467	532	710	59.5	57.9	46.8	34.9	42.1	50.3	5.6	0.0	2.9
Washington	526	585	755	31.9	30.3	32.0	65.8	67.5	66.1	2.3	2.2	1.9
West Virginia	87	119	144	42.4	40.4	32.8	55.7	59.2	67.1	2.0	0.4	0.1
Wisconsin	405	580	589	27.1	27.8	33.3	72.4	72.0	66.5	0.5	0.2	0.2
Wyoming	30	50	75	43.4	29.9	29.4	53.8	68.5	69.0	2.8	1.6	1.7

—Data not available.

[1] Central office includes administration, research, training, prevention, and other central and regional office expenditures.

[2] Series may contain substantial changes due to the consolidation and/or restructuring of State agencies and funding streams. See NRI Inc. Revenues and Expenditures Study at http://www.nri-inc.org/projects/Profiles/RevenuesExpenditures.cfm for more details.

NOTES: NRI's Revenues and Expenditures Study describes the major expenditures and funding sources of the State mental health agencies. NRI has conducted this survey every year since 1981.

The estimates in Table 119 and 120 correspond to the totals in Table 87.

SOURCE: Revenues and Expenditures Study, 2011, NRI Inc.

Table 121. State mental health agencies experiencing budget cuts, by region, FY 2009, FY 2010, and FY 2011

[Data are based on reports from State mental health agencies]

Region	Total percentage cut[1]			Total dollars cut[2] (millions of dollars)		
	FY 2009	FY 2010	FY 2011	FY 2009	FY 2010	FY 2011
New England[3]	2.9	1.1	2.0	$56.6	$20.3	$33.8
Middle Atlantic[4]	2.4	2.8	2.6	149.4	238.0	181.8
East North Central[5]	4.1	6.1	4.1	109.5	109.6	93.4
West North Central[6]	2.4	4.7	2.4	66.8	33.8	13.6
South Atlantic[7]	5.9	7.4	7.0	169.6	240.3	215.3
East South Central[8]	3.1	2.1	1.9	35.4	4.8	8.5
West South Central[9]	2.9	5.7	1.8	10.0	40.8	17.0
Mountain[10]	2.8	7.1	6.9	58.5	72.1	37.5
Pacific[11]	2.0	4.5	6.3	8.5	34.0	44.2
United States	**4.0**	**5.3**	**4.9**	**$664.3**	**$793.9**	**$645.2**

[1] Total percentage cut in State budget expressed at the regional level.

[2] Total dollars cut expressed at the regional level.

[3] Of the six States from the New England region, five responded to surveys in 2009, 2010, and 2011.

[4] Of the three States from the Middle Atlantic region, three responded to surveys in 2009, 2010, and 2011.

[5] Of the five States from the East North Central region, five responded to surveys in 2009, 2010, and 2011.

[6] Of the seven States from the West North Central region, six responded to surveys in 2009 and five responded to surveys in 2010 and 2011.

[7] Of the nine States from the South Atlantic region, eight responded to surveys in 2009 and seven responded to surveys in 2010 and 2011.

[8] Of the four States from the East South Central region, four responded to surveys in 2009 and three responded to surveys in 2010 and 2011.

[9] Of the four States from the West South Central region, four responded to surveys in 2009, 2010, and 2011.

[10] Of the eight States from the Mountain region, eight responded to surveys in 2009, 2010, and 2011.

[11] Of the five States from the Pacific region, two responded to surveys in 2009, 2010, and 2011.

NOTES: The State Mental Health Agency (SMHA) Budget Reductions Survey is conducted by the National Association of State Mental Health Program Directors (NASMHPD) and NRI Inc. The survey is a semiannual series on the impact of State budget shortages on SMHA systems. The above estimates are from the summer 2010 survey.

Regions are based on the U.S. Census Bureau's regional designations: New England (Connecticut, Maine, Massachusetts, New Hampshire, Rhode Island, Vermont), Middle Atlantic (New Jersey, New York, Pennsylvania), East North Central (Illinois, Indiana, Michigan, Ohio, Wisconsin), West North Central (Iowa, Kansas, Minnesota, Missouri, Nebraska, North Dakota, South Dakota), South Atlantic (Delaware, District of Columbia, Florida, Georgia, Maryland, North Carolina, South Carolina, Virginia, West Virginia), East South Central (Alabama, Kentucky, Mississippi, Tennessee), West South Central (Arkansas, Louisiana, Oklahoma, Texas), Mountain (Arizona, Colorado, Idaho, Montana, Nevada, New Mexico, Utah, Wyoming), and Pacific (Alaska, California, Hawaii, Oregon, Washington).

SOURCE: State Mental Health Agency Budget Reductions Survey, 2011, NRI Inc.

Table 122. Number of State psychiatric hospital residents, hospitals, and hospital beds closed or to be closed, by State, 2009 and 2010

[Data are based on reports from State mental health agencies]

State	State psychiatric hospital residents, 2010	State psychiatric hospitals, 2010[1,2]	State psychiatric hospital beds closed, 2009–2010	Plan to close or consider closing State psychiatric hospital beds in the future, 2010
Alabama	1,130	6	0	Y
Alaska	72	1	0	N
Arizona	252	1	16	N
Arkansas	203	1	0	N
California	5,153	5	0	N
Colorado	1,314	2	59	N
Connecticut	711	3	40	N
Delaware	273	1	0	N
District of Columbia	407	1	100	Y
Florida	3,242	7	27	N
Georgia	1,133	7	191	Y
Hawaii	179	1	0	N
Idaho	161	2	0	N
Illinois	1,444	4	0	Y
Indiana	962	6	0	Y
Iowa	163	4	20	N
Kansas	711	3	0	N
Kentucky	440	3	0	N
Louisiana	952	4	42	Y
Maine	146	2	0	N
Maryland	1,146	7	201	N
Massachusetts	698	4	152	N
Michigan	545	5	0	N
Minnesota	327	10	0	N
Mississippi	1,137	5	0	N
Missouri	1,340	9	250	Y
Montana	189	1	0	N
Nebraska	304	2	11	N
Nevada	310	3	28	Y
New Hampshire	187	1	8	N
New Jersey	2,060	5	87	Y
New Mexico	159	1	0	N
New York	5,236	25	450	Y
North Carolina	690	4	80	N
North Dakota	179	1	0	N
Ohio	1,048	6	0	N
Oklahoma	334	3	28	N
Oregon	732	2	0	Y
Pennsylvania	1,959	7	60	Y
Rhode Island[3]	132	03	0	N
South Carolina	485	4	0	N

(continued)

Table 122. Number of State psychiatric hospital residents, hospitals, and hospital beds closed or to be closed, by State, 2009 and 2010 *(continued)*

State	State psychiatric hospital residents, 2010	State psychiatric hospitals, 2010[1,2]	State psychiatric hospital beds closed, 2009–2010	Plan to close or consider closing State psychiatric hospital beds in the future, 2010
South Dakota	234	1	0	N
Tennessee	813	5	247	N
Texas	2,154	9	0	Y
Utah	320	1	0	N
Vermont	50	1	0	Y
Virginia	1,476	10	16	Y
Washington	1,408	3	30	Y
West Virginia	289	2	0	N
Wisconsin	470	2	55	Y
Wyoming	118	1	0	N
United States	**45,577**	**204**	**2,198**	**17**

[1] Four States (Connecticut, Florida, Massachusetts, and Missouri) reported closing one State psychiatric hospital in the past year, whereas one State (Maryland) reported closing two State psychiatric hospitals in the past year.

[2] Five States (Georgia, Illinois, Indiana, New Jersey, and Pennsylvania) reported that plans are in place, or are under consideration, for closing State psychiatric hospitals at some point in the future.

[3] Rhode Island has State-operated psychiatric inpatient beds that are part of a general hospital.

NOTE: The State Mental Health Agency (SMHA) Budget Reductions Survey is conducted by the National Association of State Mental Health Program Directors (NASMHPD) and NRI Inc. The survey is a semiannual series on the impact of State budget shortages on SMHA systems. The above estimates are from the summer 2010 survey.

SOURCES: State Mental Health Agency Budget Reductions Survey, 2011, NRI Inc.

Uniform Reporting System, 2009, Substance Abuse and Mental Health Services Administration.

Table 123. Medicaid fee-for-service (FFS) mental health (MH) beneficiaries and expenditures, by State for 13 States, 2003

[Data are based on Medicaid claims]

State	FFS MH beneficiaries[1] (number)	FFS expenditures[2] for MH beneficiaries (dollars)	FFS expenditures per FFS MH beneficiary (dollars)
Arkansas	76,974	$744,792,675	$9,676
Georgia	145,204	1,196,211,970	8,238
Idaho	28,639	331,251,194	11,566
Illinois	212,004	2,644,269,525	12,473
Indiana	120,057	1,324,755,530	11,034
Kansas	47,274	528,719,744	11,184
Maine	62,726	1,051,008,650	16,756
Montana	20,244	199,810,477	9,870
North Carolina	182,439	1,984,070,793	10,875
South Carolina	95,755	775,816,882	8,102
Texas	265,419	2,618,025,520	9,864
Vermont	26,452	220,779,874	8,346
Wyoming	9,667	100,916,045	10,439

[1] Fee-for-service (FFS) beneficiaries include beneficiaries enrolled in Medicaid, but not in comprehensive managed care or a behavioral health managed care plan, for at least 1 month during the year. FFS mental health (MH) beneficiaries include FFS beneficiaries who, during the year, (1) had at least one claim on which an MH disorder was the primary diagnosis or (2) received a clearly identifiable MH service.

[2] Expenditures are claims-based Medicaid payments, including both Federal and State shares.

NOTES: This study identified Medicaid beneficiaries using MH or substance abuse services in FFS plans in 13 States in 2003 (n = 1,380,190) and examined their use of medical services.

Estimates are limited to MH care. Table 78 aggregates the above States and shows more detail on beneficiaries and expenditures. For more information on State-level Medicaid estimates, see the source below. The study analyzed Medicaid Analytic eXtract (MAX) files of all 50 States and the District of Columbia for the year 2003. These tables display data for 13 States that were selected after examining the completeness and quality of their MAX data. "Data completeness" refers to the extent to which FFS data were available (States with a greater proportion of beneficiaries in FFS are considered to have more complete data than States with a greater proportion of beneficiaries in managed care). "Data quality" refers to technical problems, such as missing diagnosis codes, missing eligibility data, duplicate records, and missing claims. Each State's data were assigned a score from 1 to 4; scores were developed specifically for purposes of the analysis presented in *Mental Health and Substance Abuse Services in Medicaid, 2003: Charts and State Tables*, strictly to assist readers in understanding how to interpret the data presented, and were not intended to reflect the quality of the States' overall MAX data. If beneficiaries had multiple diagnoses on different claims during the year, they are included in the category that represents the most frequent diagnosis.

SOURCE: Substance Abuse and Mental Health Services Administration (SAMHSA). (2010). *Mental health and substance abuse services in Medicaid, 2003: Charts and state tables* (DHHS Publication No. SMA 10-4608). Rockville, MD: Center for Mental Health Services, SAMHSA.

Table 124. Number and percentage of Medicaid fee-for-service (FFS) mental health (MH) beneficiaries, by diagnostic categories, by State for 13 States, 2003

[Data are based on Medicaid claims]

State	FFS MH beneficiaries[1] (number)	Total MH conditions		Schizophrenia[2]		Major depression and affective psychoses[2]		Neurotic and other depressive disorders[2]		Stress and adjustment reactions[2]		Attention deficit hyperactivity disorder[2]		All other diagnoses[3]	
		Number	Percent	Number	Percent	Number	Percent	Number	Percent	Number	Percent	Number	Percent	Number	Percent
Arkansas	76,974	76,974	100.0	5,805	7.5	11,708	15.2	15,691	20.4	8,619	11.2	18,349	23.8	16,802	21.8
Georgia	145,204	145,204	100.0	12,362	8.5	22,947	15.8	28,200	19.4	16,351	11.3	38,017	26.2	27,327	18.8
Idaho	28,639	28,639	100.0	1,935	6.8	6,676	23.3	5,821	20.3	5,092	17.8	4,087	14.3	5,028	17.6
Illinois	212,004	212,004	100.0	29,469	13.9	48,484	22.9	52,734	24.9	13,302	6.3	28,997	13.7	39,017	18.4
Indiana	120,057	120,057	100.0	11,039	9.2	26,825	22.3	26,439	22.0	16,084	13.4	18,350	15.3	21,320	17.8
Kansas	47,274	47,274	100.0	4,853	10.3	10,245	21.7	8,358	17.7	6,124	13.0	6,728	14.2	10,966	23.2
Maine	62,726	62,726	100.0	2,996	4.8	12,996	20.7	19,284	30.7	11,425	18.2	6,366	10.1	9,659	15.4
Montana	20,244	20,244	100.0	1,355	6.7	5,537	27.4	4,544	22.4	2,549	12.6	2,020	10.0	4,239	20.9
North Carolina	182,439	182,439	100.0	14,795	8.1	31,777	17.4	38,807	21.3	20,735	11.4	33,188	18.2	43,137	23.6
South Carolina	95,755	95,755	100.0	8,430	8.8	12,016	12.5	20,299	21.2	11,008	11.5	24,590	25.7	19,412	20.3
Texas	265,419	265,419	100.0	22,128	8.3	60,741	22.9	51,287	19.3	36,114	13.6	49,089	18.5	46,060	17.4
Vermont	26,452	26,452	100.0	502	1.9	2,921	11.0	6,978	26.4	9,534	36.0	2,749	10.4	3,768	14.2
Wyoming	9,667	9,667	100.0	447	4.6	1,796	18.6	2,239	23.2	1,680	17.4	1,563	16.2	1,942	20.1

[1] Fee-for-service (FFS) beneficiaries include beneficiaries enrolled in Medicaid, but not in comprehensive managed care or a behavioral health managed care plan, for at least 1 month during the year. FFS mental health (MH) beneficiaries include FFS beneficiaries who, during the year, had at least one claim on which one of the MH disorders shown in this table was the primary diagnosis or who received a clearly identifiable MH service during the year.

[2] Schizophrenia (ICD-9-CM diagnosis codes beginning with 295) includes both chronic and acute schizophrenic disorders. Major depression and affective psychoses (ICD-9-CM diagnosis codes beginning with 296) includes manic, depressive, and bipolar disorders. Neurotic and other depressive disorders (ICD-9-CM diagnosis codes beginning with 300 or 311) includes anxiety states; phobic, obsessive compulsive, and other neurotic disorders; and unspecified depressive disorders. Stress and adjustment reactions (ICD-9-CM diagnosis codes beginning with 308 or 309) includes acute reaction to stress, depressive reaction, separation disorders, and conduct disturbance. Attention deficit hyperactivity disorder (ICD-9-CM diagnosis codes beginning with 314) includes attention deficit with and without hyperactivity and hyperkinesis with or without developmental delay.

[3] All other diagnoses include other psychoses, childhood psychoses, personality disorders, other mental disorders, special symptoms or syndromes, conduct disorders, emotional disturbances, mental disorders associated with childbirth, and individuals with no diagnosis. Across the 13 States, 218 people have no diagnosis.

Table 124 notes *(continued)*

NOTES: This study identified Medicaid beneficiaries using MH or substance abuse services in FFS plans in 13 States in 2003 (n = 1,380,190) and examined their use of medical services.

Table 79 aggregates the above States and shows more detail on diagnostic categories. The five diagnostic categories included in the current table are those with the most beneficiaries in Table 79. These tables display data for 13 States that were selected after examining the completeness and quality of their Medicaid Analytic eXtract (MAX) data. "Data completeness" refers to the extent to which FFS data were available (States with a greater proportion of beneficiaries in FFS are considered to have more complete data than States with a greater proportion of beneficiaries in managed care). "Data quality" refers to technical problems, such as missing diagnosis codes, missing eligibility data, duplicate records, and missing claims. Each State's data were assigned a score from 1 to 4; scores were developed specifically for purposes of the analysis presented in *Mental Health and Substance Abuse Services in Medicaid, 2003: Charts and State Tables*, strictly to assist readers in understanding how to interpret the data presented, and were not intended to reflect the quality of the States' overall MAX data. If beneficiaries had multiple diagnoses on different claims during the year, they are included in the category that represents the most frequent diagnosis.

SOURCE: Substance Abuse and Mental Health Services Administration (SAMHSA). (2010). *Mental health and substance abuse services in Medicaid, 2003: Charts and state tables* (DHHS Publication No. SMA 10-4608). Rockville, MD: Center for Mental Health Services, SAMHSA.

Table 125. Number and percentage of Medicaid fee-for-service (FFS) mental health (MH) and substance abuse (SA) beneficiaries using prescription psychotropic medications, by State for 13 States, 2003

[Data are based on Medicaid claims]

State	Total FFS beneficiaries[1] with any psychotropic[2] medication use		FFS MH beneficiaries with any psychotropic medication use		FFS SA beneficiaries with any psychotropic medication use		All other FFS beneficiaries with any psychotropic medication use	
	Number	Percent	Number	Percent	Number	Percent	Number	Percent
Arkansas	112,624	16.4	53,320	69.3	676	46.7	58,628	9.7
Georgia	268,630	16.2	105,078	72.4	4,197	48.3	159,355	10.6
Idaho	37,557	17.8	19,748	69.0	344	48.5	17,465	9.6
Illinois	301,130	14.5	152,415	71.9	8,711	43.6	140,004	7.6
Indiana	174,604	23.0	88,499	73.7	4,033	54.7	82,072	13.0
Kansas	60,943	20.6	32,565	68.9	1,307	38.7	27,071	11.0
Maine	88,708	30.2	46,602	74.3	4,127	55.9	37,979	17.0
Montana	24,936	22.4	13,035	64.4	659	38.3	11,242	12.6
North Carolina	317,068	21.4	133,357	73.1	7,969	49.6	175,742	13.7
South Carolina	163,027	16.4	66,883	69.8	2,738	42.5	93,406	10.5
Texas	401,424	13.3	177,016	66.7	3,299	34.2	221,109	8.1
Vermont	38,660	24.1	15,627	59.1	1,956	51.0	21,077	16.2
Wyoming	12,482	16.4	6,501	67.2	264	39.3	5,717	8.7

[1] Fee-for-service (FFS) beneficiaries include beneficiaries enrolled in Medicaid, but not in comprehensive managed care or a behavioral health managed care plan, for at least 1 month during the year. FFS mental health (MH) beneficiaries include FFS beneficiaries who, during the year, (1) had at least one claim on which an MH disorder was the primary diagnosis or (2) received a clearly identifiable MH service. FFS substance abuse (SA) beneficiaries include FFS beneficiaries who, during the year, had at least one claim on which an SA disorder was the primary diagnosis. If beneficiaries had at least one claim on which an MH disorder was the primary diagnosis and at least one claim on which an SA disorder was the primary diagnosis, they are included in the category that represents the diagnosis most frequently listed during the year.

[2] Psychotropic medications include antidepressants, antipsychotics, antianxiety agents, and stimulants.

Table 125 notes *(continued)*

NOTES: This study identified Medicaid beneficiaries using MH or SA services in FFS plans in 13 States in 2003 (*n* = 1,380,190) and examined their use of medical services.

Table 80 aggregates the above States and shows more detail on prescription psychotropic medication use.

The above table displays data for 13 States that were selected after examining the completeness and quality of their Medicaid Analytic eXtract (MAX) data. "Data completeness" refers to the extent to which FFS data were available (States with a greater proportion of beneficiaries in FFS are considered to have more complete data than States with a greater proportion of beneficiaries in managed care). "Data quality" refers to technical problems, such as missing diagnosis codes, missing eligibility data, duplicate records, and missing claims. Each State's data were assigned a score from 1 to 4; scores were developed specifically for purposes of the analysis presented in *Mental Health and Substance Abuse Services in Medicaid, 2003: Charts and State Tables*, strictly to assist readers in understanding how to interpret the data presented, and were not intended to reflect the quality of the States' overall MAX data. If beneficiaries had multiple diagnoses on different claims during the year, they are included in the category that represents the most frequent diagnosis.

SOURCE: Substance Abuse and Mental Health Services Administration (SAMHSA). (2010). *Mental health and substance abuse services in Medicaid, 2003: Charts and state tables* (DHHS Publication No. SMA 10-4608). Rockville, MD: Center for Mental Health Services, SAMHSA.

Table 126. Number and percentage of Medicaid fee-for-service (FFS) mental health (MH) beneficiaries using Medicaid services, by service type, by State for 13 States, 2003

[Data are based on Medicaid claims]

State	Total FFS benefi-ciaries (number)	Percent of all FFS beneficiaries using:[1]					Total FFS MH benefi-ciaries (number)	Percent of all MH FFS beneficiaries using:[1,2]				
		Physician or other practi-tioner	Prescrip-tion medi-cations	Lab and X-ray	Outpatient hospital	Inpatient hospital		Physician or other practi-tioner	Prescrip-tion medi-cations	Lab and X-ray	Outpatient hospital	Inpatient hospital
Arkansas	685,199	67.2	59.0	46.6	33.0	11.7	76,974	88.5	89.0	63.1	49.9	14.9
Georgia	1,655,020	70.9	66.2	49.3	41.0	13.7	145,204	90.5	91.3	69.8	58.5	15.4
Idaho	211,563	70.7	65.3	49.7	33.8	11.3	28,639	89.0	90.5	70.9	50.8	12.4
Illinois	2,181,601	58.0	61.2	45.3	32.3	11.5	212,004	86.5	91.6	69.5	54.0	26.8
Indiana	949,303	63.5	60.8	44.9	37.5	13.1	120,057	88.7	88.7	66.4	56.6	18.5
Kansas	329,864	59.2	57.7	38.3	20.1	12.4	47,274	77.4	84.8	55.6	32.0	16.0
Maine	293,529	63.6	72.1	49.1	44.5	7.7	62,726	81.1	92.9	65.5	61.9	10.3
Montana	111,457	67.8	63.5	44.1	32.7	14.5	20,244	85.7	85.5	60.9	46.4	16.2
North Carolina	1,488,991	75.1	70.7	57.6	42.0	15.6	182,439	90.3	92.9	72.9	57.1	19.1
South Carolina	1,033,446	57.8	63.2	43.7	31.0	11.2	95,755	81.1	90.7	60.1	48.2	14.7
Texas	3,728,699	68.9	67.9	59.8	25.7	16.1	265,419	90.4	90.6	81.1	37.1	18.5
Vermont	160,518	68.1	71.0	47.5	33.0	6.3	26,452	87.6	87.5	68.8	49.6	10.2
Wyoming	75,958	70.5	63.9	47.8	38.0	13.8	9,667	90.3	89.5	68.6	54.5	16.0

[1] Fee-for-service (FFS) beneficiaries include beneficiaries enrolled in Medicaid, but not in comprehensive managed care or a behavioral health managed care plan, for at least 1 month during the year. FFS mental health (MH) beneficiaries include FFS beneficiaries who, during the year, (1) had at least one claim on which an MH disorder was the primary diagnosis or (2) received a clearly identifiable MH service.

[2] Claims in the Medicaid Analytic eXtract (MAX) files are classified into 1 of 31 types of service (TOS) categories based on State and local service or procedure codes. States may vary in how they categorize similar claims into TOS categories. The psychiatric TOS includes both MH and substance abuse (SA) services. In some cases, treatments classified in the psychiatric TOS in the MAX may be received by beneficiaries who are not identified as MH or SA beneficiaries in these tables.

Table 126 notes *(continued)*

NOTES: This study identified Medicaid beneficiaries using MH or SA services in FFS plans in 13 States in 2003 (*n* = 1,380,190) and examined their use of medical services.

Estimates for "all FFS beneficiaries" include estimates for general medical, MH, and SA services. The MH estimates are depicted separately under "MH FFS beneficiaries" and are only for MH. Table 81 aggregates the above States and shows more detail on service type. The five service types included in the current table are the four services with the highest proportion of all beneficiaries across the 13 States in Table 81 as well as inpatient hospital services. These tables display data for 13 States that were selected after examining the completeness and quality of their Medicaid Analytic eXtract (MAX) data. "Data completeness" refers to the extent to which FFS data were available (States with a greater proportion of beneficiaries in FFS are considered to have more complete data than States with a greater proportion of beneficiaries in managed care). "Data quality" refers to technical problems, such as missing diagnosis codes, missing eligibility data, duplicate records, and missing claims. Each State's data were assigned a score from 1 to 4; scores were developed specifically for purposes of the analysis presented in *Mental Health and Substance Abuse Services in Medicaid, 2003: Charts and State Tables*, strictly to assist readers in understanding how to interpret the data presented, and were not intended to reflect the quality of the States' overall MAX data. If beneficiaries had multiple diagnoses on different claims during the year, they are included in the category that represents the most frequent diagnosis.

SOURCE: Substance Abuse and Mental Health Services Administration (SAMHSA). (2010). *Mental health and substance abuse services in Medicaid, 2003: Charts and state tables* (DHHS Publication No. SMA 10-4608). Rockville, MD: Center for Mental Health Services, SAMHSA.

Table 127. Average annual expenditures of all and mental health (MH) Medicaid fee-for-service (FFS) beneficiaries, by service type, by State for 13 States, 2003

[Data are based on Medicaid claims]

State	Total FFS benefi-ciaries (number)	All FFS beneficiaries (dollars)[1,2]					Total FFS MH benefi-ciaries (number)	MH FFS beneficiaries (dollars)[1,2,3]				
		Physician or other practi-tioner	Prescrip-tion medi-cations	Lab and X-ray	Outpatient hospital	Inpatient hospital		Physician or other practi-tioner	Prescrip-tion medi-cations	Lab and X-ray	Outpatient hospital	Inpatient hospital
Arkansas	685,199	$484	$847	$203	$226	$2,999	76,974	$606	$1,783	$270	$265	3,134
Georgia	1,655,020	460	941	371	718	4,739	145,204	565	2,178	514	977	6,639
Idaho	211,563	447	1,032	193	819	5,226	28,639	584	2,455	290	1,077	6,240
Illinois	2,181,601	366	1,124	201	428	8,675	212,004	538	2,710	277	507	10,435
Indiana	949,303	402	1,442	257	395	4,026	120,057	610	2,780	341	468	5,076
Kansas	329,864	388	1,399	154	173	4,316	47,274	430	2,631	201	197	5,902
Maine	293,529	340	1,337	302	1,525	14,782	62,726	447	2,178	388	2,023	19,174
Montana	111,457	523	1,277	331	526	3,909	20,244	628	2,308	410	656	4,754
North Carolina	1,488,991	514	1,282	278	609	3,945	182,439	662	2,467	399	806	5,655
South Carolina	1,033,446	463	941	144	241	4,060	95,755	526	1,819	206	303	5,934
Texas	3,728,699	446	843	291	366	4,253	265,419	615	2,257	456	507	5,845
Vermont	160,518	398	1,167	254	690	4,532	26,452	496	1,548	317	827	6,263
Wyoming	75,958	576	934	251	377	4,163	9,667	718	2,008	341	476	5,142

[1] Fee-for-service (FFS) beneficiaries include beneficiaries enrolled in Medicaid, but not in comprehensive managed care or a behavioral health managed care plan, for at least 1 month during the year. FFS mental health (MH) beneficiaries include FFS beneficiaries who, during the year, (1) had at least one claim on which an MH disorder was the primary diagnosis or (2) received a clearly identifiable MH service.

[2] Expenditures are claims-based Medicaid payments, including both Federal and State share.

[3] Claims in the Medicaid Analytic eXtract (MAX) files are classified into 1 of 31 types of service (TOS) categories based on State and local service or procedure codes. States may vary in how they categorize similar claims into TOS categories. The psychiatric TOS includes both MH and substance abuse (SA) services. In some cases, treatments classified in the psychiatric TOS in the MAX may be received by beneficiaries who are not identified as MH or SA beneficiaries in these tables.

Table 127 notes *(continued)*

NOTES: This study identified Medicaid beneficiaries using MH or SA services in FFS plans in 13 States in 2003 (n = 1,380,190) and examined their use of medical services.

Estimates for "all FFS beneficiaries" include estimates for general medical, MH, and SA services. The MH estimates are depicted separately under "MH FFS beneficiaries" and are only for MH. Table 81 aggregates the above States and shows more detail on service type. The five service types included in the current table are the four services with the highest proportion of all beneficiaries across the 13 States in Table 81 as well as inpatient hospital services. These tables display data for 13 States that were selected after examining the completeness and quality of their Medicaid Analytic eXtract (MAX) data. "Data completeness" refers to the extent to which FFS data were available (States with a greater proportion of beneficiaries in FFS are considered to have more complete data than States with a greater proportion of beneficiaries in managed care). "Data quality" refers to technical problems, such as missing diagnosis codes, missing eligibility data, duplicate records, and missing claims. Each State's data were assigned a score from 1 to 4; scores were developed specifically for purposes of the analysis presented in *Mental Health and Substance Abuse Services in Medicaid, 2003: Charts and State Tables*, strictly to assist readers in understanding how to interpret the data presented, and were not intended to reflect the quality of the States' overall MAX data. If beneficiaries had multiple diagnoses on different claims during the year, they are included in the category that represents the most frequent diagnosis.

SOURCE: Substance Abuse and Mental Health Services Administration (SAMHSA). (2010). *Mental health and substance abuse services in Medicaid, 2003: Charts and state tables* (DHHS Publication No. SMA 10-4608). Rockville, MD: Center for Mental Health Services, SAMHSA.

Table 128. Estimated Medicare expenditures in mental health/substance abuse units of community hospitals, United States and by State, selected years 1997–2007

[Data are from Medicare Cost Reports]

State	Expenditures (in thousands of dollars)				
	1997	2001	2005	2006	2007[1]
Alabama	$108,980	$94,088	$126,763	$131,124	$150,843
Alaska	2,434	2,124	3,116	3,194	3,644
Arizona	48,686	52,918	123,307	104,175	94,752
Arkansas	62,071	74,699	68,679	61,545	60,005
California	433,006	594,772	682,510	712,818	720,655
Colorado	62,456	70,463	71,394	71,989	71,979
Connecticut	109,515	156,143	203,308	212,543	226,815
Delaware	14,009	11,631	13,484	13,447	7,552
District of Columbia	20,365	20,525	23,973	26,276	26,772
Florida	252,441	302,164	322,175	337,892	338,132
Georgia	84,933	114,483	145,974	156,253	156,733
Hawaii	718	4,960	5,374	5,202	5,623
Idaho	11,746	17,435	24,239	16,204	14,740
Illinois	308,660	326,803	345,315	370,013	363,526
Indiana	102,954	124,512	132,610	134,976	127,920
Iowa	68,277	67,111	76,043	78,625	83,984
Kansas	41,852	58,509	55,512	57,743	58,230
Kentucky	66,375	77,720	90,600	93,679	92,868
Louisiana	143,290	127,751	148,779	117,728	115,516
Maine	21,406	20,417	30,412	30,225	25,647
Maryland[2]	—	—	—	—	—
Massachusetts	218,537	238,014	326,689	294,960	304,641
Michigan	328,921	282,069	301,122	319,465	299,161
Minnesota	68,756	106,249	131,736	131,715	122,515
Mississippi	94,003	94,856	124,791	126,118	120,924
Missouri	135,800	165,352	165,897	162,756	160,738
Montana	6,560	6,667	10,140	7,312	7,343
Nebraska	29,322	17,357	30,678	29,121	30,823
Nevada	14,551	17,532	15,697	16,316	16,286
New Hampshire	56,043	49,169	53,472	62,902	65,623
New Jersey	188,954	236,193	286,166	296,147	281,227
New Mexico	29,366	28,850	46,772	53,762	55,285
New York	776,967	1,152,799	1,495,095	1,540,297	1,563,199
North Carolina	166,039	176,149	213,266	237,782	250,060
North Dakota	14,517	16,012	20,015	20,630	20,567
Ohio	257,784	291,701	320,059	312,817	312,676
Oklahoma	70,158	66,986	77,319	75,979	78,053
Oregon	39,475	51,803	67,983	71,631	69,781
Pennsylvania	421,686	446,798	478,369	487,859	488,764
Rhode Island	16,875	20,572	39,995	42,128	44,018
South Carolina	84,098	82,530	104,368	109,504	113,874

(continued)

Table 128. Estimated Medicare expenditures in mental health/substance abuse units of community hospitals, United States and by State, selected years 1997–2007 *(continued)*

State	Expenditures (in thousands of dollars)				
	1997	2001	2005	2006	2007[1]
South Dakota	$17,134	$17,167	$18,573	$27,393	$29,145
Tennessee	102,228	148,168	164,370	168,773	214,206
Texas	231,642	187,134	160,865	186,145	206,376
Utah	20,580	19,973	28,715	28,856	29,619
Vermont	12,105	13,014	18,683	8,804	8,993
Virginia	141,240	145,566	173,991	193,002	198,095
Washington	59,349	78,887	93,181	88,715	94,609
West Virginia	30,927	44,971	56,586	61,018	70,403
Wisconsin	65,746	74,725	59,890	64,515	66,429
Wyoming	6,159	6,033	8,852	8,921	9,666
United States	**$5,669,694**	**$6,602,526**	**$7,786,900**	**$7,970,997**	**$8,079,038**

— Data not available.

[1] 2007 data are preliminary.

[2] Maryland hospitals do not provide specialty unit data on the Medicare Cost Reports.

NOTES: The Medicare Cost Report is based on annual financial information reported to the Centers for Medicare & Medicaid Services. The Cost Report contains provider information, such as facility characteristics, utilization data, cost and charges by cost center (in total and for Medicare), Medicare settlement data, and financial statement data.

Number of beds in other State and local government hospitals can be found in Table 113.

Dollar estimates are not adjusted for inflation.

SOURCE: Medicare Cost Reports, 1997, 2001, 2005, 2006, and 2007, Centers for Medicare & Medicaid Services.

Table 129. Medicare fee-for-service (FFS) expenditures for mental health (MH) claimants, United States and by State, 2007

[Data are based on Medicare claims data]

State	MH claimants (number)	FFS expenditures (dollars) for MH claimants[1]			
		All services	All services per MH claimant	MH services	MH services per MH claimant
Alabama	65,920	$1,061,495,100	$16,103	$123,946,647	$1,880
Alaska	5,540	72,786,435	13,138	5,406,048	976
Arizona	50,400	762,962,355	15,138	76,715,100	1,522
Arkansas	49,760	674,085,620	13,547	79,156,835	1,591
California	329,020	6,009,086,432	18,264	653,807,241	1,987
Colorado	44,460	649,821,210	14,616	49,929,493	1,123
Connecticut	77,300	1,494,083,461	19,328	127,524,395	1,650
Delaware	13,980	280,046,141	20,032	16,181,754	1,157
District of Columbia	7,540	156,071,324	20,699	12,421,549	1,647
Florida	308,640	6,813,923,676	22,077	586,553,135	1,900
Georgia	109,460	1,576,354,148	14,401	154,225,134	1,409
Hawaii	13,200	130,526,489	9,888	14,242,364	1,079
Idaho	17,320	196,814,225	11,363	18,451,094	1,065
Illinois	203,120	3,993,960,791	19,663	328,778,479	1,619
Indiana	112,080	1,802,044,660	16,078	133,119,688	1,188
Iowa	60,720	661,721,493	10,898	52,270,434	861
Kansas	51,740	706,579,758	13,656	62,773,344	1,213
Kentucky	85,100	1,188,805,142	13,970	82,534,790	970
Louisiana	57,280	1,151,672,021	20,106	222,561,655	3,886
Maine	37,840	409,642,555	10,826	39,732,353	1,050
Maryland	80,220	1,753,316,817	21,856	136,926,745	1,707
Massachusetts	157,800	2,859,103,643	18,119	278,433,019	1,764
Michigan	183,280	3,389,872,593	18,496	223,367,161	1,219
Minnesota	76,760	937,405,026	12,212	97,852,888	1,275
Mississippi	52,920	870,444,039	16,448	114,067,675	2,155
Missouri	112,020	1,621,213,497	14,473	153,119,663	1,367
Montana	16,480	165,063,249	10,016	14,754,988	895
Nebraska	29,580	391,333,742	13,230	37,429,109	1,265
Nevada	20,600	414,266,543	20,110	41,276,081	2,004
New Hampshire	31,260	431,208,995	13,794	37,889,307	1,212
New Jersey	135,840	3,137,738,929	23,099	229,481,141	1,689
New Mexico	24,880	283,537,958	11,396	26,567,163	1,068
New York	315,960	6,058,782,362	19,176	562,586,530	1,781
North Carolina	143,940	2,092,882,265	14,540	165,592,162	1,150
North Dakota	13,200	131,893,720	9,992	10,661,339	808
Ohio	212,960	3,595,158,985	16,882	276,377,673	1,298
Oklahoma	59,180	955,823,972	16,151	88,344,640	1,493
Oregon	40,120	403,224,809	10,050	47,210,388	1,177
Pennsylvania	197,920	3,564,510,072	18,010	263,022,826	1,329
Rhode Island	20,540	326,085,907	15,876	36,033,275	1,754
South Carolina	69,800	966,663,393	13,849	89,860,790	1,287

(continued)

Table 129. Medicare fee-for-service (FFS) expenditures for mental health (MH) claimants, United States and by State, 2007 *(continued)*

State	MH claimants (number)	FFS expenditures (dollars) for MH claimants[1]			
		All services	All services per MH claimant	MH services	MH services per MH claimant
South Dakota	15,040	$163,375,918	$10,863	$11,973,301	$796
Tennessee	112,020	1,821,712,652	16,262	158,543,805	1,415
Texas	270,660	5,408,193,094	19,982	412,963,827	1,526
Utah	21,860	247,286,426	11,312	21,574,591	987
Vermont	14,520	179,223,676	12,343	16,589,983	1,143
Virginia	115,280	1,491,305,641	12,936	131,282,180	1,139
Washington	80,220	1,029,651,788	12,835	84,343,242	1,051
West Virginia	47,240	543,359,878	11,502	40,199,006	851
Wisconsin	99,200	1,344,950,676	13,558	98,036,132	988
Wyoming	6,720	81,071,545	12,064	6,449,971	960
United States	**4,478,440**	**$76,452,144,845**	**$17,071**	**$6,753,142,132**	**$1,508**

[1] ICD-9 diagnostic codes for mental health diagnoses categories are as follows: schizophrenia (295), major depression (296.2, 296.3), bipolar disorders and manic disorders (296.0, 296.1, 296.4–296.99), other psychoses (293, 294, 297, 298, 299), stress and adjustment disorders (308, 309), anxiety disorders and other mood disorders (300, 301.13, 311), and all other mental disorders (302, 306, 307, 310, 312, 313, 314, 316, 301 w/o 301.13).

NOTES: The Medicare Standard Analytical Files (SAF) is a nationally representative claims database that consists of a randomly selected 5 percent sample of U.S. Medicare beneficiaries. The database includes claims across various care settings, including inpatient, outpatient, skilled nursing, home health, and hospice, as well as for durable medical equipment. These estimates do not include expenditures on prescription medications.

Estimates for the United States only include data for the 50 U.S. States and exclude U.S. territories and foreign/unknown; as a result, the cumulative estimates shown here may differ from national estimates reported in Table 84.

SOURCES: Medicare 5 Percent Standard Analytical Files, 2007, Centers for Medicare & Medicaid Services.

Table 130. Medicare fee-for-service (FFS) expenditures on major depression claimants, United States and by State, 2007

[Data are based on Medicare claims data]

State	Major depression claimants (number)	FFS expenditures (dollars) for major depression claimants[1]			
		All services	All services per major depression claimant	MH services	MH services per major depression claimant
Alabama	12,860	$162,861,701	$12,664	$22,970,402	$1,786
Alaska	700	7,030,611	10,044	531,897	760
Arizona	7,280	97,652,627	13,414	7,187,464	987
Arkansas	6,920	97,926,505	14,151	11,356,995	1,641
California	67,480	1,314,798,281	19,484	128,637,392	1,906
Colorado	5,480	75,110,621	13,706	4,104,349	749
Connecticut	13,660	207,792,345	15,212	23,819,772	1,744
Delaware	2,980	52,962,799	17,773	4,657,510	1,563
District of Columbia	880	25,499,429	28,977	1,109,199	1,260
Florida	79,520	2,029,758,913	25,525	217,944,358	2,741
Georgia	22,800	316,792,512	13,894	25,283,096	1,109
Hawaii	2,060	15,914,959	7,726	1,870,921	908
Idaho	1,900	20,980,414	11,042	2,200,983	1,158
Illinois	38,320	695,417,106	18,148	65,348,150	1,705
Indiana	19,480	289,903,272	14,882	22,877,728	1,174
Iowa	9,700	112,350,066	11,582	11,033,407	1,137
Kansas	8,700	119,823,865	13,773	13,645,290	1,568
Kentucky	13,640	160,137,947	11,740	14,239,992	1,044
Louisiana	12,860	285,933,795	22,234	65,755,875	5,113
Maine	5,020	50,277,468	10,015	7,489,078	1,492
Maryland	15,640	312,620,212	19,989	27,549,812	1,761
Massachusetts	35,100	606,892,817	17,290	66,574,419	1,897
Michigan	33,240	602,499,205	18,126	40,720,762	1,225
Minnesota	12,820	147,862,707	11,534	18,737,327	1,462
Mississippi	8,620	146,431,967	16,987	24,162,837	2,803
Missouri	25,680	395,196,014	15,389	35,145,761	1,369
Montana	1,740	18,242,911	10,484	2,660,919	1,529
Nebraska	4,040	60,040,296	14,861	6,707,007	1,660
Nevada	3,380	65,688,287	19,434	5,102,390	1,510
New Hampshire	5,800	80,249,781	13,836	8,167,149	1,408
New Jersey	27,040	539,174,173	19,940	33,220,627	1,229
New Mexico	3,800	39,267,740	10,334	4,866,029	1,281
New York	54,940	964,692,441	17,559	82,504,485	1,502
North Carolina	24,680	306,601,282	12,423	29,955,600	1,214
North Dakota	1,240	11,046,841	8,909	1,084,713	875
Ohio	32,180	526,156,035	16,350	38,102,112	1,184
Oklahoma	9,560	160,248,099	16,762	14,279,817	1,494
Oregon	5,060	52,936,769	10,462	5,412,929	1,070
Pennsylvania	37,640	682,554,033	18,134	54,398,618	1,445
Rhode Island	3,640	41,484,101	11,397	6,454,481	1,773
South Carolina	11,580	126,961,198	10,964	10,424,261	900

(continued)

Table 130. Medicare fee-for-service (FFS) expenditures on major depression claimants, United States and by State, 2007 *(continued)*

State	Major depression claimants (number)	FFS expenditures (dollars) for major depression claimants[1]			
		All services	All services per major depression claimant	MH services	MH services per major depression claimant
South Dakota	1,540	$14,764,987	$9,588	$1,905,507	$1,237
Tennessee	28,100	467,655,238	16,643	43,734,034	1,556
Texas	51,500	985,694,000	19,140	87,479,876	1,699
Utah	3,940	43,007,762	10,916	4,975,338	1,263
Vermont	2,080	21,010,570	10,101	3,782,674	1,819
Virginia	22,360	294,944,206	13,191	25,103,282	1,123
Washington	11,000	138,929,337	12,630	12,050,678	1,096
West Virginia	9,500	85,624,924	9,013	5,585,360	588
Wisconsin	14,080	173,727,189	12,339	14,276,385	1,014
Wyoming	720	6,117,792	8,497	330,955	460
United States	**834,480**	**$14,257,248,151**	**$17,085**	**$1,367,520,005**	**$1,639**

[1] ICD-9 diagnostic codes for the major depression category (296.2, 296.3) include major depressive disorder—single episode and major depressive disorder—recurrent episode.

NOTES: The Medicare Standard Analytical Files (SAF) is a nationally representative claims database that consists of a randomly selected 5 percent sample of U.S. Medicare beneficiaries. The database includes claims across various care settings, including inpatient, outpatient, skilled nursing, home health, and hospice, as well as for durable medical equipment. These estimates do not include expenditures on prescription medications.

Estimates for the United States only include data for the 50 U.S. States and exclude U.S. territories and foreign/ unknown; as a result, the cumulative estimates shown here may differ from national estimates reported in Table 84.

SOURCES: Medicare 5 Percent Standard Analytical Files, 2007, Centers for Medicare & Medicaid Services.

Table 131. Medicare fee-for-service (FFS) expenditures on mental health (MH) claimants and MH expenditures for claimants aged 0 to 64, United States and by State, 2007

[Data are based on Medicare claims data]

State	MH claimants (number)	FFS expenditures (dollars)			
		All services	All services per claimant	MH services	MH services per claimant
Alabama	28,800	$321,695,823	$11,170	$62,424,365	$2,168
Alaska	2,620	18,700,830	7,138	3,184,426	1,215
Arizona	19,340	197,143,343	10,194	27,373,623	1,415
Arkansas	21,240	192,802,305	9,077	34,459,513	1,622
California	132,680	1,704,424,704	12,846	403,092,938	3,038
Colorado	17,080	157,181,506	9,203	22,246,629	1,302
Connecticut	27,660	374,139,000	13,526	72,517,730	2,622
Delaware	5,080	69,317,677	13,645	6,636,536	1,306
District of Columbia	2,660	48,382,131	18,189	8,899,710	3,346
Florida	95,020	1,504,288,290	15,831	258,766,694	2,723
Georgia	46,640	488,173,642	10,467	70,603,418	1,514
Hawaii	5,700	27,946,643	4,903	5,438,684	954
Idaho	6,760	57,955,464	8,573	9,902,121	1,465
Illinois	70,380	926,363,134	13,162	175,791,330	2,498
Indiana	43,300	441,278,652	10,191	57,438,852	1,327
Iowa	22,280	172,746,860	7,753	30,321,568	1,361
Kansas	18,640	165,482,640	8,878	29,009,240	1,556
Kentucky	39,380	363,676,828	9,235	40,444,907	1,027
Louisiana	22,740	339,185,809	14,916	116,762,787	5,135
Maine	16,480	121,543,233	7,375	22,237,186	1,349
Maryland	27,180	448,414,864	16,498	82,403,359	3,032
Massachusetts	68,160	821,579,392	12,054	168,516,012	2,472
Michigan	73,080	955,692,575	13,077	117,798,249	1,612
Minnesota	35,060	330,783,770	9,435	63,952,936	1,824
Mississippi	23,920	280,353,710	11,720	53,260,227	2,227
Missouri	49,840	507,720,127	10,187	89,483,542	1,795
Montana	5,580	38,220,551	6,850	6,454,802	1,157
Nebraska	10,760	101,901,481	9,470	22,426,298	2,084
Nevada	8,700	119,326,065	13,716	19,103,116	2,196
New Hampshire	11,720	113,055,058	9,646	18,640,213	1,590
New Jersey	46,240	695,332,262	15,037	128,736,057	2,784
New Mexico	10,820	98,373,860	9,092	14,095,594	1,303
New York	120,640	1,478,884,680	12,259	334,178,978	2,770
North Carolina	60,600	665,789,625	10,987	82,128,253	1,355
North Dakota	4,000	34,858,833	8,715	6,257,135	1,564
Ohio	78,020	936,093,815	11,998	132,459,800	1,698
Oklahoma	23,100	235,354,938	10,189	38,812,420	1,680
Oregon	16,520	140,133,385	8,483	19,721,700	1,194
Pennsylvania	67,720	756,654,785	11,173	118,655,423	1,752
Rhode Island	8,900	97,124,242	10,913	22,021,603	2,474
South Carolina	30,580	302,205,893	9,882	43,710,822	1,429

(continued)

Table 131. Medicare fee-for-service (FFS) expenditures on mental health (MH) claimants and MH expenditures for claimants aged 0 to 64, United States and by State, 2007 *(continued)*

State	MH claimants (number)	FFS expenditures (dollars)			
		All services	All services per claimant	MH services	MH services per claimant
South Dakota	4,600	$39,848,948	$8,663	$6,111,038	$1,328
Tennessee	50,200	558,460,329	11,125	84,551,302	1,684
Texas	95,760	1,402,651,663	14,648	206,056,952	2,152
Utah	9,940	79,157,676	7,964	13,217,201	1,330
Vermont	6,260	68,893,058	11,005	11,183,355	1,786
Virginia	44,820	399,402,409	8,911	70,056,795	1,563
Washington	33,020	309,286,324	9,367	53,803,395	1,629
West Virginia	22,680	184,757,185	8,146	21,373,170	942
Wisconsin	35,940	348,668,338	9,701	49,303,611	1,372
Wyoming	2,380	21,639,736	9,092	4,007,546	1,684
United States	**1,731,220**	**$20,263,048,089**	**$11,704**	**$3,560,033,166**	**$2,056**

NOTES: The Medicare Standard Analytical Files (SAF) is a nationally representative claims database that consists of a randomly selected 5 percent sample of U.S. Medicare beneficiaries. The database includes claims across various care settings, including inpatient, outpatient, skilled nursing, home health, and hospice, as well as for durable medical equipment. These estimates do not include expenditures on prescription medications.

Estimates for the United States only include data for the 50 U.S. States and exclude U.S. territories and foreign/unknown; as a result, the cumulative estimates shown here may differ from national estimates reported in Table 84.

SOURCES: Medicare 5 Percent Standard Analytical Files, 2007, Centers for Medicare & Medicaid Services.

Table 132. Medicare fee-for-service (FFS) expenditures on mental health (MH) claimants and MH expenditures for claimants aged 65 or older, United States and by State, 2007

[Data are based on Medicare claims data]

State	MH claimants (number)	FFS expenditures (dollars)			
		All services	All services per claimant	MH services	MH services per claimant
Alabama	37,120	$739,799,278	$19,930	$61,522,281	$1,657
Alaska	2,920	54,085,605	18,522	2,221,622	761
Arizona	31,060	565,819,011	18,217	49,341,476	1,589
Arkansas	28,520	481,283,314	16,875	44,697,322	1,567
California	196,340	4,304,661,728	21,925	250,714,303	1,277
Colorado	27,380	492,639,704	17,993	27,682,864	1,011
Connecticut	49,640	1,119,944,461	22,561	55,006,665	1,108
Delaware	8,900	210,728,463	23,677	9,545,218	1,072
District of Columbia	4,880	107,689,193	22,067	3,521,839	722
Florida	213,620	5,309,635,387	24,856	327,786,441	1,534
Georgia	62,820	1,088,180,506	17,322	83,621,716	1,331
Hawaii	7,500	102,579,846	13,677	8,803,680	1,174
Idaho	10,560	138,858,761	13,150	8,548,973	810
Illinois	132,740	3,067,597,657	23,110	152,987,149	1,153
Indiana	68,780	1,360,766,008	19,784	75,680,836	1,100
Iowa	38,440	488,974,632	12,720	21,948,866	571
Kansas	33,100	541,097,118	16,347	33,764,104	1,020
Kentucky	45,720	825,128,314	18,047	42,089,883	921
Louisiana	34,540	812,486,212	23,523	105,798,867	3,063
Maine	21,360	288,099,322	13,488	17,495,167	819
Maryland	53,040	1,304,901,953	24,602	54,523,385	1,028
Massachusetts	89,640	2,037,524,251	22,730	109,917,007	1,226
Michigan	110,200	2,434,180,018	22,089	105,568,913	958
Minnesota	41,700	606,621,256	14,547	33,899,952	813
Mississippi	29,000	590,090,328	20,348	60,807,448	2,097
Missouri	62,180	1,113,493,371	17,908	63,636,121	1,023
Montana	10,900	126,842,698	11,637	8,300,185	761
Nebraska	18,820	289,432,262	15,379	15,002,811	797
Nevada	11,900	294,940,477	24,785	22,172,964	1,863
New Hampshire	19,540	318,153,937	16,282	19,249,094	985
New Jersey	89,600	2,442,406,667	27,259	100,745,084	1,124
New Mexico	14,060	185,164,098	13,170	12,471,569	887
New York	195,320	4,579,897,682	23,448	228,407,552	1,169
North Carolina	83,340	1,427,092,639	17,124	83,463,909	1,001
North Dakota	9,200	97,034,887	10,547	4,404,205	479
Ohio	134,940	2,659,065,169	19,706	143,917,873	1,067
Oklahoma	36,080	720,469,035	19,969	49,532,220	1,373
Oregon	23,600	263,091,424	11,148	27,488,688	1,165
Pennsylvania	130,200	2,807,855,288	21,566	144,367,403	1,109
Rhode Island	11,640	228,961,665	19,670	14,011,673	1,204
South Carolina	39,220	664,457,500	16,942	46,149,967	1,177

(continued)

Table 132. Medicare fee-for-service (FFS) expenditures on mental health (MH) claimants and MH expenditures for claimants aged 65 or older, United States and by State, 2007 *(continued)*

State	MH claimants (number)	FFS expenditures (dollars)			
		All services	All services per claimant	MH services	MH services per claimant
South Dakota	10,440	$123,526,971	$11,832	$5,862,263	$562
Tennessee	61,820	1,263,252,323	20,434	73,992,503	1,197
Texas	174,900	4,005,541,432	22,902	206,906,874	1,183
Utah	11,920	168,128,749	14,105	8,357,390	701
Vermont	8,260	110,330,618	13,357	5,406,627	655
Virginia	70,460	1,091,903,232	15,497	61,225,384	869
Washington	47,200	720,365,464	15,262	30,539,847	647
West Virginia	24,560	358,602,693	14,601	18,825,836	767
Wisconsin	63,260	996,282,338	15,749	48,732,520	770
Wyoming	4,340	59,431,809	13,694	2,442,425	563
United States	**2,747,220**	**$56,189,096,756**	**$20,453**	**$3,193,108,965**	**$1,162**

NOTES: The Medicare Standard Analytical Files (SAF) is a nationally representative claims database that consists of a randomly selected 5 percent sample of U.S. Medicare beneficiaries. The database includes claims across various care settings, including inpatient, outpatient, skilled nursing, home health, and hospice, as well as for durable medical equipment. These estimates do not include expenditures on prescription medications.

Estimates for the United States only include data for the 50 U.S. States and exclude U.S. territories and foreign/unknown; as a result, the cumulative estimates shown here may differ from national estimates reported in Table 84.

SOURCES: Medicare 5 Percent Standard Analytical Files, 2007, Centers for Medicare & Medicaid Services.

7.5 References

Achenbach, T. M. (1991). *Manual for the Child Behavior Checklist/4-18 and 1991 profile.* Burlington, VT: University of Vermont, Department of Psychiatry.

Achenbach, T. M., & Rescorla, L. A. (2001). *Manual for the ASEBA School-Age Forms & Profiles.* Burlington, VT: University of Vermont, Research Center for Children, Youth, & Families.

American Psychiatric Association (APA). (1994). *Diagnostic and statistical manual of mental disorders* (4th ed.). Washington, DC: APA.

Aron, L., Honberg, R., Duckworth, K., Kimball, A., Edgar, E., Carolla, B., ... & Fitzpatrick, M. (2009). *Grading the States 2009: A report on America's health care system for adults with serious mental illness.* Arlington, VA: National Alliance on Mental Illness.

Bazelon Center for Mental Health Law. (2008). *Following the rules: A report on Federal rules and State actions to cover mental health services under Medicaid.* Washington, DC: Judge David L. Bazelon Center for Mental Health Law. Retrieved from http://www.bazelon.org/LinkClick.aspx?fileticket=zeqlTk_ltSk%3D&tabid=104

Beck, A. J., & Maruschak, L. M. (2001). *Mental health treatment in State prisons, 2000* (NCJ 188215). Washington, DC: U.S. Department of Justice, Office of Justice Programs, Bureau of Justice Statistics. Retrieved from http://bjs.ojp.usdoj.gov/content/pub/pdf/mhtsp00.pdf

Bray, R. M., Pemberton, M. R., Hourani, L. L., Witt, M., Rae Olmsted, K. L., Brown, J. M., ... Bradshaw, M. R. (2009). *2008 Department of Defense survey of health related behaviors among active duty military personnel.* Report prepared for TRICARE Management Activity, Office of the Assistant Secretary of Defense (Health Affairs) and U.S. Coast Guard. Retrieved from http://www.tricare.mil/2008HealthBehaviors.pdf

Brener, N. D., Weist, M., Adelman, H., Taylor, L., & Vernon-Smiley, M. (2007). Mental health and social services: Results from the School Health Policies and Programs Study 2006. *Journal of School Health, 77*(8), 486–499.

Casanueva, C., Ringeisen, H., Wilson, E., Smith, K., & Dolan, M. (2011). *NSCAW II baseline report: Child well-being* (OPRE Report #2011-27b). Washington, DC: Office of Planning, Research and Evaluation, Administration for Children and Families, U.S. Department of Health and Human Services. Retrieved from http://www.acf.hhs.gov/programs/opre/abuse_neglect/nscaw/reports/nscaw2_child/nscaw2_child.pdf

Ellis, A. R., Konrad, T. R., Thomas, K. C., & Morrissey, J. P. (2009). County-level estimates of mental health professional supply in the United States. *Psychiatric Services, 60*(10), 1315–1322.

Goodman, R. (1999). The extended version of the Strengths and Difficulties Questionnaire as a guide to child psychiatric caseness and consequent burden. *Journal of Child Psychology and Psychiatry, 40*(5), 791–799.

Horgan, C. M., Garnick, D. W., Merrick, E. L., & Hodgkin, D. (2009). Changes in how health plans provide behavioral health services. *The Journal of Behavioral Health Services & Research, 36*(1), 11–24.

Hourani, L. L., Bray, R. M., Marsden, M. E., Witt, M. B., Vandermaas-Peeler, R., Scheffler, S., ... Strange, L. B. (2007, September). *2006 Department of Defense survey of health related behaviors among the Guard and Reserve force.* Report prepared for TRICARE Management Activity. Retrieved from http://www.tricare.mil/hpae/_docs/RC_2006 Reserve Component_FR_9-07.pdf

James, D. J., & Glaze, L. E. (2006). *Mental health problems of prison and jail inmates* (NCJ-213600). Washington, DC: U.S. Department of Justice, Office of Justice Programs, Bureau of Justice Statistics. Retrieved from http://bjs.ojp.usdoj.gov/content/pub/pdf/mhppji.pdf

Kaiser Family Foundation/Health Research & Educational Trust (2000). *Employer health benefits, 2000.* Menlo Park, CA: Kaiser Family Foundation. Retrieved from http://www.kff.org/insurance/loader.cfm?url=/commonspot/security/getfile.cfm&PageID=13512

Kaiser Family Foundation/Health Research & Educational Trust (2008). *Employer health benefits, 2008.* Menlo Park, CA: Kaiser Family Foundation. Retrieved from http://ehbs.kff.org/pdf/7790.pdf

Kaiser Family Foundation/Health Research & Educational Trust (2010). *Employer health benefits, 2010 annual survey.* Menlo Park, CA: Kaiser Family Foundation. Retrieved from http://ehbs.kff.org/pdf/2010/8085.pdf

Kessler, R. C., & Ustün, T. B. (2004). The World Mental Health (WMH) Survey Initiative Version of the World Health Organization (WHO) Composite International Diagnostic Interview (CIDI). *International Journal of Methods in Psychiatric Research, 13*(2), 93–121.

Kessler, R. C., Andrews, G., Colpe, L. J., Hiripi, E., Mroczek, D. K., Normand, S. L., Walters, E. E., & Zaslavsky, A. M. (2002). Short screening scales to monitor population prevalences and trends in non-specific psychological distress. *Psychological Medicine, 32*(6), 959–976.

Kessler, R. C., Chiu, W. T., Demler, O., Merikangas, K. R., & Walters, E. E. (2005). Prevalence, severity, and comorbidity of 12-month DSM-IV disorders in the National Comorbidity Survey Replication. *Archives of General Psychiatry, 62*(6), 617–627.

Konrad, T. R., Ellis, A. R., Thomas, K. C., Holzer, C. E., & Morrissey, J. P. (2009). County-level estimates of need for mental health professionals in the United States. *Psychiatric Services, 60*(10), 1307–1314.

Manderscheid, R. W., Atay, J. E., & Crider, R. A. (2009). Changing trends in State psychiatric hospital use from 2002 to 2005. *Psychiatric Services, 60*(1), 29–34.

Mark, T. L., Vandivort-Warren, R., Owens, P. L., Buck, J. A., Levit, K. R., Coffey, R. M., & Stocks, C. (2010). Psychiatric discharges in community hospitals with and without psychiatric units: How many and for whom? *Psychiatric Services, 61*(6), 562–568.

Merikangas, K. R., He, J.-P., Brody, D., Fisher, P. W., Bourdon, K., & Koretz, D. S. (2010). Prevalence and treatment of mental disorders among US children in the 2001–2004 NHANES. *Pediatrics, 125*(1), 75–81.

Morrissey, J. P., Thomas, K. C., Ellis, A. R., & Konrad, T. R. (2007). *Development of a new method for designation of mental health professional shortage areas* (Contract No. HHSH-230200532038C). Prepared with the Bureau of Health Professions, Health Resources and Services Administration, U.S. Department of Health and Human Services.

Morton, J. D., & Aleman, P. (April 2005). Trends in employer-provided mental health and substance abuse benefits. *Monthly Labor Review*, 25–35.

Radloff, L. S. (1977). The CES-D Scale: A self-report depression scale for research in the general population. *Applied Psychological Measurement, 1*, 385–401.

Robins, L. N., Helzer, J. E., Croughan, J., & Ratcliff, K. S. (1981). National Institute of Mental Health Diagnostic Interview Schedule: Its history, characteristics, and validity. *Archives of General Psychiatry, 38*(4), 381–389.

Sondik, E. J., Madans, J. H., & Gentleman, J. F. (2010). Summary health statistics for U.S. children: National Health Interview Survey, 2009. *Vital and Health Statistics, 10*(247). Hyattsville, MD: National Center for Health Statistics.

Spitzer, R. L., Kroenke, K., & Williams, J. B. (1999). Validation and utility of a self-report version of PRIME-MD: The PHQ primary care study. Primary care evaluation of mental disorders. Patient Health Questionnaire. *Journal of the American Medical Association, 282*(18), 1737–1744.

Substance Abuse and Mental Health Services Administration (SAMHSA). (2008). *Results from the 2007 National Survey on Drug Use and Health: National findings* (DHHS Publication No. SMA 08-4343, NSDUH Series H-34). Rockville, MD: SAMHSA, Office of Applied Studies.

Substance Abuse and Mental Health Services Administration (SAMHSA). (2010). *Mental Health, United States, 2008* (DHHS Publication No. SMA 10-4590). Rockville, MD: Center for Mental Health Services, SAMHSA.

Substance Abuse and Mental Health Services Administration (SAMHSA). (2010). *Mental health and substance abuse services in Medicaid, 2003: Charts and state tables* (DHHS Publication No. SMA 10-4608). Rockville, MD: Center for Mental Health Services, SAMHSA.

Substance Abuse and Mental Health Services Administration (SAMHSA). (2010). *National expenditures for mental health services and substance abuse treatment, 1986–2005* (DHHS Publication No. SMA 10-4612). Rockville, MD: Center for Mental Health Services and Center for Substance Abuse Treatment, SAMHSA.

Teich, J. L., & Buck, J. A. (2007). Mental health benefits in employer-sponsored health plans, 1997–2003. *Journal of Behavioral Health Services Research, 34*(3), 343–348.

Tejada-Vera, B., & Sutton, P. D. (2010). Births, marriages, divorces, and deaths: Provisional data for 2009. *National Vital Statistics Report, 58*(25). Hyattsville, MD: National Center for Health Statistics.

Thomas, C. R., & Holzer, C. E. III (2006). The continuing shortage of child and adolescent psychiatrists. *Journal of the American Academy of Child and Adolescent Psychiatry, 45*(9), 1023–1031.

Thomas, K. C., Ellis, A. R., Konrad, T. R., Holzer, C. E., & Morrissey, J. P. (2009). County-level estimates of mental health professional shortage in the United States. *Psychiatric Services, 60*(10), 1323–1328.

Thomas, K. C., Ellis, A. R., & Morrissey, J. P. (2010). Where are the psychiatric physician assistants? Reply. *Psychiatric Services, 61*(1), 95–96.

Wang, P. S., Lane, M., Olfson, M., Pincus, H. A., Wells, K. B., & Kessler, R. C. (2005). Twelve-month use of mental health services in the United States: Results from the National Comorbidity Survey Replication. *Archives of General Psychiatry, 62*(6), 629–640.

Weathers, F. W., Litz, B. T., Huska, J. A., & Keane, T. M. (1994). *The PTSD checklist-civilian version (PCL-C)*. Boston, MA: National Center for PTSD.

Wells, R., Morrissey, J. P., Lee, I.-H., & Radford, A. (2010). Trends in behavioral health care service provision by community health centers, 1998–2007. *Psychiatric Services, 61*(8), 759–764.

World Health Organization (WHO). (1977). *International classification of diseases, ninth revision (ICD-9)*. Geneva, Switzerland: WHO.

World Health Organization (WHO). (1991). *International classification of diseases, 10th revision (ICD-10)*. Geneva, Switzerland: WHO.

Xu, J. Q., Kochanek, K. D., Murphy, S. L., & Tejada-Vera, B. (2010). Deaths: Final data for 2007. *National Vital Statistics Reports, 58*(19). Hyattsville, MD: National Center for Health Statistics.

Zuvekas, S. H. (2005). Prescription drugs and the changing patterns of treatment for mental disorders, 1996–2001. *Health Affairs, 24*(1), 195–205.

APPENDIX A: DATA SOURCE DESCRIPTIONS

Data Source *(Sponsor)*	Description
American Hospital Association Annual Survey *(American Hospital Association)*	The American Hospital Association Annual Survey is completed online by most U.S. hospitals and profiles more than 6,500 hospitals throughout the United States. The overall response rate for fiscal year 2007 was 78 percent, but this rate varied among subgroups of hospitals depending on size, ownership, service, geographical location, and membership status. The survey covers hospital organization structure, service lines, staffing, expenses, physician organization structures, beds, and utilization.
Annual Census of Admission and Resident Patient Characteristics *(Substance Abuse and Mental Health Services Administration)*	The Annual Census of Admission and Resident Patient Characteristics, State and County Mental Hospital 24-Hour Services, collects annual aggregate data from each State on age, sex, race, and ethnicity, by diagnosis, for annual admissions and year-end residents.
Area Resource File (ARF) *(Health Resources and Services Administration)*	The Area Resource File (ARF) contains more than 6,000 variables for each of the Nation's counties. ARF includes information on health facilities, health professions, measures of resource scarcity, health status, economic activity, health training programs, and socioeconomic and environmental characteristics.
Brandeis Health Plan Survey on Alcohol, Drug Abuse, and Mental Health Services *(Brandeis University)*	The Brandeis Health Plan Survey on Alcohol, Drug Abuse, and Mental Health Services is a nationally representative survey that tracks trends in how alcohol, drug abuse, and mental health services are provided for the more than 200 million privately insured individuals in 1999 ($n = 434$; 92 percent response) and 2003 ($n = 368$; 83 percent response).
Census of State and Federal Adult Correctional Facilities *(Bureau of Justice Statistics)*	The 2005 Census of State and Federal Adult Correctional Facilities provides information on facilities, inmates, programs, and staff of State and Federal correctional facilities throughout the Nation, and of private correctional facilities housing State or Federal inmates. Data were gathered from 1,821 separate institutions (prisons; prison boot camps; reception, diagnostic, and classification centers; prison forestry camps and farms; prison hospitals; youthful offender facilities [except in California]; facilities for alcohol and drug treatment; work release and prerelease; and State-operated local detention facilities in Alaska, Connecticut, Delaware, Hawaii, Rhode Island, and Vermont).
Decision Support System *(Veterans Health Administration)*	The Veterans Health Administration (VHA) Decision Support System is a managerial cost accounting system that interacts with Department of Veterans Affairs' national databases to provide data elements on VHA costs to VHA products (goods and services provided during patient care).
Department of Defense Survey of Health Related Behaviors Among Active Duty Personnel *(Department of Defense)*	The 2008 Department of Defense Survey of Health Related Behaviors Among Active Duty Personnel provides representative estimates on substance use and abuse, mental well-being, stress and coping, combat exposure experience, deployment experience, and selected general health topics for all active duty personnel. The final sample consisted of 28,546 military personnel (5,927 Army; 6,637 Navy; 5,117 Marine Corps; 7,009 Air Force; and 3,856 Coast Guard) who completed self-administered questionnaires anonymously.

(continued)

Data Source *(Sponsor)*	Description
Department of Defense Survey of Health Related Behaviors Among the Guard and Reserve Force *(Department of Defense)*	The 2006 Department of Defense Survey of Health Related Behaviors Among the Guard and Reserve Force provides representative estimates on substance use; stress and mental health; healthy behaviors and lifestyles; and other specific issues, such as injuries and injury prevention, sleep habits, and risk taking for all Reserve component personnel. The final sample consisted of 18,342 military personnel (2,796 Army National Guard; 1,665 Army Reserve; 3,215 Navy Reserve; 1,159 Marine Corps Reserve; 6,656 Air Force Reserve; and 2,851 Air National Guard) who completed self-administered questionnaires anonymously.
Employer Health Benefits Survey *(Henry J. Kaiser Family Foundation and Health Research & Educational Trust)*	The Henry J. Kaiser Family Foundation and Health Research & Educational Trust Employer Health Benefits Survey is an annual survey of employers that provides a detailed look at trends in employer-sponsored health coverage, including changes in premiums, employee contributions, cost-sharing policies, and other relevant information. The 2008 survey included 2,832 randomly selected public and private firms with three or more employees, and the 2000 survey included 1,887 randomly selected public and private firms with three or more employees.
International Survey of Clubhouses *(International Center for Clubhouse Development)*	The International Survey of Clubhouses was conducted in 2010 by the International Center for Clubhouse Development (ICCD). The survey contains information about clubhouse characteristics, governance and administration, membership, staffing and staff credentials, unit structure, employment, housing activities, services, and participation in clubhouse training. In 2010, there were 197 ICCD clubhouses in the United States; however, data were only available for 114 of them.
Medicaid Analytic eXtract (MAX) *(Centers for Medicare & Medicaid Services)*	The Medicaid Analytic eXtract (MAX) is a set of person-level data files on Medicaid eligibility, service utilization, and payments. The data are extracted from the Medicaid Statistical Information System (MSIS). The MAX development process combines MSIS initial claims, interim claims, voids, and adjustments for a given service into final action events.
Medical Expenditure Panel Survey (MEPS) *(Agency for Healthcare Research and Quality)*	The Medical Expenditure Panel Survey (MEPS) is a set of large-scale surveys of families and individuals, their medical providers (e.g., doctors, hospitals, pharmacies), and employers across the United States. Since 1996, MEPS has collected data on the specific health services that Americans use, how frequently they use them, the cost of these services, and how they are paid for, as well as data on the cost, scope, and breadth of health insurance held by and available to U.S. workers.
Medicare Cost Report *(Centers for Medicare & Medicaid Services)*	The Medicare Cost Report is based on annual financial information reported to the Centers for Medicare & Medicaid Services. The Cost Report contains provider information such as facility characteristics, utilization data, cost and charges by cost center (in total and for Medicare), Medicare settlement data, and financial statement data.
Medicare Standard Analytical Files (SAF) *(Centers for Medicare & Medicaid Services)*	The Medicare Standard Analytical Files (SAF) is a nationally representative claims database that consists of a randomly selected 5 percent sample of U.S. Medicare beneficiaries. The database includes claims across various care settings, including inpatient, outpatient, skilled nursing, home health, and hospice, as well as for durable medical equipment.
Mercer National Survey of Employer-Sponsored Health Plans *(Mercer)*	Established in 1986, the Mercer National Survey of Employer-Sponsored Health Plans is an annual survey that collects information on a wide range of health care issues regarding employer health plans, including costs, strategic planning, and the scope and limitations of coverage. Nearly 3,000 employers participated in the 2003 survey.
National Vital Statistics Report *(Centers for Disease Control and Prevention)*	The National Vital Statistics Report presents detailed data on U.S. deaths and death rates according to a number of social, demographic, and medical characteristics. In 2007, 2,423,712 deaths were reported in the United States.

(continued)

Data Source *(Sponsor)*	Description
National Ambulatory Medical Care Survey (NAMCS) *(Centers for Disease Control and Prevention)*	The National Ambulatory Medical Care Survey is a national probability sample survey of visits to office-based physicians.
National Comorbidity Survey Replication (NCS-R) *(National Institute of Mental Health)*	The National Comorbidity Survey Replication (NCS-R) is a nationally representative household survey of 9,282 English speakers in 2001 aged 18 or older in the United States. The survey collected diagnostic and other information on people with mental illness.
National Compensation Survey *(Bureau of Labor Statistics)*	The Bureau of Labor Statistics National Compensation Survey provides comprehensive measures of occupational wages, employment cost trends, benefit incidence, and detailed plan provisions from more than 361 metropolitan statistical areas and 573 micropolitan statistical areas in the United States, as defined by the Office of Management and Budget. A component of the survey in 1997 reports on benefits provided to employees in establishments with 100 or more workers in all private nonfarm industries. The survey included a national sample of 1,945 U.S. employers with more than 100 workers. Because smaller employers generally offer less generous health benefits packages, the estimates likely represent the upper limits on rates of mental health coverage by employer-based health insurance in the United States. Between 1979 and 1986, the survey provided benefits data on full-time employees in medium and large establishments, those with either 100 or 250 employees or more, depending on the industry; coverage in the service industries was limited.
National Expenditures for Mental Health Services and Substance Abuse Treatment *(Substance Abuse and Mental Health Services Administration)*	National Expenditures for Mental Health Services and Substance Abuse Treatment (otherwise known as the Spending Estimates Project) presents a broad overview of spending on mental health services and substance abuse treatment. The project is modeled on the National Health Expenditures published by the Centers for Medicare & Medicaid Services and uses data from 15 national sources to produce estimates.
National Health and Nutrition Examination Survey (NHANES) *(Centers for Disease Control and Prevention)*	The National Health and Nutrition Examination Survey (NHANES) is a nationally representative probability sample of noninstitutionalized U.S. civilians. The survey contains detailed information on the health and nutritional status of adults and children.
National Health Interview Survey (NHIS) *(Centers for Disease Control and Prevention)*	The National Health Interview Survey (NHIS) provides national estimates for a broad range of health measures for the U.S. civilian noninstitutionalized population. It is an annual, ongoing survey. The interviewed sample for 2009 consisted of 33,856 households, which yielded 88,446 persons in 34,640 families.
National Home and Hospice Care Survey *(Centers for Disease Control and Prevention)*	The National Home and Hospice Care Survey is a continuing series of nationally representative sample surveys of U.S. home health and hospice agencies. It is designed to provide descriptive information on home health and hospice agencies, their staffs, their services, and their patients. The survey was first conducted in 1992 and was repeated in 1993, 1994, 1996, 1998, and 2000, and most recently in 2007.
National Nursing Home Survey *(Centers for Disease Control and Prevention)*	The National Nursing Home Survey is a nationally representative probability sample of 1,500 nursing homes, their residents, and their staff. The survey is continuing, and data are available for 1995, 1997, 1999, and 2004.
National Survey of Child and Adolescent Well-Being II (NSCAW II) *(Administration for Children and Families)*	The National Survey of Child and Adolescent Well-Being II (NSCAW II) includes a longitudinal, national probability sample of 5,873 children from birth to 17 years of age who became involved with the child welfare system in 2008 when reported for child maltreatment.
National Survey of Children's Health *(Centers for Disease Control and Prevention)*	The National Survey of Children's Health is a nationally representative survey of 91,642 noninstitutionalized children aged 0 to 17 and provides a range of children's health and well-being information.

(continued)

Data Source *(Sponsor)*	Description
National Survey of Mental Health Treatment Facilities *(Substance Abuse and Mental Health Services Administration)*	The National Survey of Mental Health Treatment Facilities includes approximately 15,000 point-of-contact facilities nationwide representing approximately 4,400 mental health organizations nationwide. Data are available for 2008.
National Survey on Drug Use and Health (NSDUH) *(Substance Abuse and Mental Health Services Administration)*	The National Survey on Drug Use and Health (NSDUH) is a nationally representative survey of the civilian, noninstitutionalized population of the United States aged 12 or older. The survey interviews approximately 67,500 persons each year.
Nationwide Emergency Department Sample (NEDS) *(Agency for Healthcare Research and Quality)*	The Nationwide Emergency Department Sample (NEDS) database provides national estimates of emergency department visits.
Revenues and Expenditures Study *(NRI Inc.)*	NRI's Revenues and Expenditures Study describes the major expenditures and funding sources of State mental health agencies. NRI has conducted this survey every year since 1981.
School Health Policies and Programs Study (SHPPS) *(Centers for Disease Control and Prevention)*	The School Health Policies and Programs Study (SHPPS) is a nationally representative survey of State education agency personnel in all 50 States plus the District of Columbia; school districts ($n = 538$); elementary, middle, and high schools ($n = 1{,}103$); teachers of classes covering required health instruction in elementary schools and required health education courses in middle and high schools ($n = 912$); and teachers of required physical education classes and courses ($n = 1{,}194$).
State Inpatient Databases *(Agency for Healthcare Research and Quality)*	The State Inpatient Databases consist of data from 43 States on the number of community hospitals as well as discharges from those hospitals, accounting for approximately 90 percent of all community hospital discharges.
State Mental Health Agency Budget Reductions Survey *(NRI Inc.)*	The State Mental Health Agency (SMHA) Budget Reductions Survey is conducted by the National Association of State Mental Health Program Directors (NASMHPD) and NRI Inc. The survey is a semiannual series on the impact of State budget shortages on SMHA systems.
Survey of Inmates in State and Federal Correctional Facilities, and the Survey of Inmates in Local Jails *(Bureau of Justice Statistics)*	The Survey of Inmates in State and Federal Correctional Facilities, 2004, and the Survey of Inmates in Local Jails, 2002, included a modified structured clinical interview for the *Diagnostic and Statistical Manual of Mental Disorders, Fourth Edition* (DSM-IV). The interviewed sample included 681,600 State prison inmates, 56,600 Federal prison inmates, and 398,800 local jail inmates.
Survey of Mental Health Organizations (SMHO) *(Substance Abuse and Mental Health Services Administration)*	The Survey of Mental Health Organizations (SMHO) was a biennial survey with two phases. In the first phase, limited data were collected from all mental health organizations. In the second phase, more detailed data were collected from a sample of specialty mental health organizations. The survey changed names during its course, and data are available for 1986, 1990, 1992, 1994, 1998, 2000, 2002, and 2004.
Survey of Youth in Residential Placement (SYRP) *(Office of Juvenile Justice and Delinquency Placement)*	The Survey of Youth in Residential Placement (SYRP) is a nationally representative survey of offender youth aged 10 to 20 in State and local facilities. The final sample consisted of 7,073 youth who were interviewed using an audio computer-assisted self-interview system.
Uniform Data System *(Health Resources and Services Administration)*	The Uniform Data System is a set of electronic files compiled by the Health Resources and Services Administration from reports submitted annually by all U.S. federally funded community health centers on administration, patient population, demographic characteristics, utilization, and finances.

APPENDIX B: GLOSSARY

Any mental illness (AMI). Among adults aged 18 or older, defined as having a diagnosable mental, behavioral, or emotional disorder (excluding developmental and substance use disorders), regardless of functional impairment level. Estimates of AMI are provided annually in the National Survey on Drug Use and Health.

Behavioral health. A state of mental/emotional being and/or choices and actions that affect wellness. Behavioral health problems include substance abuse or misuse, alcohol and drug addiction, serious psychological distress, suicide, and mental and substance use disorders.

Children's Health Insurance Program (CHIP). A program by which States insure low-income children who are ineligible for Medicaid but whose families cannot afford private insurance. States receive Federal matching dollars to help provide for this coverage.

Child welfare system. The social service system that receives and investigates reports of possible child abuse and neglect; provides services to families that need assistance in the protection and care of their children; arranges for children to live with kin or with foster families when they are not safe at home; and arranges for reunification, adoption, or other permanent family connections for children leaving foster care.

Clubhouse. An organization hosting a specific model of care that helps people with mental illness participate in the broader community. A clubhouse provides a membership of several people an array of nonmedical services, many of which focus on education and employment. Members themselves often participate in service provision.

Community health center (CHC). An organization that serves populations with limited access to health care, usually because of limited financial resources. These centers are public and private nonprofit health care organizations that meet certain criteria under the Medicare and Medicaid programs.

Community hospital. Any non-Federal, short-term general or other specialty hospital, including academic medical centers or other teaching hospitals that are non-Federal short-term hospitals. The term typically excludes hospitals not accessible by the general public, such as prison hospitals or college infirmaries. See also **general hospital.**

Complementary and alternative medicine (CAM). A broad class of services that are not traditionally provided as billable services in the treatment system. Includes services from several types of healers, participation in an Internet support group, or participation in a self-help group. The most commonly used CAM services are those from spiritual advisors, relaxation techniques, and use of multivitamins and herbs.

Emergency department. A section of an institution that is staffed and equipped to provide immediate care, particularly for sudden, acute illness and trauma.

Emotional disturbance. An emotional or behavioral health condition that prevents a child or adolescent from performing everyday tasks. This condition is characterized by an inability to build or maintain relationships, inappropriate behaviors or feelings under normal circumstances, a pervasive mood of unhappiness or depression, or a tendency to develop physical symptoms or fears related to personal or school problems.

Functional impairment. A level of disability or distress in daily life that is attributable to symptoms of mental illness.

General hospital. A community medical/surgical or specialty hospital (other than a mental health and substance abuse specialty hospital) providing diagnostic and medical treatment to inpatients, including inpatient psychiatric care in a specialized treatment unit of a general hospital and other mental health treatment services. See also **community hospital.**

Health maintenance organization (HMO). A type of managed care organization that provides a variety of services. Typically, services are provided for a set flat fee per patient. In some HMOs, a primary care provider directs access to other medical services. Usually, providers agree to treat patients in accordance with the HMO's guidelines and restrictions.

Home health care. A set of services provided in the patient's residence by private and public freestanding agencies or home health agencies. Freestanding means that the agency is not based in a hospital, nursing home, or other type of provider whose primary mission is something other than home health services.

Hospice. A form of care that provides palliative and supportive care services, including physical, psychological, social, and spiritual care for dying persons, their families, and other loved ones. Hospice services are available in home and inpatient settings.

Inpatient. Care provided in an acute medical care unit, usually a hospital, and treatment typically requires an overnight stay.

Insurance administration. The set of activities used to run health care insurance programs.

Major depressive episode (MDE). A period of at least 2 weeks when a person experienced a depressed mood or loss of interest or pleasure in daily activities and had a majority of specified depression symptoms. MDE is one of the components of the diagnostic criteria for major depressive disorder (MDD). MDD is a serious mental disorder that can result in impairment and societal costs, including work disability and lost productivity. Estimates of MDE are provided annually in the National Survey on Drug Use and Health.

Medicaid. A program jointly funded by Federal and State governments that provides health care coverage to certain classes of persons with limited income and resources. Within Federal guidelines, State governments set eligibility standards, determine optional services provided, set reimbursement rates, and administer the program. Income and resources are only two factors in determining eligibility, so not all persons with limited income in a State are necessarily covered by this program.

Medicare. A Federal government program that provides health insurance coverage to eligible adults aged 65 or older and disabled persons. It has four parts: Part A, which covers institutional services, including inpatient hospital services, nursing home care, initial home health visits, and hospice care; Part B, which covers physicians and other professional services, outpatient clinic or hospital services, laboratory services, rehabilitation therapy, and home health visits not covered by Part A, among other services; Part C, the Medicare Advantage program, which is managed by private companies for a flat fee per patient per month; and Part D, which began in 2006 and covers medication.

Mood disorder. A collection of disorders where a disturbance of mood is the main underlying feature. Includes depressive or bipolar disorders as defined in the *Diagnostic and Statistical Manual of Mental Disorders, Fourth Edition* (DSM-IV).

Nursing home care. A set of services provided in private and public freestanding nursing home facilities. Freestanding means that the nursing home is not based in a hospital, nursing home, or other type of provider whose primary mission is something other than nursing home care. The facility includes nursing and rehabilitative services, generally for an extended period of time by staff of registered or licensed practical nurses with physician consultation or oversight.

Out-of-pocket payment. Direct expenditure by consumers for health care goods and services, including coinsurance, deductibles, and any amounts paid for health care services that are not covered by insurance. Depending on the data source, health insurance premiums may or may not be included.

Outpatient. Care provided in an ambulatory setting and treatment does not require an overnight stay. Unless otherwise specified, this setting may include a hospital outpatient department; an emergency room; physician's or other medical professional's (private therapist, psychologist, psychiatrist, social worker, or counselor) office or clinic; mental health clinic or center; partial day hospital or day treatment program; and in-home therapist, counselor, or family preservation worker.

Prescription drug or prescription medication. A medication available through primary or specialty providers; retail outlets, such as community pharmacies; pharmacies in mass merchandise stores, grocery stores, and department stores; mail order pharmacies; hospitals; exclusive-to-patient health maintenance organizations; and nursing home pharmacies.

Primary diagnosis. The main or principal diagnosis that most typically has led to the admission of an individual to a hospital or to receive outpatient treatment. In an outpatient care setting, the condition may be referred to as the first-listed diagnosis. In an inpatient setting, the condition may be the most serious and/or resource intensive during that hospitalization.

Private health insurance. Third-party coverage not provided by government sources.

Psychiatric hospitals. Facilities that typically specialize in treating people with serious mental illness and vary widely in their size and function. Many specialize in the temporary or permanent care of residents who require routine assistance, treatment, or a controlled environment.

Psychiatrist. Independently billing private or group practice of health practitioners having the degree of M.D. or D.O. who are primarily engaged in the practice of psychiatry or psychoanalysis.

Psychotropic medication. Medication used to treat mental health symptoms and disorders. Although there are several ways to categorize such medications, this report includes the following categories: antianxiety, antidepressant, antimanic, antipsychotic, anticonvulsant, and stimulant.

Residential services. Services provided in a 24-hour care setting that provide therapeutic care to patients using licensed behavioral health professionals.

Retail prescription drug or retail prescription medication. Prescription medication that excludes prescription medication sold through hospitals, exclusive-to-patient health maintenance organizations, or nursing home pharmacies.

Scatter bed. A general medical bed in a hospital dedicated to providing inpatient psychiatric care. Psychiatric care in scatter beds may occur even in hospitals with separate psychiatric units.

Serious mental illness (SMI). Among adults aged 18 or older, defined as having a diagnosable mental, behavioral, or emotional disorder (excluding developmental and substance use disorders) that has resulted in serious functional impairment, which substantially interferes with or limits one or more major life activities. Estimates of SMI are provided annually in the National Survey on Drug Use and Health.

Serious psychological distress (SPD). The presence of mental health symptoms in the past 30 days that may negatively affect an adult's ability to participate in family, community, and work life. SPD is not a diagnosis and does not represent a specific mental disorder. This construct is measured annually in the National Health Interview Survey.

State Mental Health Agency (SMHA). A State government organization responsible for directing resources for people in need of mental health services. For example, an SMHA typically applies for and administers Federal Community Mental Health Services Block Grant funding for its State.

Substance abuse. A pattern of substance use that leads to clinically significant impairment and includes symptoms such as failure to fulfill major role obligations, legal problems, use in situations that are physically hazardous, and continued use despite persistent social or interpersonal problems.

Substance dependence. A pattern of substance use that leads to clinically significant impairment and includes symptoms such as drug taking in larger amounts than intended, inability to cut down on drug use, a great deal of time spent on activities necessary to obtain the drug, and continued use despite knowledge of health or social problems caused by the drug.

Substance disorder/Substance use disorder. Disorder that is characterized by substance abuse and/or dependence.

APPENDIX C: MEDICATION LISTS

This appendix lists the mental health and/or substance abuse medications for each medication class presented in Exhibits 9, 13, 19, and 20 and in Tables 30, 31, 62, 63, 95, and 96.

Medications for Mental Health Disorders

Antianxiety, Sedative, Hypnotic		
Alprazolam	Diazepam	Methylprylon
Amobarbital	Droperidol	Oxazepam
Amobarbital-Secobarbital	Estazolam	Pentobarbital
Buspirone	Ethchlorvynol	Phenobarbital
Butabarbital	Flurazepam	Prazepam
Butalbital	Glutethimide	Quazepam
Chloral hydrate	Halazepam	Secobarbital
Chlordiazepoxide	Hexobarbital	Temazepam
Chlordiazepoxide-Clidinium	Hydroxyzine	Triazolam
Chlormezanone	Lorazepam	Zaleplon
Clonazepam	Mephobarbital	Zolpidem
Clorazepate	Meprobamate	

Antidepressant		
Amitriptyline	Duloxetine	Nortriptyline
Amitriptyline-Chlordiazepoxide	Escitalopram	Paroxetine
Amoxapine	Fluoxetine	Phenelzine
Bupropion	Fluvoxamine	Protriptyline
Citalopram	Imipramine	Sertraline
Clomipramine	Isocarboxazid	Tranylcypromine
Desipramine	Maprotiline	Trazodone
Desvenlafaxine	Mirtazapine	Trimipramine
Doxepin	Nefazodone	Venlafaxine

Medications for Mental Health Disorders *(continued)*

Antimanic or Anticonvulsant		
Carbamazepine	Lithium	Topiramate
Divalproex sodium	Oxcarbazepine	Valproate
Gabapentin	Tiagabine	Valproic acid
Lamotrigine		

Antipsychotic		
Amitriptyline-Chlordiazepoxide	Mesoridazine	Quetiapine
Amitriptyline-Perphenazine	Methotrimeprazine	Risperidone
Aripiprazole	Molindone	Thioridazine
Chlorpromazine	Olanzapine	Thiothixene
Clozapine	Paliperidone	Trifluoperazine
Fluoxetine-Olanzapine	Perphenazine	Triflupromazine
Fluphenazine	Pimozide	Ziprasidone
Haloperidol	Prochlorperazine	
Loxapine	Promazine	

Stimulant		
Amphetamine	Lisdexamfetamine	Methylphenidate
Amphetamine-Dextroamphetamine	Extroamphetamine	Modafinil
Atomoxetine	Methamphetamine	Pemoline
Dexmethylphenidate		

Medications for Substance Use Disorders

Acamprosate	Disulfiram	Naltrexone
Buprenorphine	Methadone	

Medications for Alzheimer's Disease

Donepezil	Memantine	Rivastigmine
Galantamine	Physostigmine	Tacrine

SOURCE: National Institute on Mental Health. (2011). Mental health medications. Retrieved from http://www.nimh.nih.gov/health/publications/mental-health-medications/alphabetical-list-of-medications.shtml

ADDITIONAL ACKNOWLEDGMENTS

The following people contributed to this edition of *Mental Health, United States*: Alexander Cowell (project director), Heather Ringeisen, Leyla Stambaugh, David Kaiser, Natalie Hodges, Justin Landwehr, and Valerie Hoffman (RTI International); Tami Mark, Elizabeth Stranges, and Katharine Levit (Thomson Reuters); Dominic Hodgkin and Elizabeth Merrick (Brandeis University); Ted Lutterman (NRI Inc.); Barbara Burns and Marvin Swartz (Duke University); and Carla Linkous (Cloudburst Consulting Group).

Additionally, a number of individuals prepared and contributed data that were crucial to the completion of *Mental Health, United States, 2010*: Anita Bercovitz (National Center for Health Statistics), Donald Cherry (National Center for Health Statistics), Joseph Gfroerer (CBHSQ), Lauren Glaze (Bureau of Justice Statistics), Sarra Hedden (CBHSQ), Art Hughes (CBHSQ), Michael Jones (CBHSQ), Colleen McKay (Center for Mental Health Services Research, University of Massachusetts Medical School), Laura Milazzo-Sayre (CBHSQ), Ryan Mutter (Agency for Healthcare Research and Quality), Catherine Simile (National Center for Health Statistics), Mark Smith (Veterans Health Administration), Peter Tice (CBHSQ), and Samuel Zuvekas (Agency for Healthcare Research and Quality).

The following individuals served as external reviewers for the volume: Lisa Colpe (National Institute of Mental Health), Rachel Garfield (Kaiser Commission on Medicaid and the Uninsured), Darcy Gruttadaro (National Alliance on Mental Illness), Kevin Hennessy (SAMHSA), Chris Koyanagi (Judge David L. Bazelon Center for Mental Health Law), Lisa Patton (Assistant Secretary for Planning & Evaluation, HHS), Marvin Swartz (Duke University), Mohini Venkatesh (National Council for Community Behavioral Healthcare), and Capt. Elise Young (Health Resources and Services Administration).

Finally, particular recognition is due to Marceline Murawski, Susan Murchie, Pamela Prevatt, and E. Andrew Jessup, along with other members of the publications staff at RTI International, who provided expert editorial services.

MENTAL HEALTH, UNITED STATES, 2010
EXPERT ADVISORY PANEL

The structure and content of the report were guided by the suggestions of an Expert Advisory Panel that was convened on February 24, 2010:

Panel Member	Affiliation
Amy Bernstein	Centers for Disease Control and Prevention
William Clark	Centers for Medicare & Medicaid Services
Lisa Colpe	National Institute of Mental Health
John Drabek	Assistant Secretary for Planning and Evaluation, HHS
William Gardner	Nationwide Children's Hospital
Olinda Gonzalez	SAMHSA
Kevin Martone	New Jersey Department of Human Services
Joseph Morrissey	University of North Carolina at Chapel Hill
Alexander Ross	Health Resources and Services Administration
David Shern	Mental Health America
Shawn Terrell	Office on Disability, HHS
Virginia Trotter Betts	Department of Mental Health and Developmental Disabilities
Mohini Venkatesh	National Council for Community Behavioral Healthcare
Samuel Zuvekas	Agency for Healthcare Research and Quality

Substance Abuse and Mental Health Services Administration

SAMHSA

www.samhsa.gov • 1-877-SAMHSA-7 (1-877-726-4727)

www.ingramcontent.com/pod-product-compliance
Ingram Content Group UK Ltd.
Pitfield, Milton Keynes, MK11 3LW, UK
UKHW051040091026
15624UKWH00011B/594

9 781782 662082